Ocu
Reconst
M

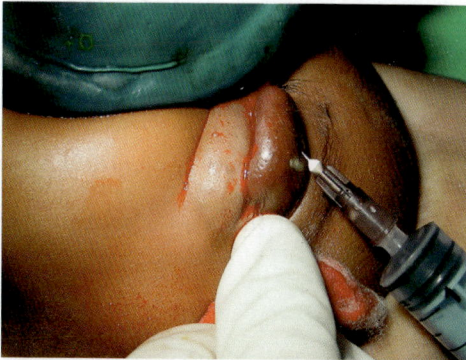

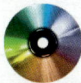

System requirement:
- **Windows XP or above**
- **Power DVD player (Software)**
- **Windows media player 10.0 version or above (Software)**

Accompanying DVD ROM is playable only in Computer and not in DVD player.

Kindly wait for few seconds for DVD to autorun. If it does not autorun then please do the following:
- Click on my computer
- Click the **drive labelled JAYPEE** and after opening the drive, kindly double click the file **Jaypee**

DVD Contents

Oculoplasty and Reconstructive Surgery Made Easy®

Editors

Ashok Garg MS PhD FIAO (Bel) FRSM FAIMS ADM FICA
International and National Gold Medalist
Chairman and Medical Director
Garg Eye Institute and Research Centre
235-Model Town, Dabra Chowk, Hisar 125 005 (India)

Essam El Toukhy MD FRCOph
Deputy Director
National Eye Institute, Egypt
Associate Professor of Ophthalmology
Cairo University, 14-A, El Sobki Street No. 23
Dokki, Cairo, Egypt 12311

Belquiz A Nassaralla MD FRCOph
Consultant Ophthalmic Surgeon
Department of Cornea and Refractive Surgery
Goiania Eye Institute, Goiania, GO, Brazil

Forewords
Frank Goes
Pelin Kaynak-Hekimhan

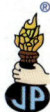

JAYPEE BROTHERS MEDICAL PUBLISHERS (P) LTD

New Delhi • Ahmedabad • Bengaluru • Chennai • Hyderabad • Kochi
Kolkata • Lucknow • Mumbai • Nagpur • St Louis (USA)

Published by

Jitendar P Vij

Jaypee Brothers Medical Publishers (P) Ltd

Corporate Office

4838/24 Ansari Road, Daryaganj, **New Delhi** - 110002, India, Phone: +91-11-43574357

Registered Office

B-3 EMCA House, 23/23B Ansari Road, Daryaganj, **New Delhi** - 110 002, India

Phones: +91-11-23272143, +91-11-23272703, +91-11-23282021

+91-11-23245672, Rel: +91-11-32558559, Fax: +91-11-23276490, +91-11-23245683

e-mail: jaypee@jaypeebrothers.com, Website: www.jaypeebrothers.com

Branches

- ❑ 2/B, Akruti Society, Jodhpur Gam Road Satellite
  Ahmedabad 380 015, Phones: +91-79-26926233, Rel: +91-79-32988717
  Fax: +91-79-26927094, e-mail: ahmedabad@jaypeebrothers.com

- ❑ 202 Batavia Chambers, 8 Kumara Krupa Road, Kumara Park East
  Bengaluru 560 001, Phones: +91-80-22285971, +91-80-22382956, 91-80-22372664
  Rel: +91-80-32714073, Fax: +91-80-22281761 e-mail: bangalore@jaypeebrothers.com

- ❑ 282 IIIrd Floor, Khaleel Shirazi Estate, Fountain Plaza, Pantheon Road
  Chennai 600 008, Phones: +91-44-28193265, +91-44-28194897, Rel: +91-44-32972089
  Fax: +91-44-28193231 e-mail: chennai@jaypeebrothers.com

- ❑ 4-2-1067/1-3, 1st Floor, Balaji Building, Ramkote Cross Road,
  Hyderabad 500 095, Phones: +91-40-66610020, +91-40-24758498
  Rel:+91-40-32940929, Fax:+91-40-24758499 e-mail: hyderabad@jaypeebrothers.com

- ❑ No. 41/3098, B and B1, Kuruvi Building, St. Vincent Road
  Kochi 682 018, Kerala, Phones: +91-484-4036109, +91-484-2395739
  +91-484-2395740 e-mail: kochi@jaypeebrothers.com

- ❑ 1-A Indian Mirror Street, Wellington Square
  Kolkata 700 013, Phones: +91-33-22651926, +91-33-22276404
  +91-33-22276415, Rel: +91-33-32901926, Fax: +91-33-22656075
  e-mail: kolkata@jaypeebrothers.com

- ❑ Lekhraj Market III, B-2, Sector-4, Faizabad Road, Indira Nagar
  Lucknow 226 016 Phones: +91-522-3040553, +91-522-3040554
  e-mail: lucknow@jaypeebrothers.com

- ❑ 106 Amit Industrial Estate, 61 Dr SS Rao Road, Near MGM Hospital, Parel
  Mumbai 400 012, Phones: +91-22-24124863, +91-22-24104532,
  Rel: +91-22-32926896, Fax: +91-22-24160828
  e-mail: mumbai@jaypeebrothers.com

- ❑ "KAMALPUSHPA" 38, Reshimbag, Opp. Mohota Science College, Umred Road
  Nagpur 440 009 (MS), Phone: Rel: +91-712-3245220, Fax: +91-712-2704275
  e-mail: nagpur@jaypeebrothers.com

USA Office

1745, Pheasant Run Drive, Maryland Heights (Missouri), MO 63043, USA, Ph: 001-636-6279734

e-mail: jaypee@jaypeebrothers.com, anjulav@jaypeebrothers.com

Oculoplasty and Reconstructive Surgery Made Easy®

This book has been published in good faith that the material provided by contributors is original. Every effort is made to ensure accuracy of material, but the publisher, printer and editors will not be held responsible for any inadvertent error(s). In case of any dispute, all legal matters are to be settled under Delhi jurisdiction only.

First Edition: 2009

ISBN 978-81-8448-596-7

Typeset at JPBMP typesetting unit

Printed at Replika Press Pvt. Ltd.

To

- My Respected Param Pujya Guru Sant Gurmeet Ram Rahim Singh Ji for his blessings and motivation.
- My Respected parents, teachers, my wife Dr Aruna Garg, son Abhishek and daughter Anshul for their constant support and patience during all these days of hard work.
- My dear friend Dr Amar Agarwal, a renowned International Ophthalmologist for his constant support, guidance and expertise....

—Ashok Garg

- All those who supported me during my life, to all the wonderful people in my life, my dear parents, my lovely wife and my beloved children....

—Essam El Toukhy

- To my parents Lucia and Justino, for their blessings and motivation. To my husband Joao, a greater partner at home and at work. To my children Arthur, Joao Neto and Anna Paula, who have been giving me constant support and love....

—Belquiz A Nassaralla

Contributors

AK Grover MD FRCS
Chairman
Department of Ophthalmology
Sir Ganga Ram Hospital
Rajinder Nagar
New Delhi 110 060, India

Ali Saeed Odadi Assiri MD
Egyptian Board ICO
Fellow Specialist
Raudh El-Faraj Eye Center, Egypt

Amar Agarwal
MS FRCS FRC Ophth
Consultant
Dr Agarwal's Eye Institute
19, Cathedral Road
Chennai 600 086
Tamil Nadu, India

Anil M Shah MS
Director
Suryakanta Eye Hospital
Opposite Nagar Palika
Nandurbar 425 412
Maharashtra, India

Arif Adenwala MD
Consultant
Aditya Jyot Eye Hospital
Wadala, Mumbai 400 031
Maharashtra, India

Ashok Garg MS PhD FRSM
Chairman and Medical Director
Garg Eye Institute and Research
Centre
235-Model Town, Dabra Chowk
Hisar 125 005, Haryana
India

Belquiz A Nassaralla
Consultant Ophthalmic Surgeon
Department of Cornea and
Refractive Surgery
Goiania Eye Institute
Goiania, GO, Brazil

Claudio Lucchini MD
Studio Lucchini
Via G Leopardi 21
20123, Milan
Italy

Daljit Singh MS DSc
Director
Dr Daljit Singh Eye Hospital
57, Joshi Colony
Amritsar 143 001, Punjab
India

Dhiya Ashok Kumar MS
Consultant
Dr Agarwal's Eye Institute
19, Cathedral Road
Chennai 600 086
Tamil Nadu, India

Essam El Toukhy MD FRCOph
Deputy Director
National Eye Institute
Egypt
Associate Professor of
Ophthalmology, Cairo University
Egypt

Gauri Mankekar MS
PD Hinduja National Hospital and
Medical Research Centre
Mumbai, Maharashtra
India

Hatem A Tawfik MD
Department of Ophthalmology
Ain Shams University
Cairo, Egypt

Ibrahim Mosad MD
Consultant Ophthalmologist
Cairo University Hospital
Cairo, Egypt

Jes Mortensen MD
Professor of Ophthalmology
The Eye Department
Orebro University Hospital
SE-70185, Orebro, Sweden

João J Nassaralla
Consultant Ophthalmic Surgeon
Department of Cornea and
Refractive Surgery
Goiania Eye Institute
Goiania, GO, Brazil

Kiran Tandon MD
Director Oculoplasty Services
Dr Chaudhary Eye Centre and
Laser Vision, 4802, Bharat Ram
Road, 24, Darya Ganj
New Delhi 110 002, India

Kirit Mody MS FRCS FRCO
Consulting Eye Surgeon
Salil Eye Clinic and Contact Lens
Centre, 506, Om Chambers
Kemps Corner, 123
August Kranti Marg
Mumbai 400 036, Maharashtra
India

Lobna Khazbak MD
Department of Ophthalmology
Cairo University
Cairo, Eqypt

Lucas Henrique Barbosa Dos Santos MD
Consultant Ophthalmic Surgeon
Department of Cornea and Refractive Surgery
Goiania Eye Institute
Goiania, GO, Brazil

Mahesh Dalvi MS
Consultant
Department of Pediatric Ophthalmology
Tejomay Eye Hospital
Kolhapur, Maharashtra
India

Malvika Bansal MS
Department of Ophthalmology
Sir Gangaram Hospital
Rajinder Nagar, New Delhi
India

Milind Navlakhe MS
Associate Professor
Department of Ophthalmology
KEM Hospital, Mumbai
Maharashtra, India

Mayur Moreker MS
Surya Eye Hospital, Mulund
Mumbai, Maharashtra
India

Mohamed El Badri MD
Specialist Ophthalmologist
National Eye Centre, Egypt

Murad Lala MS
PD Hinduja National Hospital and Medical Research Centre
Mumbai, Maharashtra, India

MV Kirtane MS
PD Hinduja National Hospital and Medical Research Centre
Mumbai, Maharashtra, India

Norlaila Talib MD
Department of Ophthalmology
Ain Shams University
Cairo, Egypt

Pelin Kaynak-Hekimhan MD
Director
Ophthalmic Plastic and Reconstructive Surgery Division
Istanbul
Prof R Belger Beyoglu Eye Research Hospital, Istanbul
Turkey

Quresh Maskati MS
Maskati Eye Clinic
Harishankar Building
Ist Floor, 23, M Karve Road
Opposite Charni Road, Railway
Station (E), Mumbai 400 004
Maharashtra, India

Ramesh Murthy MD
Ophthalmic Plastic Services
LV Prasad Eye Institute
LV Prasad Marg, Banjara Hills
Hyderabad 500 034
Andhra Pradesh, India

Rania Abdel Salam MD
Consultant Ophthalmologist
National Eye Center
Cairo, Egypt

Ranjit S Dhaliwal MS DOMS
Director
Eye Infirmary, Hira Mahal
Radha Soami Marg
Nabha 147 201, Punjab
India

Roshmi Gupta MD
Consultant
Ophthalmic Plastic and Ocular,
Oncology Services
LV Prasad Eye Institute
Vishakhapatnam, Orissa
India

Santosh G Honavar MD FACS
Director
Ophthalmic Plastics and Ocular
Oncology Services
LV Prasad Eye Institute
LV Prasad Marg, Banjara Hills
Hyderabad 500 034
Andhra Pradesh, India

Savari Desai MD
Ophthalmic Plastics and Ocular
Oncology Services
LV Prasad Eye Institute
LV Prasad Marg
Banjara Hills
Hyderabad 500 034
Andhra Pradesh, India

Shaloo Bageja MS
Department of Ophthalmology
Sir Ganga Ram Hospital
Rajinder Nagar
New Delhi 110 060, India

Sneha Kataria MD
OD Class 2012
New England College of
Optometry, Boston, USA

Soosan Jacob MD
Consultant
Dr Agarwal's Eye Institute
19, Cathedral Road
Chennai 600 086
Tamil Nadu, India

Sunil Moreker MS
Consultant Ophthalmologist
PD Hinduja National Hospital and
Medical Research Centre
Mumbai, Maharashtra
India

Sunil Vasani MS
Eye-r-us Clinic
Gowalia Tank
Mumbai 400 036, Maharashtra
India

Tamer Gawdat MD FRCS
Assistant Professor of
Ophthalmology
Cairo University
Cairo, Egypt

Foreword

Oculoplasty and Reconstructive Surgery Made Easy is really what Dr Ashok Garg, a proliferative writer and his co-editors—Essam El Toukhy and Dr B Nassaralla—have realized by editing this book and by offering it to the clinicians.

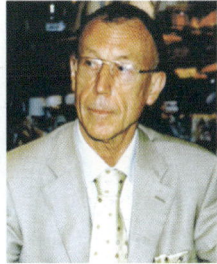

The editors of this book did a tremendous job to get an up-to-date overview on trends of oculoplasty and reconstructive surgery in external eye diseases such as congenital eyelid deformations, eye injuries, lacrymal disorders, pterygium; orbital diseases such as congenital and acquired tumors, orbital infections and injuries; and aesthetic surgery with CO_2 laser, endoscopic dacryorhinostomy, sling surgery and evidence-based update on pediatric oculoplasty have been discussed in excellent manner in this book.

Besides, accompanying DVD will guide the practitioner towards the application of the techniques proposed in this book.

The multispecialist approach enriches a book directed at the surgeons in their daily practice. The chapters are clearly written and nicely illustrated.

Indeed, Ashok Garg and the publisher M/s Jaypee Brothers Medical Publishers (P) Ltd, New Delhi, have to be congratulated for this outstanding book, and have, by doing so, contributed in an important way to the medical and surgical approach of oculoplasty and reconstructive surgery.

I do hope that the many readers of this book will experience the benefit of having access to this important volume.

Frank Goes MD
Director and Senior Eye Surgeon
Goes Eye Centre, W Klooslaan 6
B 2050 Antwerp Belgium
Tel. +32- 32193925, Fax: +32- 32196667
e-mail: frank@goes.be

Foreword

Ophthalmic plastic and reconstructive surgery is an exponentially growing field in ophthalmology. Information on new diagnostic tools, surgical techniques, treatment regimens are temptations for any academician, who would love to bind together and share the knowledge with other colleagues, however, it needs great ambition, diligent work and effort to realize it.

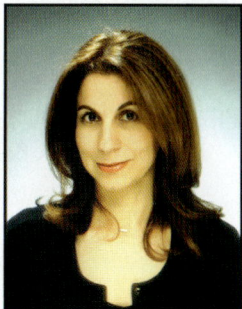

It is a great honor for me to have the opportunity to contribute to Dr Ashok Garg's and his co-editors, Dr Essam El Toukhy's and Dr B Nasaralla's, *Oculoplasty and Reconstructive Surgery Made Easy* with a chapter and it is a greater honor to receive a request to write a foreword to this book.

The tremendous work and information to publish a book in oculoplastic surgery, obviously necessitates a wide collaboration among oculoplastic surgeons from India and other countries of the world. Dr Garg and his co-editors are definitely the ophthalmologists who have this wide spectrum of national and international peers. Their great enthusiasm and dedication to ophthalmology and to the spreading of ophthalmic knowledge, brought together all of these information, experience and innovations in this new Oculoplasty Surgery Handbook, just like their previous books that helped ophthalmologists, ophthalmology residents, physicians and related health workers, and most important of all, for the patients we all value highly.

Therefore, I salute Dr Ashok Garg and all his contributing colleagues for the meticulous hard work that formed this book and presented it to our field of ophthalmic plastic and reconstructive surgery.

Pelin Kaynak-Hekimhan MD
Director
Ophthalmic Plastic and Reconstructive Surgery Division
Istanbul Prof R Belger Beyoglu Eye Research Hospital
Istanbul, Turkey
e-mail: pkaynak@superonline.com
tel:+90 532 366 8738, fax:+90 212

Preface

Oculoplasty is an important clinical branch of ophthalmology which has seen advances in the last one decade. *Oculoplasty and Reconstructive Surgery* is the surgery of eyelids, eyebrows or eye orbits. This surgery may be performed in order to improve cosmetic appearance, functions and comfort to the patients. It also refers to specialized reconstructive and aesthetic surgery of external eye abnormalities which may be present by birth or acquired later by accident, tumors or aging, etc. Oculoplasty surgeons also perform aesthetic treatments and surgery which are latest advancements and fashions to improve the cosmetic appearance. Blepharoplasty, botox injection and dermal filler injections are the excellent examples of this surgery.

This book has been written with the aim of providing latest information about various oculoplastic diseases and reconstructive procedures in a comprehensive and lucid manner. Thirty-three chapters of this book covering all aspects of eyelid disorders, lacrimal diseases, ptosis, various orbital disorders and recent advances in aesthetic ophthalmoplasty are written by international and national oculoplastic experts. Accompanying DVD will provide insight into various surgical oculoplasty procedures by the masters of this field.

We are grateful to Shri Jitendar P Vij (Chairman and Managing Director), Mr Tarun Duneja (Director-Publishing) and all staff members of M/s Jaypee Brothers Medical Publishers (P) Ltd, New Delhi who took keen interest in this project and published this unique book in a short time.

As the title of this book reflects, we hope this book will help all the keen oculoplastic surgeons worldwide in decision making and sharpen their surgical skills as well.

Editors

Contents

SECTION ONE
EXTERNAL EYE DISEASES

SECTION TWO
ORBITAL DISEASES

SECTION THREE
RECENT ADVANCES

Section *One*

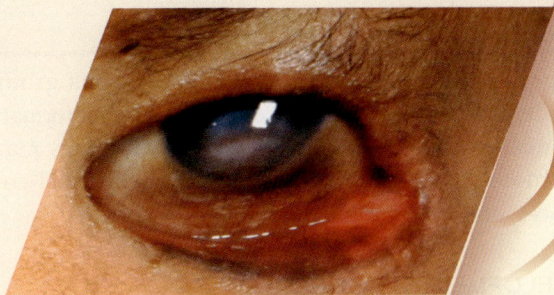

External Eye Diseases

Congenital Eyelid Anomalies

*Roshmi Gupta, Ramesh Murthy, Savari Desai,
Santosh G Honavar (India)*

INTRODUCTION

Congenital lid anomalies are a heterogeneous group of
disorders. Broadly they may be classified into malformations
and malpositions of the eyelids. Some conditions may be
innocuous, while others may have serious visual consequences, and need prompt attention.

DEVELOPMENT OF EYELIDS

The eyelids develop from lid folds that first appear in the
surface ectoderm overlying the optic vesicle in the 16 mm
stage of the embryo, and grow till the 32 mm stage. Between
the 32 to 37 mm stages of the embryo, the upper and lower
lid folds fuse together. They begin to separate at the fifth
month of gestational age, starting at the nasal side, and the
separation is completed by the sixth month.

CRYPTOPHTHALMOS

Etiology

Partial or complete failure of eyelid fold formation causes
cryptophthalmos.

Signs and Symptoms

Cryptophthalmos presents with three grades of severity.

- Complete cryptophthalmos is usually associated with other developmental anomalies, and often bilaterally symmetrical. A smooth skin passes from the forehead to the cheek. Eyebrows and lashes are usually absent **(Figure 1A)**.

- Partial cryptophthalmos shows partially formed eyelids and a disorganized anterior segment. The lids are often colobomatous. Facial skin fuses with the medial aspect of the globe **(Figure 1B)**.

- Abortive cryptophthalmos has a formed globe, with partial absence of the eyelids in some parts; symblepharon is seen at these areas. Cornea is covered by keratinised and stratified epithelium **(Figure 1C)**.

Associated ophthalmic features include microphthalmos, anterior segment anomalies such as small anterior chamber, absent trabecular meshwork, subluxated lens, posterior

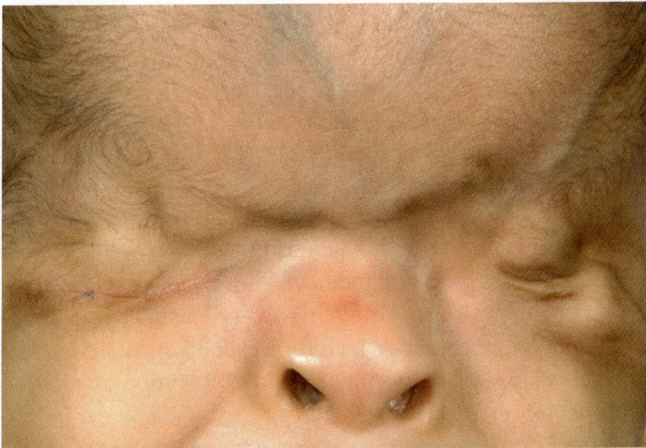

Figure 1A: Clinical photograph of bilateral complete cryptophthalmos

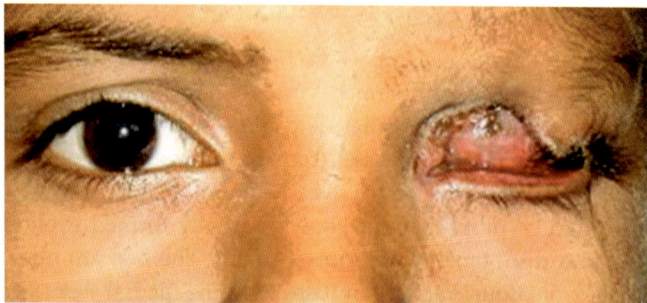

Figure 1B: Partial cryptophthalmos. There is a disorganized anterior segment and partial formation of eyelids

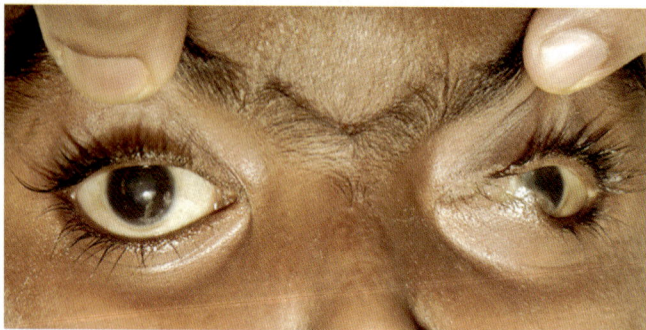

Figure 1C: Abortive cryptophthalmos, with incomplete formation of the nasal end of the eyelids, with symblepharon formation

segment anomalies like uveal coloboma, adnexal abnormalities like dermoids, supernumerary brow and absent lacrimal and accessory glands.

Cryptophthalmos may also have associated non-ophthalmic abnormalities, including cleft lip or palate, hernia, aplasia of kidneys, malformed genitalia, meningo-myelocele, and mental retardation.

Hereditary transmission of an autosomal recessive nature has been reported.

Differential Diagnosis

Complete cryptophthalmos has a characteristic appearance that is diagnostic. Incomplete cryptophthalmos needs to be differentiated from isolated lid colobomas.Causes of acquired symblepharon are to be differentiated fron abortive cryptophthalmos.

Investigation

Ultrasound B scan and computed tomography may help to assess the condition of the globe.

A thorough systemic evaluation is required to detect any associated anomalies.

Management

The management is surgical, with staged reconstruction of eyelids and the ocular surface. The visual outcome is poor.

LID COLOBOMAS

Etiology

Lid colobomas form due to delay in fusion of the mesodermal components of the fronto-nasal and maxillary processes of the face.

Signs and Symptoms

A coloboma is a partial or full thickness absence of the eyelid, which may be triangular, quadrilateral, W-shaped or irregular. The edges are rounded and covered with conjunctiva. The partial thickness coloboma may show the lid margin structures such as lashes. The upper lid colobomas are usually in the middle and the nasal third of the lid. The lower lid colobomas are often situated temporally. If situated at the medial end of the lower lid, they are associated with abnormalities of the lacrimal drainage system.

The cornea may be visible through the coloboma even when the lid is closed, and show exposure keratopathy on slit-lap examination **(Figure 2A)**.

Differential Diagnosis

Congenital colobomas need to be differentiated from acquired coloboma caused by trauma.

A coloboma may be isolated, or be a part of the Goldenhar syndrome.

Investigation

The child requires systemic evaluation to rule out other congenital abnoamalities.

Management

The urgency of surgical repair of a coloboma depends on the severity of exposure caused by it. Any coloboma larger than one-third the horizontal extent of the eyelid poses danger to the cornea, and must have early surgical correction. Any smaller one may undergo elective correction, and have conservative management with lubricants, moist chambers or bandage contact lenses. The edges of the coloboma should be manually pulled together to assess the actual size of the coloboma, to plan appropriate surgery. Smaller ones may have direct closure. Larger ones may need more extensive reconstruction. When using a lid-sharing technique, the risk of amblyopia in a young child should be remembered **(Figures 2A and B)**.

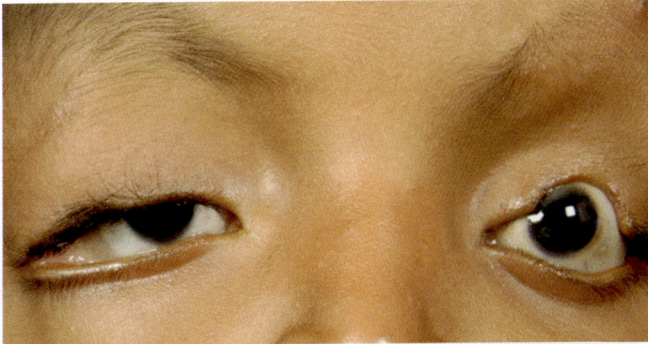

Figure 2A: Clinical photograph of patient with right eye lateral canthal ectopia, congenital ptosis, and left eye upper lid coloboma with corneal scarring due to exposure

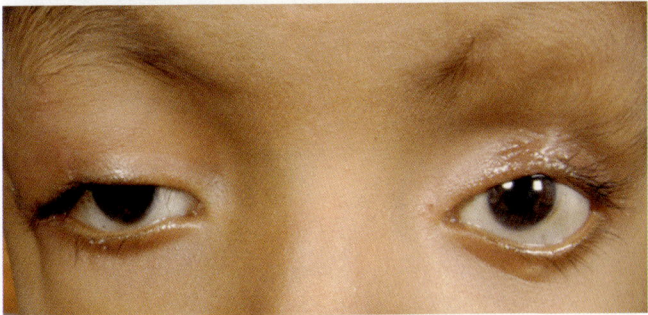

Figure 2B: Postoperative clinical photograph of the same patient, with well corrected coloboma

Goldenhar Syndrome

Lid coloboma is a common association with Goldenhar syndrome, in addition to corneal or epibulbar dermoids, and pre-auricular skin tags and external ear deformities **(Figures 3A and B).**

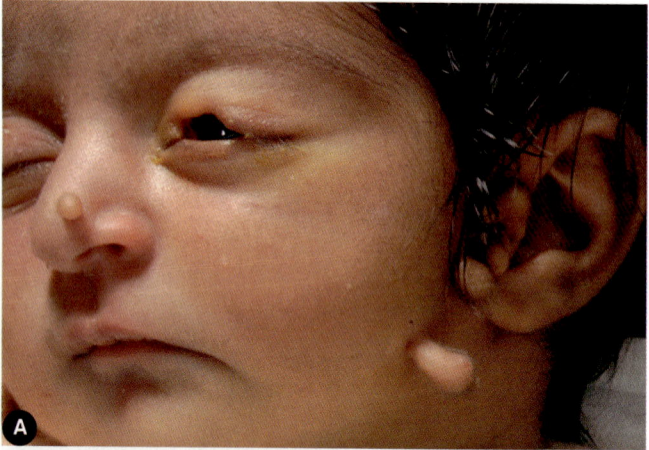

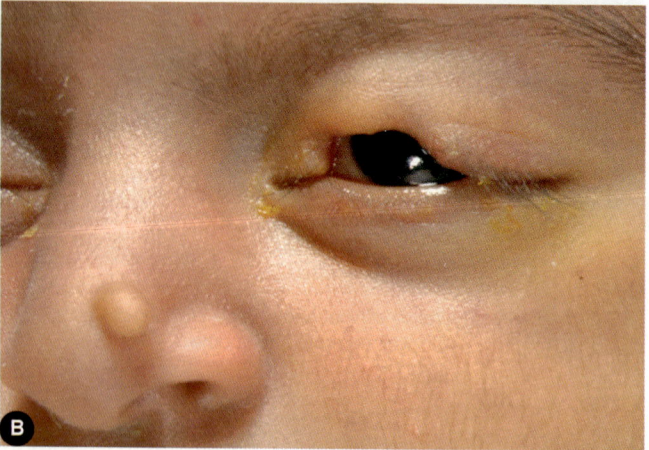

Figures 3A and B: Goldenhar syndrome with left eye upper lid coloboma and pre-auricular and external nasal skin tags

MICROBLEPHARON AND ABLEPHARON

Introduction and Signs & Symptoms

A microblepharon is a rare vertical foreshortening of the eyelid. The upper lid is more commonly affected. Apparent ablepharon may be a severe microblepharon, and one should look carefully for rudimentary eyelids. It may be associated with clinical anophthalmos. It is associated with lagophthalmos and exposure keratopathy. There may be additional ocular and systemic abnormalities **(Figure 4).**

Investigation

Evaluation should be performed for addditonal systemic and ocular abnormalities. In a microphthalmic eye, assessment for visual potential is required.

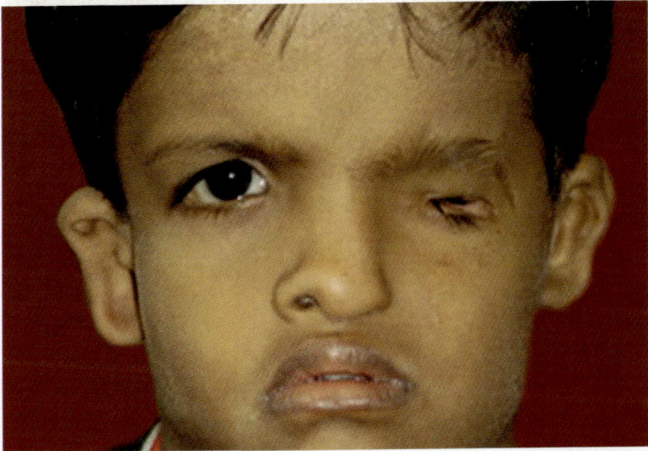

Figure 4: Patient with right eye euryblepharon, left eye clinical anophthalmos with upper and lower lid microblepharon. The eyelids are short vertically as well as horizontally

Differential Diagnosis

Microblepharon and ablepharon should be differentiated from lid colobomas.

Management

The surgical management plan depends on the visual potential and the specific features. Correction may require rotation flaps from the cheek, lid sharing procedures, pedicle flaps or skin grafts.

ANKYLOBLEPHARON

Ankyloblepharon Filiforme Adnatum

Signs and Symptoms

The condition shows fine extensile cords attaching upper and lower lids, which may be single or multiple. The cords decrease the palpebral fissure height and reduce lid excursion. It has been reported n association with trisomy 18.

This may be associated with ectodermal dysplasia and cleft lip or cleft palate – this is the autosomal dominant Hay-Well's syndrome.

Treatment

The cord is simply severed, and the epithelial tags involute.

Congenital Ankyloblepharon

Introduction

Congenital ankyloblepharon is caused by developmental arrest leading to growth aberration at either canthus, inner or outer.

Signs and Symptoms

It is caused by partial fusion of the upper and lower lid, and results in horizontal foreshortening of the palpebral fissure. The commoner external variety is at the lateral canthus, causing an appearance of pseudoexotropia. The internal ankyloblepharon at the inner canthus causes pseudo-esotropia.

Differential Diagnosis

Pseudo-eso- or exotropia must be differentiated from true strabismus.

Treatment

Ankyloblepharon requires surgical separation of the eyelids.

MEDIAL CANTHAL ECTOPIA

Introduction

Medial canthal ectopia is caused by developmental arrest in the second month of intrauterine life.

Signs and Symptoms

The medial canthal tendon is displaced inferiorly along with surrounding canthal structures. It attaches to the junction of the medial wall of the orbit and the inferior orbital rim. There may be associated nasal cleft deformities and nasolacrimal duct obstruction **(Figure 5)**.

Differential Diagnosis

The condition is to be differentiated from medial canthal dystopia acquired after trauma.

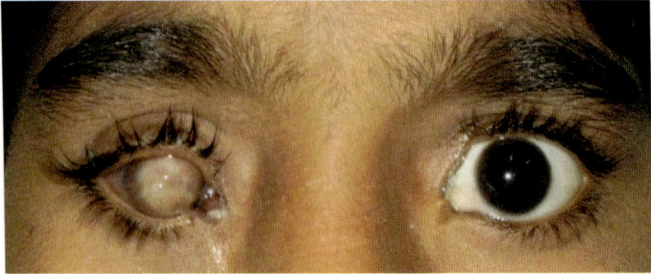

Figure 5: Clinical photograph of patient with right eye corneal dermoid, medial canthal ectopia both eyes and small colobomatous lid notching in left eye. The medial canthus is displaced downwards, and is associated with congenital nasolacrimal duct obstruction. The patient has undergone surgical correction of cleft lip and palate previously

Investigation

The child should be assessed for nas-lacrimal duct obstruction.

Treatment

The condition requires surgical supraplacement of the medial canthal tendon: a Z-plasty or a Y-V plasty may be used. The associated nasolacrimal duct obstruction should also be corrected.

EPICANTHUS

Introduction and Signs & Symptoms

Epicanthus is a semi-lunar fold of skin at the medial canthus, with its concavity directed outward. The epicanthal fold obscures the view of the medial canthal angle, the caruncle and plica. An epicanthus may be isolated or be an associated feature in a patient with congenital ptosis or Blepharophimosis syndrome. There are several varieties of epicanthus.

- Epicanthus tarsalis extends from the upper lid

- Epicanthus inversus extends from the lower lid (associated with Blepharophimosis-ptosis-epicanthus inversus syndrome—BPES)
- Epicanthus palpebralis extends from the upper lid to the lower lid
- Epicanthus superciliaris extends from below the eye-brow. Epicanthus may give an appearance of pseudoesotropia

(Figures 6A to C).

Differential Diagnosis

Any epicanthus should be examined to rule out associated BPES.

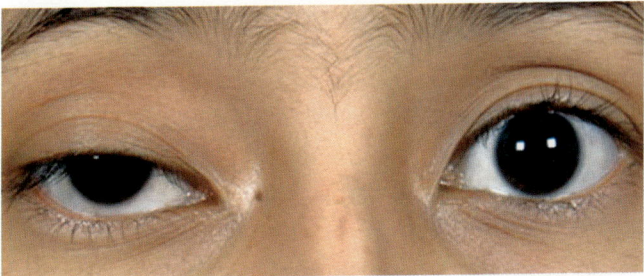

Figure 6A: Patient with right eye congenital ptosis, with epicanthus tarsalis both eyes. A fold of skin extends from the upper lid to the lower lid at the medial canthus

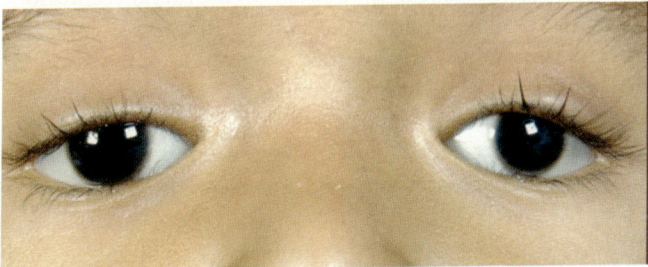

Figure 6B: Patient with bilateral congenital ptosis and bilateral epicanthus inversus. A semilunar fold of skin extends from the upper lid to the lower lid

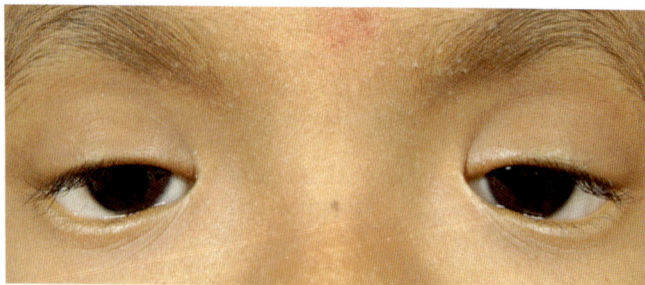

Figure 6C: Epicanthus palpebralis, with a semilunar fold of skin extending on both upper and lower lids. The epicanthal fold obscures the medial canthal structures and gives an appearance of pseudostrabismus

Treatment

Epicanthus is corrected by Mustarde double Z-plasty, modified Y-V plasty or C-U plasty.

CENTURION SYNDROME

Introduction and Signs & Symptoms

The patient of centurion syndrome has a history of epiphora since childhood, which worsens at puberty. Syringing of the nasolacrimal duct is patent. The syndrome derives its name from the resemblance of the patients to the Roman centurions in their helmets. The medial canthal tendon is taut and attached anteriorly, causing medial stand-off of the lower lid and punctum. The lacrimal punctum is displaced forward out of the lacrimal lake, causing epiphora. The facial appearance is typical, with a sharp medial canthus, long horizontal palpebral fissure and square eyebrows **(Figure 7).**

Differential Diagnosis

The condition is to be differentiated from other causes of epiphora.

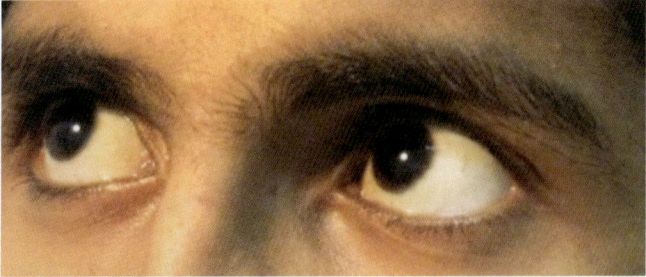

Figure 7: Patient with centurion syndrome, with sharp medial canthal angles, square eyebrows, and elongated horizontal palpebral aperture. The medial canthal tendon is prominent and attached anteriorly, not allowing proper apposition of the lacrimal punctum to the tear meniscus

Investigation

Lacrimal syringing will be patent, but dye disappearance will be delayed.

Treatment

The treatment is surgical, anterior medial canthal tendon release, with medial canthoplasty or punctoplasty.

DISTICHIASIS

Introduction and Signs & Symptoms

Distichiasis is an extra row of eyelashes behind the normal ciliary margin at the sites of meibomian glands. It may involve the whole length of the lid or only a segment. The distichiatic lashes rubbing on the ocular surface can induce epiphora or even keratopathy. Congenital distichiasis is associated with lower limb lymphedema; the gene responsible is FOXC 2 **(Figure 8).**

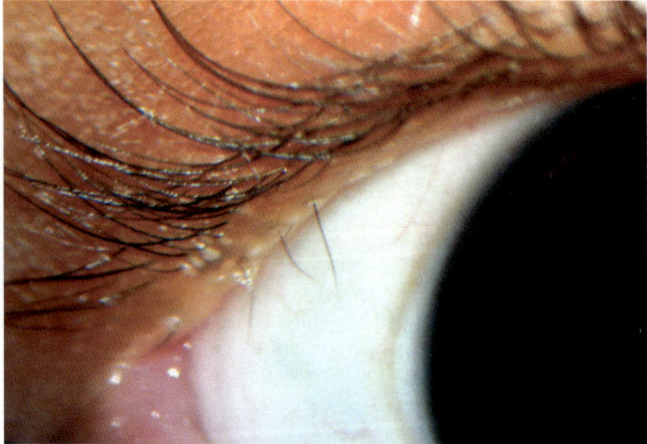

Figure 8: Incomplete row of eyelashes growing on the medial aspect of the upper lid; the lashes are at the sites of meibomian gland orifices

Differential Diagnosis

Distichiasis is to be differentiated from other conditions with abnormal positions or abnormal directions of eyelashes, such as trichiasis, epiblepharon and entropion.

Investigation

Instillation of fluorescein in the eye will help to detect early keratopathy.

Treatment

If the patient is asymptomatic, observation alone suffices. A small number of lashes may be treated by electrolysis. In extensive distichiasis, the lid can be split along the grey line and cryo applied to the posterior lamella at the roots of the distichiatic eyelashes.

EPIBLEPHARON

Introduction and Signs & Symptoms

Epiblepharon comprises a horizontal redundant lid fold of skin and orbicularis in the lower lid, causing vertical orientation of the eyelashes. There may be coexistent entropion. The eyelashes rubbing on the cornea cause epiphora, and may cause keratopathy. It is commoner in Mongolian features. It may be associated with inferior oblique weakness. Epiblepharon often resolves spontaneously by 3 years of age **(Figures 9A and B).**

Differential Diagnosis

The condition is to be differentiated from congenital entropion and distichiasis.

Investigation

Instillation of fluorescein dye will help to detect any keratopathy. Careful examination will rule out associated inferior oblique weakness.

Treatment

Epiblepharon may be treated with lubricants in the expectation of spontaneous resolution. If the cornea shows

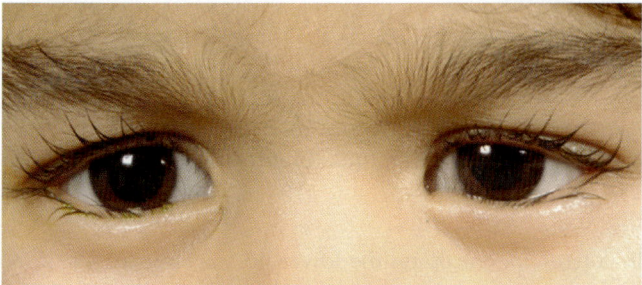

Figure 9A: Patient with bilateral epiblepharon with high tear meniscus

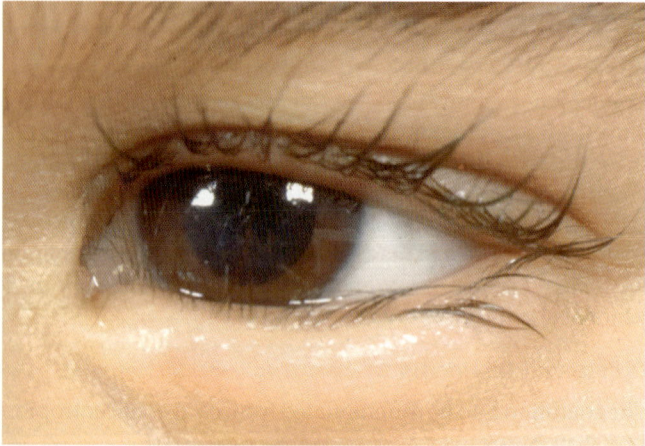

Figure 9B: Clinical photograph showing redundant horizontal fold of lower lid skin and orbicularis, with vertical orientation of eyelashes

keratopathy, surgical intervention is required. The redundant skin and orbicularis oculi muscle is excised in the form of a spindle; usually 1-3 mm of excision would suffice. In severe cases everting sutures may be used in addition.

CONGENITAL ENTROPION

Introduction

Congenital entropion affects the lower lid, and results from inadequate development of the lower lid retractors. This causes lower lid malpositions similar to that in senile entropion. The entropion is often accompanied by epiblepharon and epicanthus **(Figure 10)**.

Signs and Symptoms

In congenital entropion the lower lid rolls inwards, and the eyelashes rub on the ocular surface. The patient may be symptomatic, with epiphora and keratopathy.

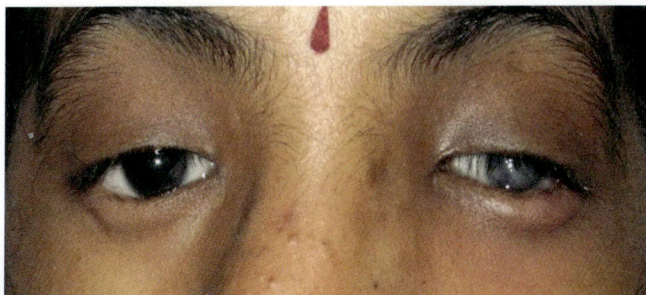

Figure 10: Clinical photograph of patient with bilateral congenital ptosis, with anti-mongoloid slant of palpebral fissures, with lower lid entropion. Left eye shows a failed corneal graft and lower lid external hordeolum

Differential Diagnosis

Congenital entropion must be distinguished from epiblepharon and distichiasis.

Management

Surgical correction is required if the patient develops keratopathy. The procedure of choice is reattachment of the lower lid retractors to the tarsus.

TARSAL KINK SYNDROME

Introduction and Signs & Symptoms

Tarsal kink syndrome is a rare entity with horizontal fold along the entire horizontal length of the tarsus. Tarsal kink results in entropion of the upper lid; in the severest cases, the child presents within a few weeks of age, and the lid margin is not visible. The patient may have absent lid crease, blepharospasm, lid edema and keratopathy. The patient commonly presents with corneal ulcer in early infancy **(Figures 11A to C).**

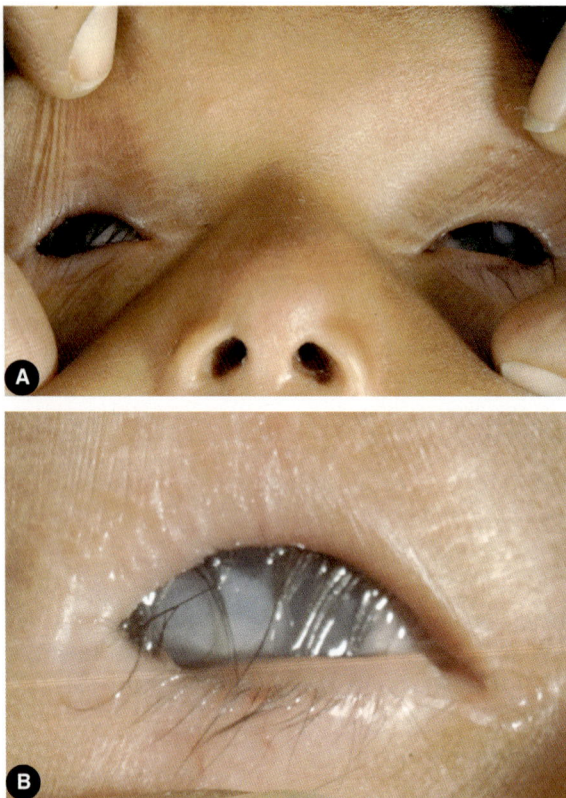

Figures 11A and B: Patient with bilateral tarsal kink and bilateral corneal ulcers. The upper lids show severe entropion, with obscuration of lid margin and absent lid crease

Differential Diagnosis

Tarsal kink syndrome with corneal infiltrate should be differentiated from patients presenting with other corneal ulcers.

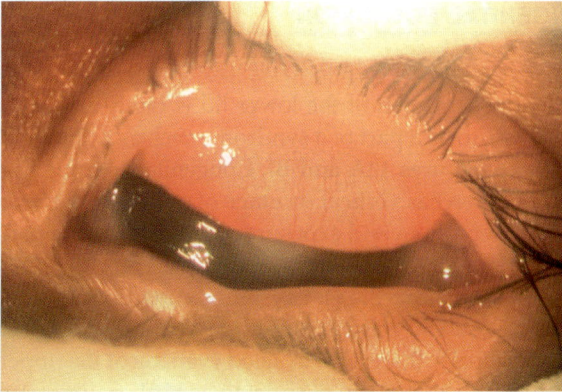

Figure 11C: The everted eyelid shows a crease in the tarsal plate along the entire horizontal length

Management

Surgical correction of the tarsal kink entails full-thickness blepharotomy the entire length of eyelid with marginal rotation. Due to the very early age of presentation and the associated corneal ulceration and scarring, amblyopia therapy is crucial after correction of the entropion **(Figure 11D).**

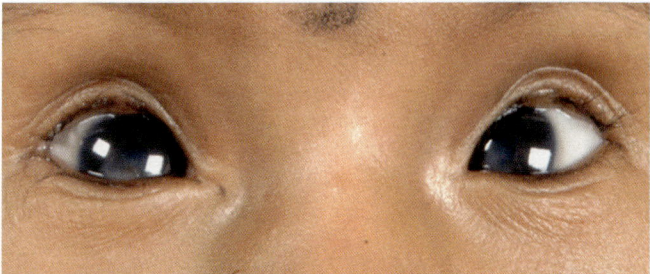

Figure 11D: The clinical photograph of the same patient after surgical correction of the entropion

CONGENITAL ECTROPION

Introduction and Signs & Symptoms

Congenital ectropion of the lower lid is rarely isolated; it is more likely to be a part of a syndrome such as Kohn Romano syndrome **(Figures 12A and B).** Congenital ectropion of the lower lid often has vertical shortage of skin. Severe ectropion will cause epiphora and exposure, and the tarsal conjunctiva may become keratinized.

Lamellar ichthyosis is a systemic condition which may result in cicatricial ectropion of upper and lower lid at birth.

Occasionally there is an isolated eversion of the upper lid, for which the etiology is postulated as birth trauma causing vascular stasis and congestion, leading to lid eversion **(Figure 13).**

Differential Diagnosis

The ectropion due to shortage of skin should be differentiated from euryblepharon, which also causes lateral ectropion of the lower lid.

Management

Congenital ectropion requires full-thickness skin grafting; the preferred donor site is the retroauricular area.

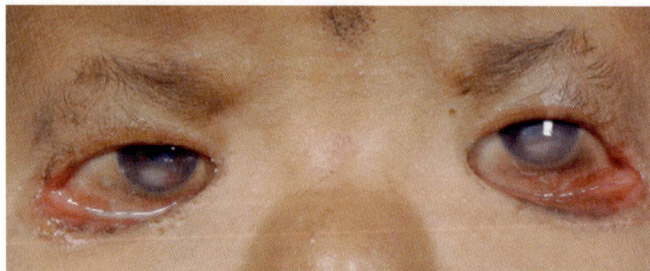

Figure 12A: Clinical photograph of patient with bilateral congenital ptosis, blepharophimosis, telecanthus and lower lid ectropion

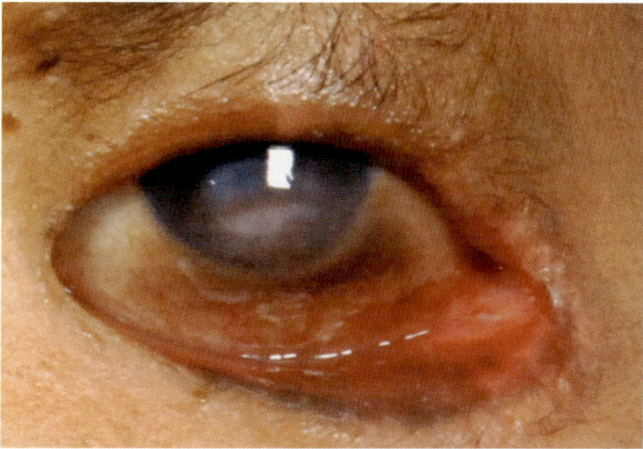

Figure 12B: The lower lid shows severe ectropion, vertical shortening of the anterior lamella, keratinization and pigmentation of the conjunctiva. The cornea shows exposure keratopathy

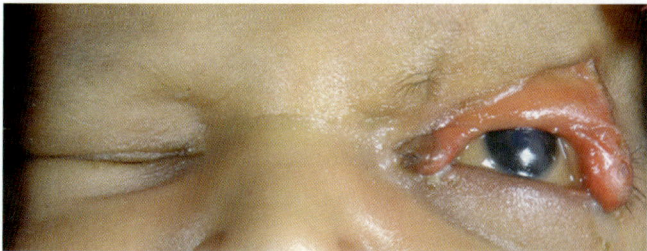

Figure 13: Left eye upper lid congenital ectropion, with complete eversion of eyelid

In lamellar ichthyosis, it may be difficult to identify any area of healthy skin as a potential donor site. Skin emollients should also be used liberally.

In the isolated upper lid eversion, one may escape surgery, and get by only with marginal traction suture to straighten the lid. If the ectropion persists, one may need to excise a part of the prolapsed conjunctiva to allow correction of the lid eversion.

EURYBLEPHARON

Introduction and Signs & Symptoms

Euryblepharon presents with bilateral symmetrical enlargement of the horizontal palpebral apertures, with vertical shortage of eyelid skin, elongated lid margins, and downward and lateral displacement of outer canthi. The horizontal palpebral fissure length is increased to approximately 35 mm from the average of 28-30 mm. There is lateral ectropion, lagophthalmos and reduced blink rate with exposure keratopathy. The exposure and reduced blink rate may cause epiphora **(Figures 14A to C).**

Differential Diagnosis

Euryblepharon should be distinguished from the congenital ectropion which has vertical shortage of skin, but not an elongated lid margin.

Other causes of epiphora in childhood should be differentiated from euryblepharon.

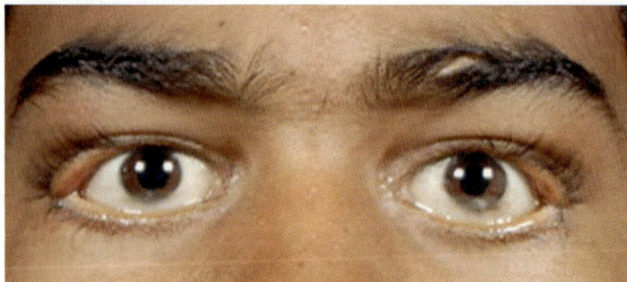

Figure 14A: Clinical photograph of patient with bilateral upper and lower lid lateral ectropion, with excess horizontal length

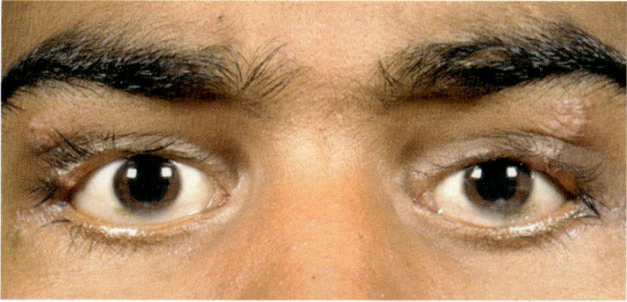

Figure 14B: Photograph of the same patient after surgical correction of the euryblepharon. The corneas are scarred due to exposure

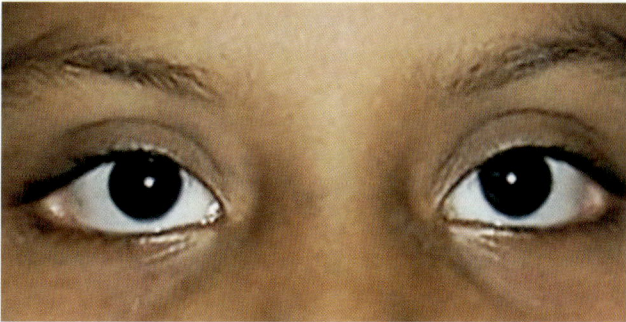

Figure 14C: Photograph of patient with mild degree of euryblepharon, with lateral ectropion of lower lid alone

Management

Mild degrees may be managed conservatively, with lubricants. Moderate degrees will require tarsorrhaphy to protect the cornea. A lateral canthoplasty with shortening of the upper and lower lids laterally may be beneficial. The severest forms may require staged correction with augmentation of the posterior lamella and anterior skin graft.

CONGENITAL LID RETRACTION

Introduction and Signs & Symptoms

Congenital retraction of the upper lid may be unilateral or bilateral. A unilateral lid retraction may simulate contralateral ptosis. The condition is non-progressive. Other systemic features are usually normal.

Differential Diagnosis

Congenital lid retraction must be differentiated from other causes of lid retraction such as thyroid abnormalities, and Marcus Gunn phenomenon. Children developing eyelid retraction must be investigated for intracranial space-occupying lesions, hydrocephalus and postencephalitic sequelae **(Figures 15A and B)**.

There has been a case report of accessory slip of levator palpebrae superioris causing lid retraction.

Investigation

Thyroid function tests may rule out endocrine-related lid retraction.

Management

Lid retraction may be treated by lid lengthening procedures.

CONGENITAL PTOSIS

Introduction and Signs & Symptoms

Congenital ptosis is the commonest of the congenital lid anomalies. The upper lid is at a lower level than normal, and the condition may be unilateral or bilateral. The affected eye may have limited elevation. A quick assessment of the severity of congenital ptosis is possible by looking at the red reflex of

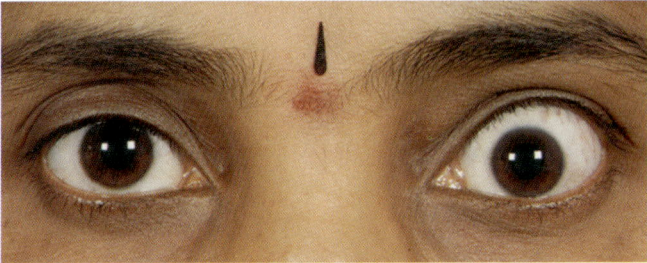

Figure 15A: Clinical photograph of patient with congenital retraction of left upper lid

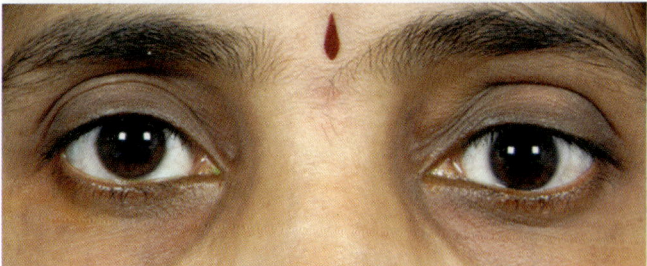

Figure 15B: Photograph of the same patient after surgical correction of the lid retraction

the pupil through distant direct ophthalmoscopy, and recording how much of the pupil is obscured by the lid. Other indicators of the severity of the ptosis are over-action of the frontalis muscles and chin elevation on inspection of the face. A greater palpebral fissure height in down gaze is seen in the unilateral ptosis, since the defective levator palpebrae muscle is also deficient in ability to relax. A faint upper lid crease indicates weak levator action. Marcus Gunn phenomenon, i.e. synkinetic elevation of the ptotic lid with jaw movement should be looked for. Amblyopia may develop due to visual deprivation, refractive error or associated strabismus **(Figures 16A and B).**

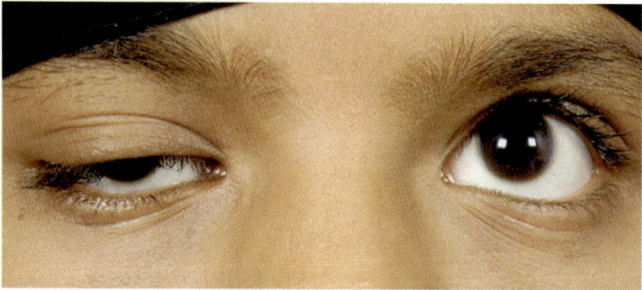

Figure 16A: Patient with right eye congenital ptosis

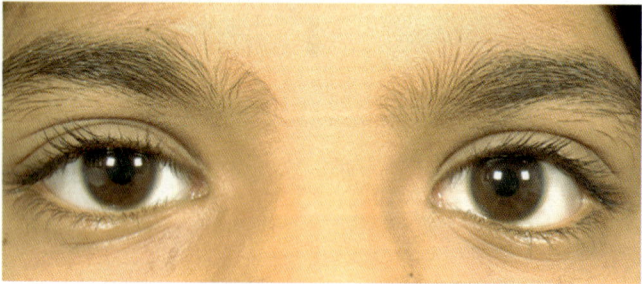

Figure 16B: Photograph of same patient after ptosis correction by frontalis suspension

Differential Diagnosis

Careful examination will rule out other causes of ptosis in the young.

Myasthenia gravis may rarely occur in a child. Variable ptosis, involvement of extraocular muscles and fatigability indicate myasthenic ptosis. The diagnosis may be confirmed by edrophonium test.

Chronic progressive external ophthalmoplegia may have an onset in the first decade of life, and show associated limitation of ocular movements.

Congenital ocular fibrosis presents with ptosis along with strabismus. The ocular movements are severely restricted.

Ptosis may be associated with weakness of the third cranial nerve.

Investigation

The child with ptosis requires careful cycloplegic refraction. Ice test and edrophomnium test help to rule out ocular myasthenia.

Management

Severe ptosis with high risk of amblyopia should be corrected early in life. Milder disease is corrected as the child reaches the school-going age. Severe ptosis with poor levator action is treated by a tarso-frontal sling; the material of the sling may be biogenic such as autogenous or preserved fascia lata or bovine pericardium, or synthetic such as mersilene, silicone, PTFE or poly-propylene. Any associated strabismus requires correction before correction of the ptosis.

Ptosis with associated Marcus Gunn phenomenon needs special consideration. Disinsertion of the levator aponeurosis from the tarsal attachment bilaterally with bilateral tarsofrontal sling has been advocated. An alternative is to disinsert the levator of the affected side alone, with bilateral sling surgery.

After correction of the ptosis, refractive error should be reassessed and correction provided. Amblyopia therapy should be instituted if required.

BLEPHAROPHIMOSIS SYNDROME

Introduction and Signs & Symptoms

Blepharophimosis syndrome presents as a combination of several features.

Blepharophimosis is characterized by a short horizontal palpebral fissure, 18-22 mm as opposed to the average of 28-30 mm. *Blepharoptosis* is severe, with poor levator function, absent lid crease and characteristic head posture with chin elevation and over-action of the frontalis. *Epicanthus inversus* shows a semilunar fold of skin at the medial canthus, extending from the lower lid to the upper lid. *Telecanthus* is an increased distance between the orbits. The inter-medial canthal distance is greater than half the inter-pupillary distance. The tetrad of Blepharophimosis, blepharoptosis, epicanthus inversus and telecanthus together comprise the Kohn Romano syndrome. Blepharophimosis syndrome may, in addition, have inferiorly slanted palpebral apertures and lateral ectropion.

The Blepharophimosis, Ptosis, Epicanthus inversus Syndrome (BPES syndrome) has been identified to be autosomal dominant. There are two types of this syndrome: BPES Type I is associated with infertility, while BPES Type II is not. The gene involved in BPES Type I is FOXL2.

The Callahan classification of blepharophimosis is based on the particular combination of clinical features at presentation:

Blepharophimosis type I: Blepharoptosis, blepharophimosis, epicanthus inversus, telecanthus.

Blepharophimosis type II: Blepharophimosis and blepharoptosis, without epicanthus and normally spaced orbits

Blepharophimosis type III: Blepharophimosis and blepharoptosis, with shortage of skin and palpebral apertures slanted inferiorly, with wide spaced orbits.

Differential Diagnosis

Blepharophimosis syndrome is to be differentiated from isolated congenital ptosis.

Management

Blepharophimosis syndrome requires staged repair. The epicanthus is corrected first, by Mustarde's double Z-plasty or by modified Y-V plasty. Any lateral ectropion causing lagophthalmos and exposure is corrected by lateral canthoplasty, and skin grafting if necessary. The ptosis is corrected by a tarsofrontal sling surgery **(Figures 17A to C).**

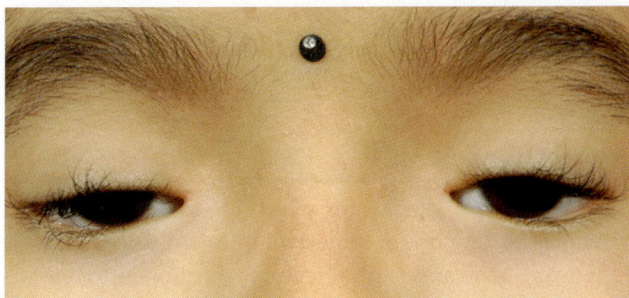

Figure 17A: Blepharophimosis syndrome type 1, with ptosis, blepharophimosis, telecanthus and epicanthus inversus

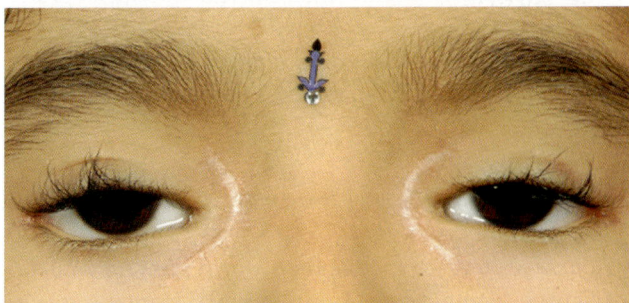

Figure 17B: Same patient after surgical correction of the epicanthus by C-U plasty

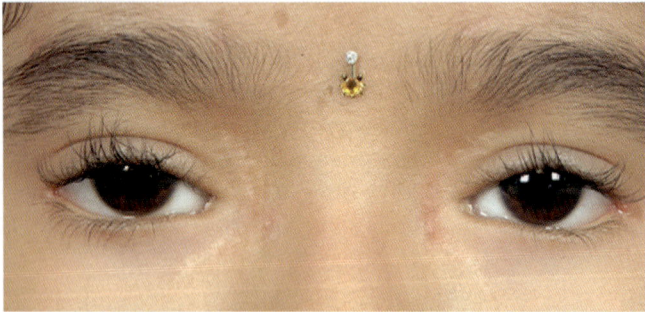

Figure 17C: Final surgical outcome of the same patient after ptosis correction

OTHER SYNDROMES

There are several syndromes which are associated with lid anomalies. A few of the important ones are listed, with the responsible gene and clinical features mentioned in brief.

Prader Willi Syndrome

- *Gene responsible*—SNRP small nuclear ribonucleoprotein polypeptide)
- *Clinical features*—almond shaped palpebral fissures, obesity, hypogonadism, mental retardation

Noonan Syndrome

- *Gene responsible* PTPN 11 (protein tyrosinase phosphatase non-receptor type).
- *Clinical features*—hypertelorism, down slanting palpebral fissures, webbing neck, pulmonary stenosis, pectus excavatum.

Rubinstein Taybi Syndrome

- *Gene responsible*—CRE binding protein
- *Clinical features*—heavy arched eyebrows, down slanting palpebral fissures, broad thumbs and toes, mental retardation.

Fraser Syndrome

- *Gene responsible*—FRAS1(ECM protein)
- *Clinical features*—cryptophthalmos, renal agenesis, syndactyly, laryngeal stenosis.

Apert Syndrome

- *Gene responsible*—FGFR2
- *Clinical features*—severe craniostenosis, syndactyly, hypertelorism, proptosis, strabismus.

Crouzon Syndrome and Related Syndromes (Pfeiffer and Jackson Weis syndrome)

- *Gene responsible*—FGFR2-FGFR
- *Clinical features*—craniostenosis, limb anomalies (absent in JWS, PS), hypertelorism, proptosis, orbital asymmetry.

Saethre-Chotzen Syndrome

- *Gene responsible*—TWIST
- *Clinical features*—craniostenosis, limb and ear anomalies, ptosis.

Waardenburg Syndrome

- *Gene responsible*—PAX3 (WS1), MITF (WS2)
- *Clinical features*—iris heterochromia, deafness, white forelock, dystopia canthorum (WS1)

Treacher Collins Syndrome

- *Gene responsible*—TCOF1
- *Clinical features*—first branchial arch syndrome, down slanting palpebral fissures, eyelid colobomas.

Coffin Lowry Syndrome

- *Gene responsible*—RPS6KA3
- *Clinical features*—X linked mental retardation syndrome, hypertelorism, down slanting palpebral fissures.

Stickler

- *Gene responsible*—COL2A1, COL11A1, COL11A2
- *Clinical features*—midfacial hypoplasia, cleft palate, hearing loss, spondyloepiphyseal dysplasia, proptosis.

BIBLIOGRAPHY

1. Bernardini FP, Kersten RC, de Conciliis C, Devoto MH. Unilateral microblepharon. Ophthal Plast Reconstr Surg. 2004 Nov; 20(6):467-9.
2. Dawodu OA. Total eversion of the upper eyelids in a newborn. Niger Postgrad Med J. 2001 Sep; 8(3):145-7.
3. DN, Ferrell RE, Meisler DM. Lymphedema-distichiasis syndrome and FOXC2 gene mutation. Am J Ophthalmol. 2002 Oct; 134(4):592-6.
4. Dollfus H, Verloes A. Dysmorphology and the orbital region: a practical clinical approach. Surv Ophthalmol. 2004 Nov-Dec; 49(6):547-61.
5. Egier D, Orton R, Allen L, Siu VM. Bilateral complete isolated cryptophthalmos: a case report. Ophthalmic Genet. 2005 Dec; 26(4):185-9.
6. Jain S, Atkinson AJ, Hopkisson B. Ankyloblepharon filiforme adnatum.Br J Ophthalmol. 1997 Aug; 81(8):708.
7. Kao YS, Lin CH, Fang RH. Epicanthoplasty with modified Y-V advancement procedure. Plast Reconstr Surg. 1998 Nov; 102(6):1835-41.

8. Khwarg SI, Choung HK. Epiblepharon of the lower eyelid: technique of surgical repair and quantification of excision according to the skin fold height. Ophthalmic Surg Lasers. 2002 Jul-Aug; 33(4):280-7.

9. Naik MN, Honavar SG, Bhaduri A, Linberg JV. Congenital horizontal tarsal kink: a single-center experience with 6 cases. Ophthalmology. 2007 Aug; 114(8):1564-8.

10. Nouby G. Congenital upper eyelid coloboma and cryptophthalmos. Ophthal Plast Reconstr Surg. 2002 Sep; 18(5):373-7.

11. Oculoplastic, Orbital and Reconstructive Surgery. Edition 1. Albert Hornblass Ed. Williams and Wilkins, 1988, Baltimore.

12. Ptosis, Edition 3. C Beard. CV Mosby Company, 1981, St Louis.

13. Samlaska CP. Congenital lymphedema and distichiasis. Pediatr Dermatol. 2002 Mar-Apr; 19(2):139-41.

14. Sires BS. Congenital horizontal tarsal kink: clinical characteristics from a large series. Ophthal Plast Reconstr Surg. 1999 Sep; 15(5):355-9.

15. Spierer A, Bourla N. Primary congenital upper eyelid retraction in infants and children. Ophthal Plast Reconstr Surg. 2004 May; 20(3):246-8.

16. Sujatha Y, Sathish S, Stewart WB. Centurion syndrome and its surgical management. Ophthal Plast Reconstr Surg. 1999 Jul; 15(4):243-4.

17. Sullivan TJ, Welham RA, Collin JR. Centurion syndrome. Idiopathic anterior displacement of the medial canthus. Ophthalmology. 1993 Mar; 100(3):328-33.

18. Traboulsi EI, Al-Khayer K, Matsumoto M, Kimak MA, Crowe S, Wilson SE, Finegold

19. Tüysüz B, Ilikkan B, Vural M, Perk Y. Ankyloblepharon filiforme adnatum (AFA) associated with trisomy 18. Turk J Pediatr. 2002 Oct-Dec; 44(4):360-2.

20. Wylen EL, Brown MS, Rich LS, Hesse RJ. Supernumerary orbital muscle in congenital eyelid retraction. Ophthal Plast Reconstr Surg. 2001 Mar; 17(2):120-2.

Pediatric Eyelid Abnormalities

2

AK Grover, Shaloo Bageja (India)

INTRODUCTION

Eyelids are essential in maintaining the integrity of the ocular system as it helps to keep the cornea moist by distribution of tears and protects eyeball against injury. The child may presents with an abnormality of eyelid or symptoms due to it. Ophthalmologist should be able to make an accurate diagnosis and plan the management accordingly.

EMBRYOLOGY OF THE EYELID

Eyelids are derived from the ectodermal tissue. At 4th to 5th week of gestation, the surface ectoderm overlying the cornea differentiates into cranial and caudal folds with a core of mesenchyme. Both folds move closer together. The mesenchyme differentiates into orbital septum anteriorly and tarsus posteriorly. The lid margins fuse together by 3rd month of gestation. The fused eyelids separate by 5th-6th month of gestation.

The eyelid abnormalities are broadly divided into two groups:

  i. Congenital
 ii. Acquired

CONGENITAL DISORDERS

Congenital eyelid disorders may be *isolated* or may be associated with other *facial or systemic anomalies.*

Congenital anomalies were classified by Duke-Elder based on chronological fetal development.

1. Abnormalities from abnormal development of lid-folds occur between 3rd and 5th month of fetal development- Cryptophthalmos, coloboma.
2. Anomalies in the differentiation of lid-margins, which occur between 5th and 6th month of development– Ankyloblepharon, Congenital ectropion and entropion
3. Anomalies in the differentiation of the tissues of the lids: Epiblepharon, Distichiasis, Euryblepharon, Telecanthus, Congenital Ptosis

Cryptophthalmos

It is a rare congenital anomaly, occurs due to failure of development of lid folds. Surface epithelium which normally differentiates to form cornea and conjunctiva, becomes part of skin. Continuous skin is seen from forehead to cheek **(Figures 1A to D)**. The underlying eye is usually under-developed and visual potential is poor. There may be

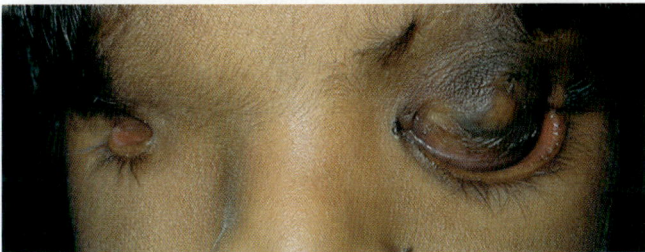

Figure 1A: 5-year-old child presented with right eye clinical anophthalmos and left eye incomplete cryptophthalmos

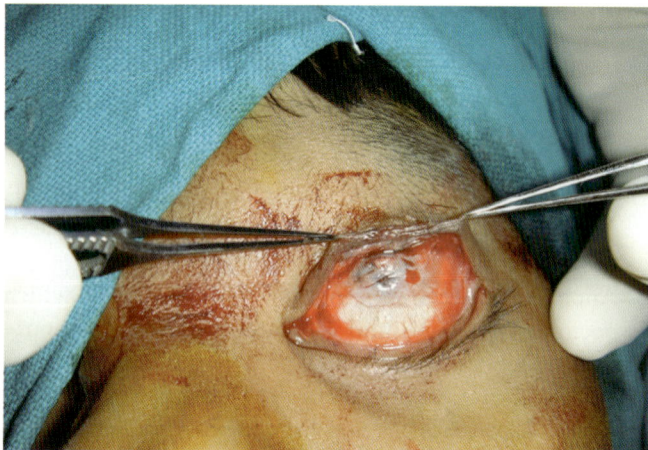

Figure 1B: Skin tissue dissected away globe and cornea

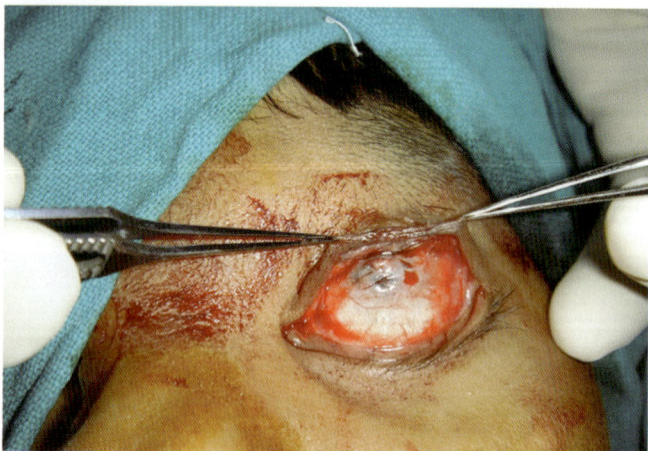

Figure 1C: Buccal covering formed by mucous membrane graft

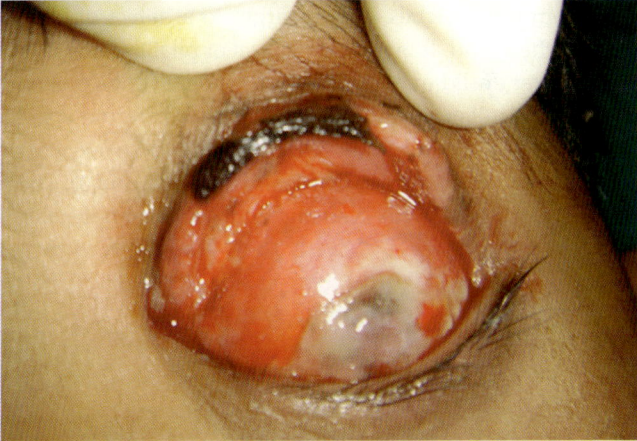

Figure 1D: Postoperative photograph showing adequate superior fornix

complete or incomplete cryptophthalmos. There is a variable deficiency in the development of eyebrows, eyelids and adhesion of eyelids to the globe. It may also be associated with systemic anomalies like facial abnormalities or renal anomalies.

Management

Lid sharing procedure may be attempted in cases of incomplete cryptophthalmos, where one may suspect some visual potential.

Coloboma

Congenital colobomas of the eyelid is a form of facial clefting. It occurs when there is a defect in the eyelid margin due to inability of fusion of surface ectoderm to form lid folds or following mechanical trauma from amniotic bands. They may vary from tiny notches in the margin to a defect of half or more of the eyelid. It may be unilateral or bilateral, the upper or the lower eyelid may be involved. Upper eyelid coloboma are usually unilateral and medial. It may vary from a small notch to large coloboma which can lead to exposure keratopathy and require early repair **(Figures 2 and 3).** These may be associated with systemic and ocular abnormalities

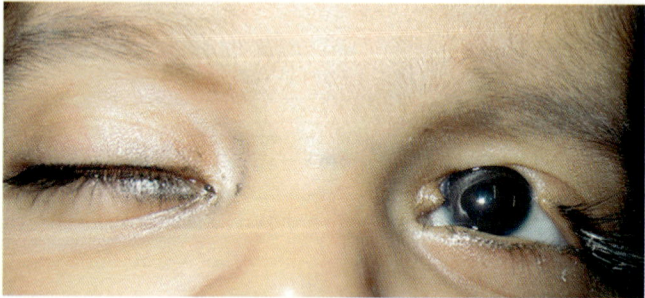

Figure 2: An 8-month-old infant with congenital upper eyelid coloboma

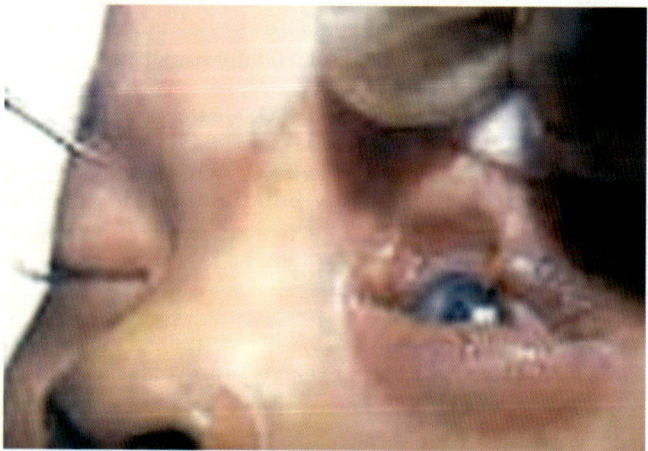

Figure 3: Congenital upper eyelid coloboma with exposure keratopathy

most common is the Goldenhar syndrome (limbal dermoids and dermal lipomas). Lower lid coloboma are unilateral – usually isolated and occur laterally. Bilateral coloboma are usually associated with a systemic syndrome like Treacher Collin syndrome.

Management

Surgical management in cases of coloboma without exposure keratopathy is deferred till 3-4 years of age.

Principles of management of eyelid reconstruction:
1. Direct suturing with or without cantholysis—for small defects upto 25% of full thickness
2. Tenzel's flap for upper lid colobomas—for defects up to 40-50% of the upper lid.
3. Lid sharing procedures—for defects more than 55% **(Figures 4A to F).**

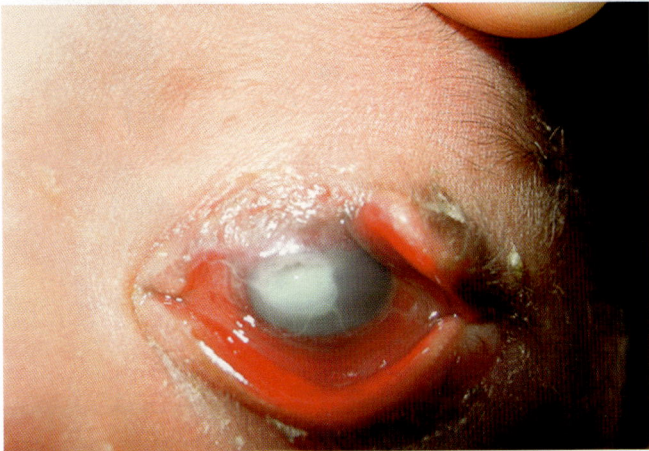

Figure 4A: 9-day-old infant with upper lid coloboma with exposure keratopathy

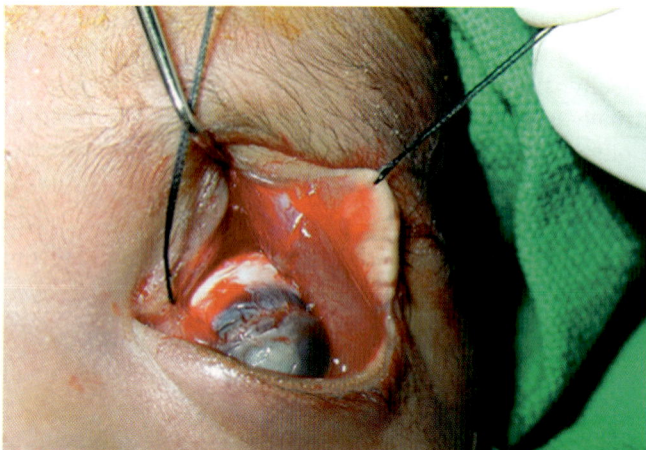

Figure 4B: Lid dissected away from cornea and globe

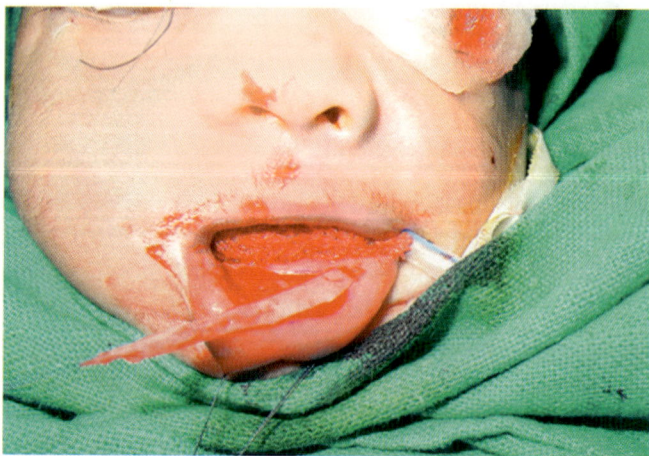

Figure 4C: Mucous membrane graft taken from buccal mucosa

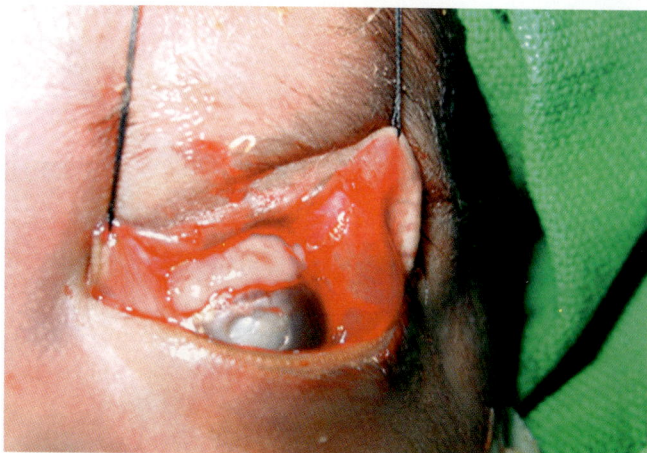

Figure 4D: Graft forming the bulbar covering and fornix

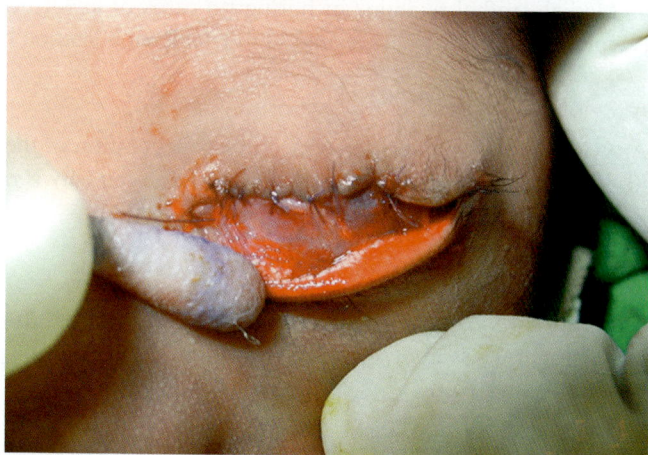

Figure 4E: Skin-muscle sutured conjunctiva inferiorly

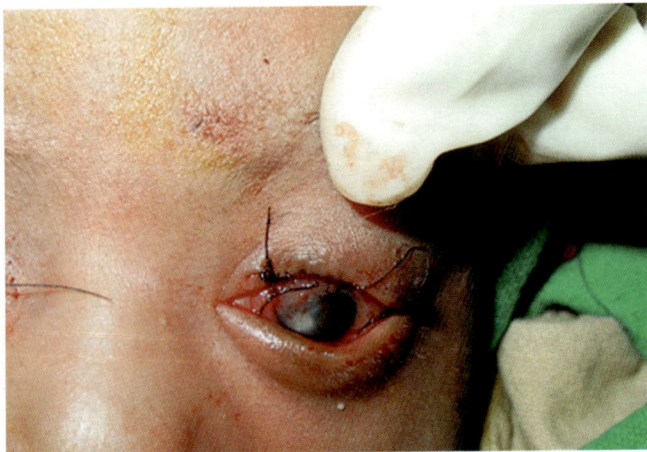

Figure 4F: Separation of flaps after 2 months

4. Medial canthal fixation/anchoring (in cases of lower lid colobomas) usually associated with lateral mobilization

Ankyloblepharon

Ankyloblepharon results from incomplete separation of the fused lid folds. It may be filiform or broad adhesion between the two lids **(Figure 5).**

Management

The adhesions can be surgically divided to increase the interpalpebral fissure.

Congenital Ectropion

Ectropion is eversion of the eyelid more so in lateral portion of the eyelid **(Figure 6).** It rarely occur as an isolated entity and is associated with congenital ptosis, blepharophimosis, microphthalmos or buphthalmos.

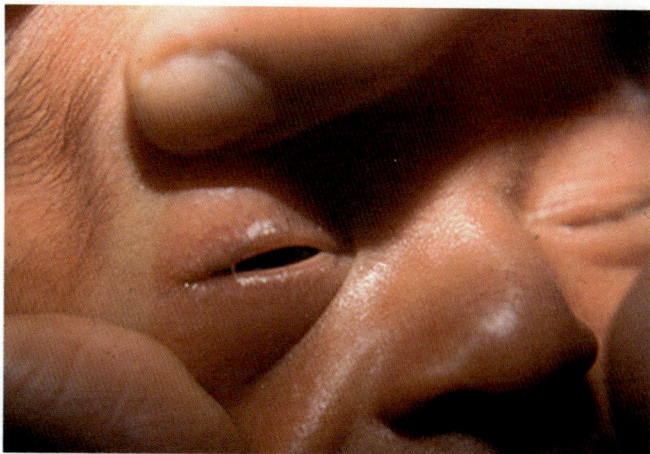

Figure 5: An infant with filiform ankyloblepharon

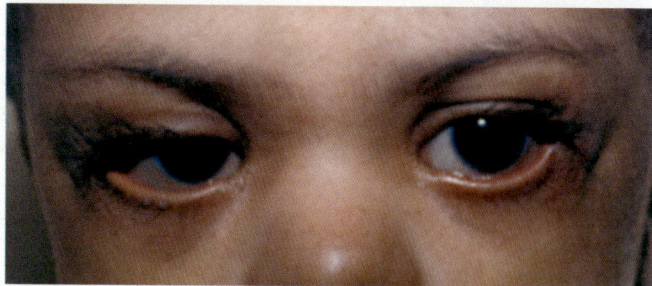

Figure 6: Congenital ectropion

Management

Management may vary depending on the degree of ectropion. In case of severe ectropion skin grafting is indicated. Full thickness graft is required in case of lower lid and partial thickness for upper lid ectropion.

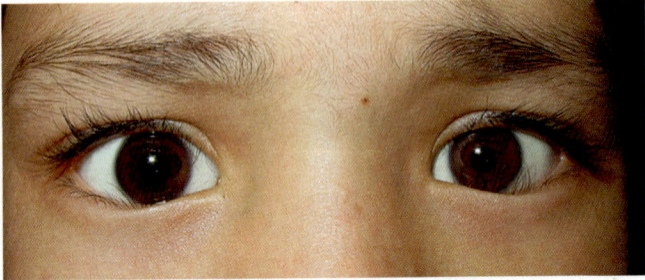

Figure 7: A young girl with congenital entropion

Congenital Entropion

It is inward turning of the eyelid margin **(Figure 7)**. It is due to absence of taral plate or hypertrophy of the marginal portion of orbicularis. Rarely it occurs as an isolated condition. Entropion may be associated with epiblepharon, epicanthus or enophthalmos.

Management

It may resolve spontaneously or may require Skin – muscle resection or tarsal fixation of the inturned tarsus or tightening of lower lid etractors.

Epiblepharon

It is a congenital condition where extra fold of skin causes the inward turning of the eyelashes with the globe **(Figures 8A to D)**. It may regress spontaneously by the age of 5 to 10 years with the growth of facial bones.

Management

No treatment is required, if asymptomatic. A conservative skin muscle resection in cases with significant discomfort or keratitis.

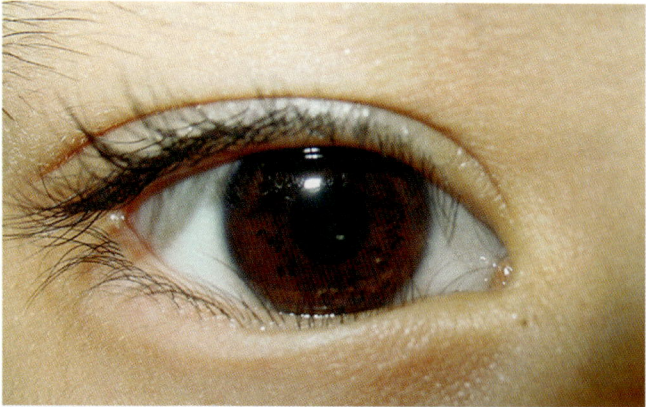

Figure 8A: Showing epiblepharon of right eye, eyelashes are not rubbing against the globe

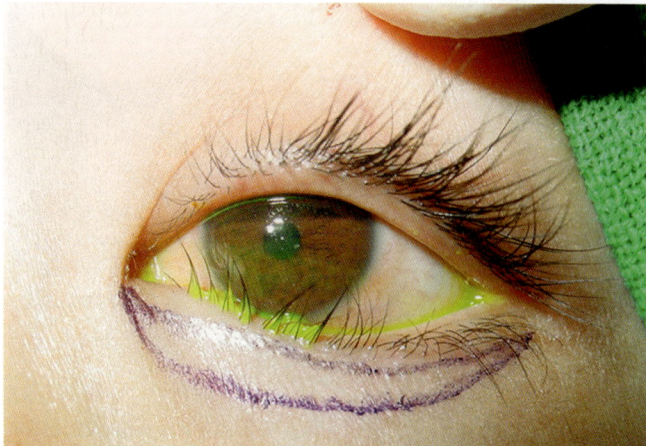

Figure 8B: Marking for skin-muscle resection

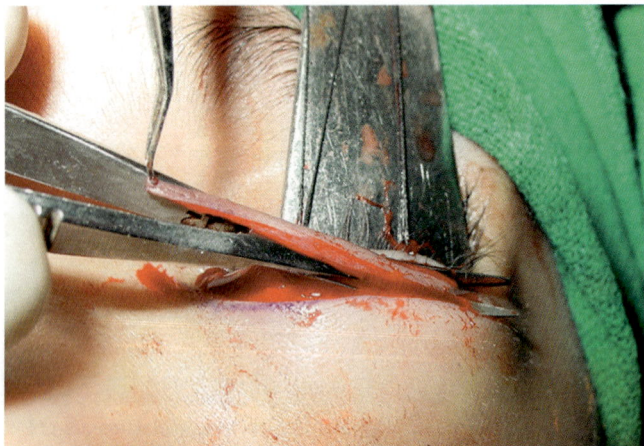

Figure 8C: Skin-muscle resection

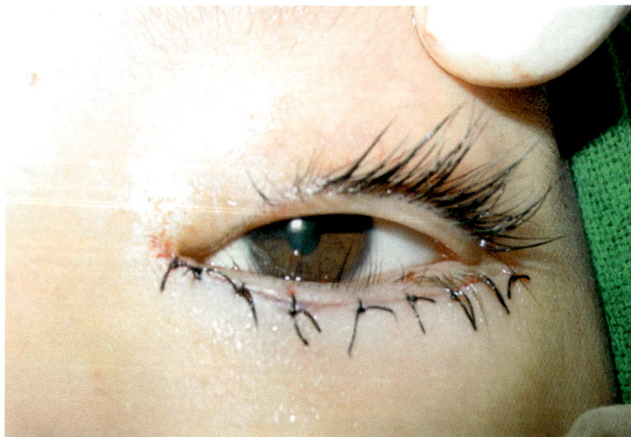

Figure 8D: Postoperative photograph

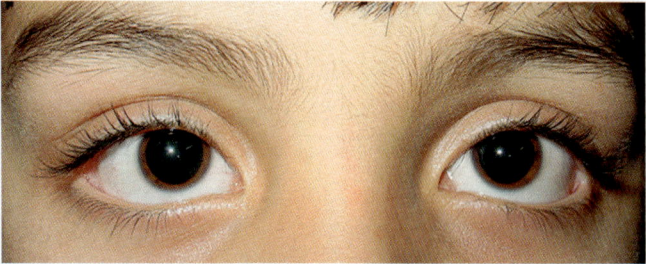

Figure 9: 7-year-old boy showing euryblepharon

Euryblepharon

In this condition there is horizontal enlargement of the palpebral aperture, more so in the lateral part. Lateral canthus is displaced downward along with downward displacement of temporal half of lower eyelid **(Figure 9).**

Management

Surgical treatment may vary depending on the downward displacement. One may treat with tarsorrhaphy or tarsal or skin graft.

Epicanthus

Epicanthal folds are redundant vertical folds of skin in the region of medial canthus, with their concavity directed towards the inner canthus.

Types of epicanthus:
1. Epicanthus tarsalis
2. Epicanthus inversus - originates in the lower lid and extends upwards to the medial canthal area. It does not resolve on its own **(Figure 10).**
3. Epicanthus palpebralis

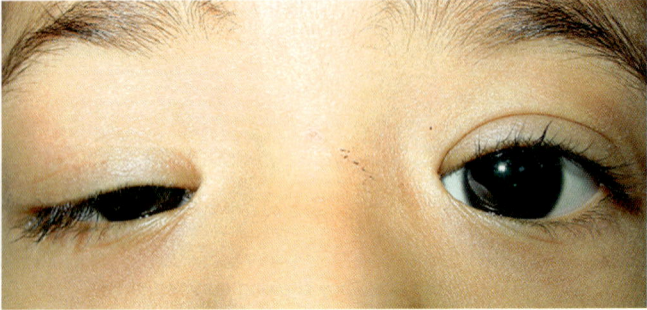

Figure 10: A 5-year-old child presented with severe ptosis with epicanthus inversus with telecanthus

It may occasionally be a isolated condition or may be associated with Blepharophimosis syndrome or Down's syndrome. In many instances, epicanthus may resolve with growing age.

Management

Mustarde's double "Z" plasty is the procedure of choice for epicanthus inversus. Some of the other options include "Y-V" plasty, Spaeth and Blair procedures.

Telecanthus

Normally the distance between the medial canthi is half the interpupillary distance. In telecanthus the intercanthal distance is more than half the interpupillary distance. It occurs due to increase length of medial canthal tendons resulting in increased distance between medial canthi. It is important to differentiate it from hypertelorism in that the distance between the medial wall of orbit is increased resulting in increased distance between the eyeballs. The natural course of telecanthus remains unchanged with age.

Management

The condition should be repaired by either MPL placation / resection or transnasal wiring.

Congenital Ptosis

Ptosis occurs due to developmental dystrophy of unknown etiology, affecting the levator muscle.

Congenital ptosis may be classified as:
- Congenital simple ptosis **(Figure 11)**
- With oculomotor abnormalities
- With blepherophimosis syndrome **(Figure 12)**

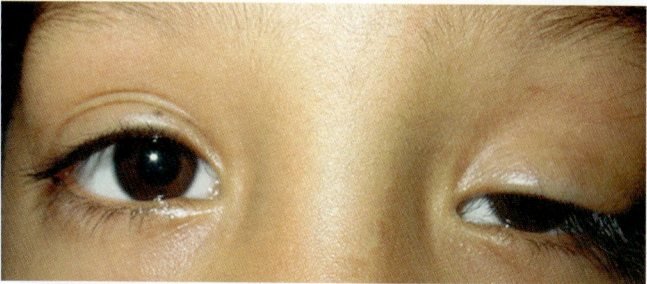

Figure 11: A child with left eye congenital simple severe ptosis

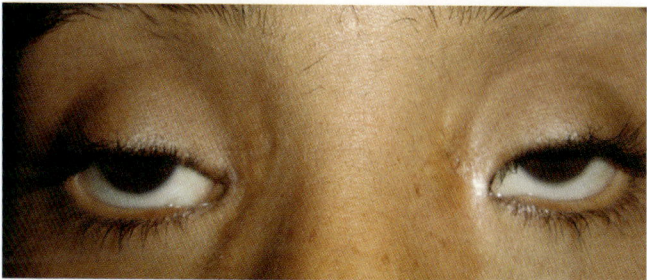

Figure 12: Blepharophimosis syndrome showing clinical features

- Synkinetic ptosis
  - Marcus Gunn Jaw winking
  - Misdirected third nerve ptosis.

Management

It is advisable to wait till 3-4 years of age as better assessment is possible at this age. Tissues are better developed to withstand surgical trauma and better postoperative care is possible due to better cooperation. However, one should not delay in surgical management in cases of severe ptosis where pupil is obstructed as it may cause amblyopia and where child is likely to develop bad postural habits like head tilt, brow wrinkling, eyebrow arching. In these cases a temporary procedure may be opted early on followed by definitive surgery later.

Choice of Surgical Procedure

Choice is determined by **(Table 1)**:
- Whether the ptosis is unilateral or bilateral
- Severity of ptosis
- Levator action
- Simple ptosis or associated anomalies

Table 1: Indications for the choice of different surgical procedures

Ptosis	Levator action	Surgery
Mild	> 10 mm	Fasanella Servat
	< 10 mm	Levator resection
Moderate	Fair to Good	Levator resection
	Poor (rare)	Whitnall's sling or Brow suspension
Severe	Fair	Levator resection or Brow suspension ptosis repair
	Poor	Brow suspension ptosis repair

Commonly Performed Surgeries

- Fasanella Servat operation
- Levator resection
- Brow suspension ptosis repair.

Congenital Tumors

Pigmented Lesions

Nevi (Figure 13)

These are benign congenital tumors. They may vary in size and may be sessile or pedunculated. The commonest location is along the lid border. Risk of malignancy is low. However, in large tumors, there will be 4-6% risk of malignant transformation. Sudden increase in size and increase in pigmentation suggests concern regarding malignant transformation and requires excision.

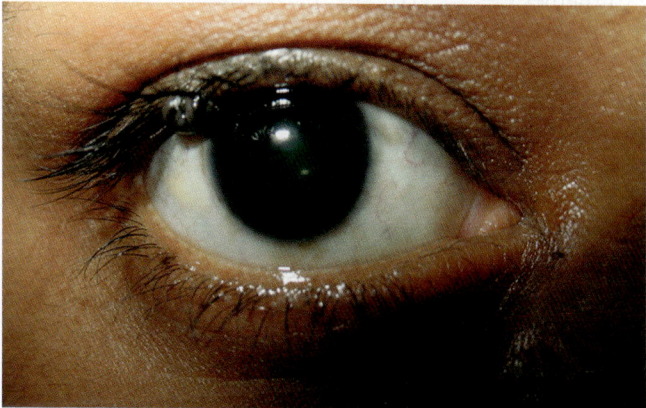

Figure 13: Showing nevus in upper eyelid

Management

If naevi involves the lid margin – shave off flush with the lid margin.

If naevus does not involve the lid margin – Excision with direct repair with margin repair.

Naevus of Ota (Oculodermal melanocytosis)

It is characterized by patchy bluish or brownish pigmentation of periocular skin and sclera. The lesion is composed of dermal melanocytes and has malignant potential. Increased intraocular pigmentation contributes to risk of glaucoma. It is occasionally associated with Sturge-Weber syndrome.

Management: Ruby laser has been tried to lighten the cutaneous component.

Angiomatous Tumors

Portwine Stain (Nevus Flammeus)

This condition is characterized by telengectesia of the deeper skin capillaries. It involves the part of the face which is innervated by the trigeminal nerve. It is often associated with Sturge-Weber syndrome. Congenital glaucoma and choroidal haemangioma have strong association. It is important to recognize such condition because of the possibility of development of above mentioned complications.

Strawberry (Capillary) Hemangioma (Figure 14)

These are benign tumors present at birth. 90% of these clinically manifest by age of 1 month. Histopathologically, these are proliferations of endothelial cells. Most commonly they involve the upper eyelid with variable extension into orbit.

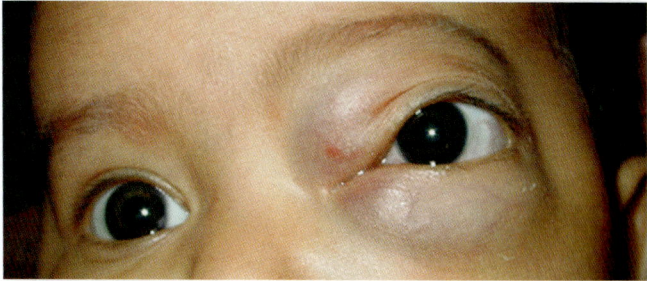

Figure 14: An infant with capillary hemangioma

These tumor grow for 3-6 months after birth and slowly regresses by second year of life. Spontaneous resolution occurs in 40% by 4 years of age and 80% by 8 years.

Management

Surgery is indicated in cases of total ptosis obscuring the visual axis and induced astigmatism and for better cosmesis.

Intralesional injection of 1-2 ml of corticosteroid. Betamethasone 6 mg/ml and Triamcinolone 40 mg/cc combined in 1:1 concentration and is injected all around the lesion with 26G needle deep into the lesion **(Figure 15).** Rapid shrinkage occurs in first two weeks and then continues slowly for several months. Injection may be repeated after 6 weeks in case of residual mass. Depigmentation of overlying skin, eyelid necrosis and rarely central retinal artery occlusion are few complications seen with steroid injection.

Dermoid and Epidermoid Cyst

Abnormal sequestration of surface ectoderm beneath the skin during embryonic development results in the cyst formation. Lids are usually secondarily involved due to extension of the tumor from the orbits.

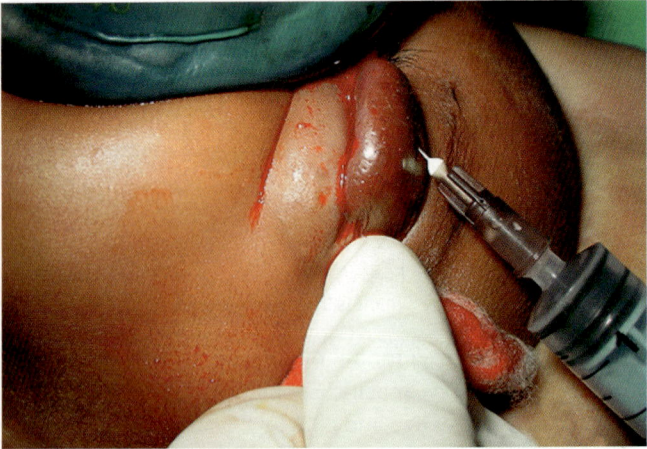

Figure 15: Injecting corticosteroid in the hemangioma

They are clinically evident by first year of life. Most common location is superonasal. On palpation, these are firm in consistency, non-tender and are attached to underlying periosteum. Imaging is necessary to know the extension.

Management

Surgical excision is required in case of progressive enlargement of mass or to prevent inflammation following rupture of the cyst.

Plexiform Neurofibroma

Involvement of the lid with plexiform neuroma in cases of neurofibromatosis **(Figure 16).** Café au lait spots are characteristic of neurofibromatosis.

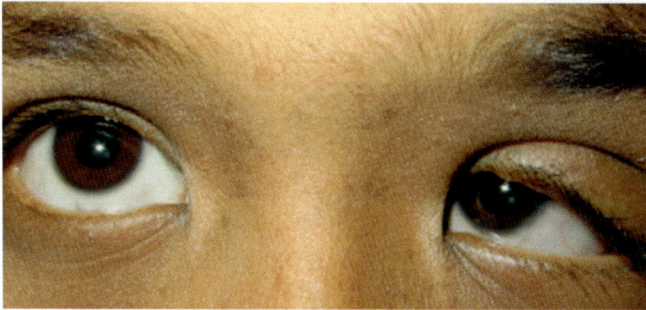

Figure 16: Showing plexiform neurofibroma of let upper lid

Management

Surgery is indicated in cases of significant mechanical ptosis and to improve cosmesis. Surgical debulking of the mass along with ptosis correction and lateral shortening may be performed in single stage or in two stages.

ACQUIRED DISORDERS

Acquired abnormalities of eyelid can be due to –

    Eyelid trauma and its sequelae

    Inflammatory and infective disorders.

Eyelid Trauma in Children

These are commonly encountered following birth injuries, automobile accidents, fall, sports injuries, child abuse and Chemical Injuries. Following injury the child may present with lid laceration with or without marginal involvement, canalicular injuries, canthal injuries, avulsion of the eyelid, coloboma, misalignments of eyelids and many others.

Management

It is important to properly evaluate the wound. Repair of injury depends on the time of presentation. In patients presenting within 24 hours of the injury primary repair of the wound is undertaken immediately. The primary repair affords the chance for best cosmetic and functional results. n cases where patient presents more than 24 hours after injury or in cases where there is marked lid edema or infection, a delayed primary repair is performed after 3 to 4 days. During this waiting period, cold saline compresses, anti-inflammatory and antibiotics are administered to reduce tissue edema and to control infection. In cases where the child presents a long time after injury or in cases of chemical and thermal burns healing by second intention must be allowed to take place. In such cases, atleast wait for a minimum of 5 to 6 months before planning a secondary wound repair **(Figure 17).**

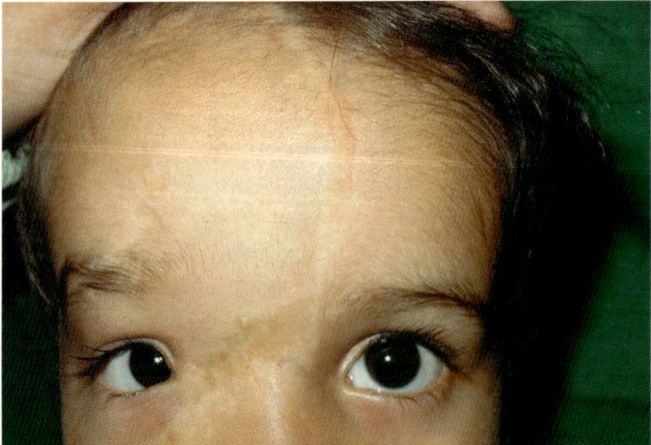

Figure 17: Traumatic telecanthus of right eye
following road traffic accidents

Inflammatomy Disorders

Blepharitis

It is a condition of inflammation of eyelid margins. It causes redness, discharge, irritation and discomfort. Commonly associated with scalp dandruff.

Management: This condition is managed by antibiotic with steroid ointment and 3% soda bicarbonate for eye lashes cleaning. Antidandruff shampoo is also advised twice weekly.

Stye

It is an acute inflammation of fat sweating glands of the eyelids (Zeis or Moll). Here a painful swelling and occurred in the lid margin **(Figure 18)**.

Management: It is managed by hot formentation, antibiotic cream and analgesics. Sometime incision and drainage of pus may be required

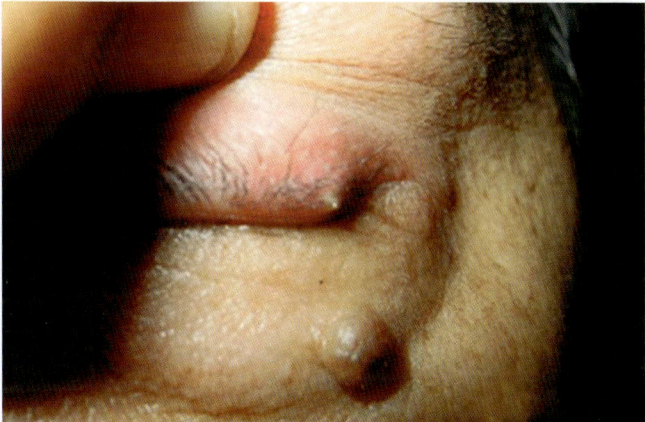

Figure 18: Stye of left upper lid

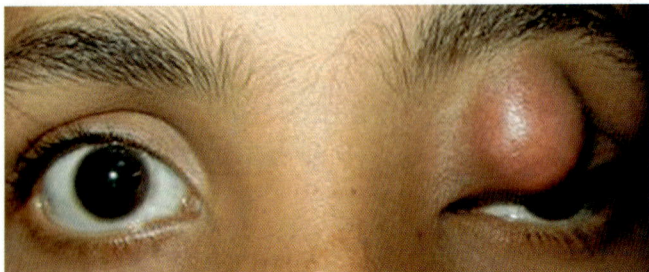

Figure 19: Chalazion of left upper lid causing mechanical ptosis

Chalazion

It is a chronic granulomatous (non-infective) inflammation of the fat secreting meibomian glands of the eyelid. It causes a painless swelling near the eyelid margin **(Figure 19).**

Management: It is managed by hot formentation, antibiotic drops, analgesic, intralesional injection of triamcinolona (5 mg per ml) and Incision and curettage.

Internal Hordeolum

It is a inflammation of the meibomian gland associated with blockage of the duct. Here pain is more intense and swelling is away from the lid margin.

Management: It is managed by hot fomentation , antibiotic drops and oral antibiotics if associated with pre-septal cellulitis.

Molluscum Contagiosum

It is a viral infection (Pox virus). Multiple, pale, waxy, umbellicated swellings are found over the skin of the eylid **(Figure 20).**

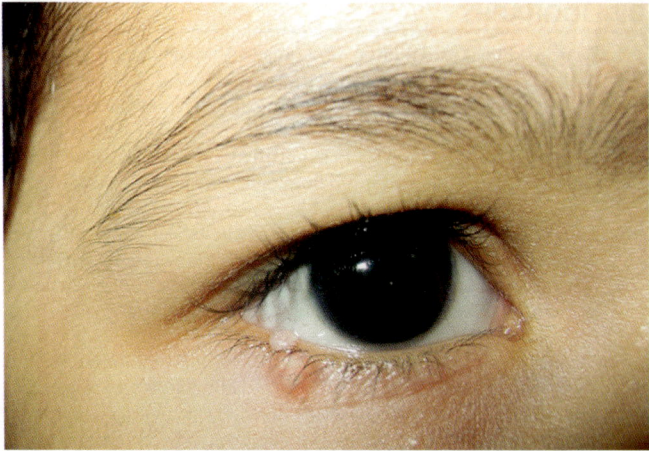

Figure 20: Molluscum contagiosum of right lower lid

Management: It is managed by Incision and curettage with tincture/iodine/pure carbolic acid and cryotherapy

Viral warts, herpes simplex or Herpes zoster infection of the eyelid along with contact dermatitis may also be encountered.

To conclude, pediatric abnormalities poses challenges for an ophthalmologist. Patient's cooperation is a limitation for adequate assessment in pediatric age group. Careful planning of management is required as pathology may change with the growing age. In conditions of eyelid abnormalities like coloboma, where there is risk of loss of vision or, where obstruction of vision may prove amblyogenic needs to be managed immediately. Cosmetic consideration is also critical for child's psychological development. It is important to carefully assess and plan the technique of intervention for gratifying results.

BIBLIOGRAPHY

1. Beard C: Ptosis, 3rd edition. St. Louis : CV Mosby Company 1981.
2. Duke-Edler S. System of Ohthalmology. Vol 3. Normal and Abnormal development. Part II: Congenital Deformities. St. Louis, C.V. Mosby Co., 1963 p.827.
3. Grover AK, Gupta AK. Proceedings of the Golden Jubilee Conference of All India Ophthalmological Society, New Delhi 1992; 54-56.
4. Grover AK, Mittal Sanjay. A Clinico-pathological study of levator muscle for Congenital Ptosis. Thesis is submitted to Delhi University.
5. Mustarde JC. Colobomas of the eyelids. Repair and reconstruction in the orbital region, 2nd Edition, pp 364-372. Edinburgh. Churchill Livingstone 1980.
6. Mustarde JC. Epicanthus and telecanthus. Int. Ophthalmol Cli. 4: 1964
7. Mustrade JC. Colobomas of the eyelids . Plastic Siurgery in infancy and childhood. 2nd ed. pp243-249. Edinburgh. Churchill livingstone 1978.
8. Saunders DH, Flanagan JC. Disorders of the lids.Pediatric Ophthalmology. 3rd edition. Pp 334-354.W.B. Saunders company.
9. Troutman RC, Converse JM, Smith B. Plastic and Reconstructive Surgery of the eye and Adnexa. Washington DC, Butterworths, 1962.

Eyelid Disorders

**Essam El Toukhy, Mohamed ElBadri
Ali Saeed Odadi Assiri (Egypt)**

Entropion

INTRODUCTION

Entropion or turning of the lid margin is one of the most Common lid malpositions encountered in clinical practice .

The most common type of entropion is involutional entropion.

CLINICAL PICTRURE

- Irritation, tearing and scaring.
- Ulceration of conjuctiva or cornea.
- It can eventually lead to visual loss from corneal opacities.

CLASSIFICATION

- Involutional entropion.
- Congenital entropion.
- Spastic entropion.
- Cicatricial entropion.

CONGENITAL ENTROPION

- Is a rare entity that is present at birth.
- The entire lower lid and lashes turn inward.
- There is absence of the lower lid crease.

Pathophysiology

- It is due to disinsertion of the lower lid retractors.
- Or secondary overaction of marginal orbicularis muscle.

Treatment

Reattaching or plicating of the lower lid retractors.

Differential Diagnosis

Epiblepharon in which a fold of skin pushes the lashes against the globe and tends to correct itself with growth of facial bones

SPASTIC ENTROPION

Causes

1. Recent ocular surgery.
2. Inflammatory eye condition.

Pathophysiology

Acute lid swelling and orbicularis spasm.

In which preseptal orbicularis muscle overrides pretarsal orbicularis and lid margin turns inward.

Treatment

- Treatment of inflammatory eye by antibiotic and steroids.
- Taping of lid.
- Local anesthesia infiltration.
- Botulinum injection in orbicularis muscle will break the cycle of ocular irritation and orbicularis spasm and lid malposition will resolve.

Prognosis

- Botulinum toxin treatment has proven successful in temporarily
- Elimination of the spasm.

CICATRICIAL ENTROPION

Pathophysiology

Caused by contracture in the conjunctiva and the tarsus or both leading to shortning of posterior lamella of lid.

Causes

Secondary to:
- Acids and alkali.
- Burns.
- Trachoma.
- Steven-Johnson syndrome .
- Mechanical trauma.
- Cicatricial pemphigoid.
- Viral

Clinical Picture

- Blepharo conjuctivitis
- Meibomitis
- Rounding of posterior lid border and posterior migration and keratinized epithelium and secondary trichiasis.
- Keratoconjunctivitis sicca.

Treatment of Cicatrizing Entropion

- Trichiasis is treated by electrolysis, cryosurgery, argon laser therapy or excision of lash follicles.
- Cicatricial entropion is treated by mucous membrane graft.

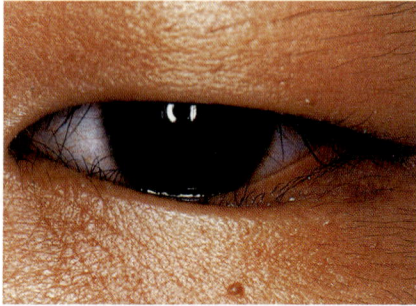

Figure 1: Epiblepharon

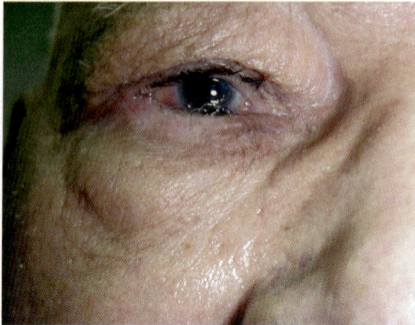

Figure 2: Involutional entropion

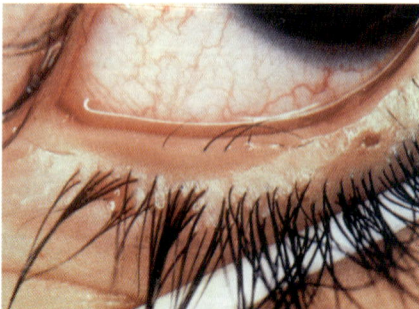

Figure 3: Distichiasis

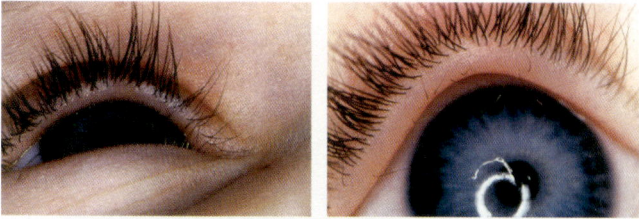

Figure 4: Trichiasis without entropion

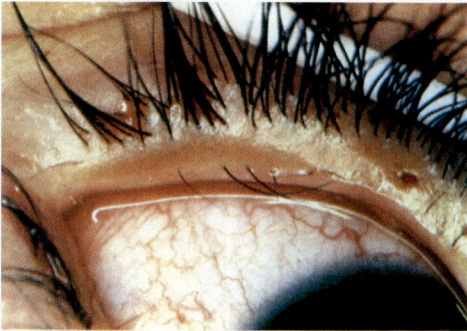

Figure 5: Trichiasis

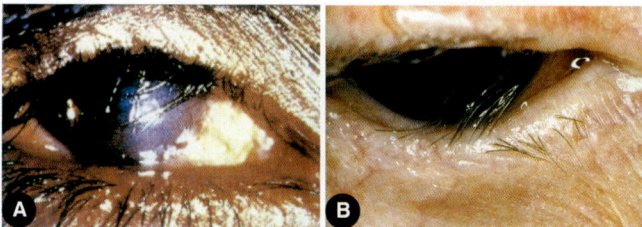

Figure 6: Upper and lower lid entropion

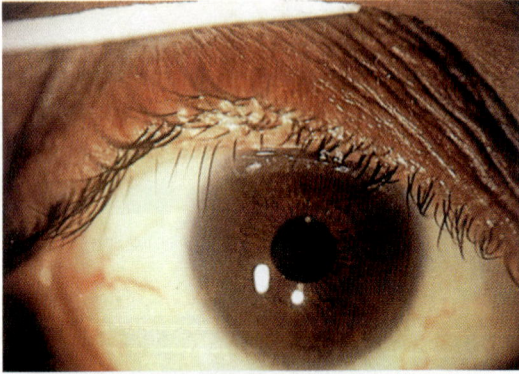

Figure 7: Upper lid entropion

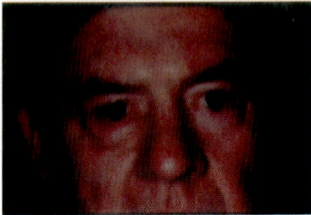

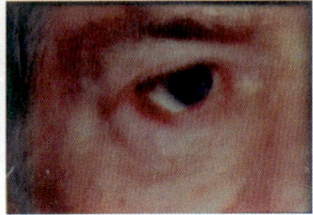

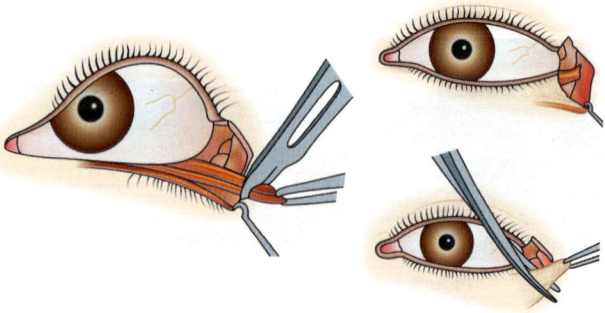

Figure 8: Lateral tarsal strip procedure

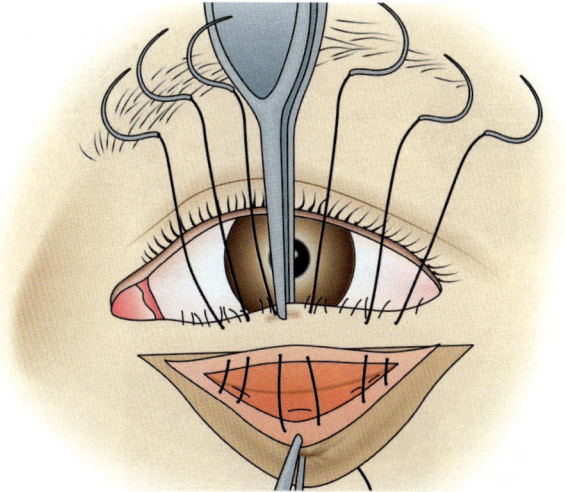

Figure 9: Weis procedure 1

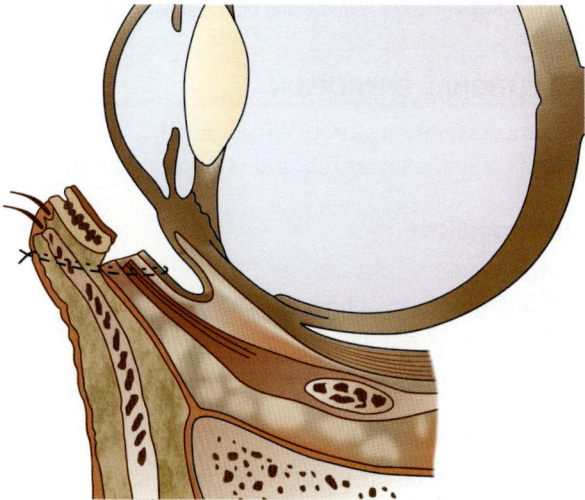

Figure 10: Weis procedure 2

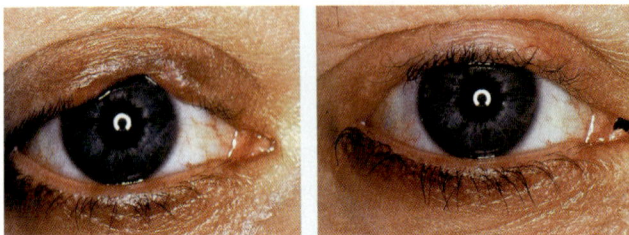

Figure 11: Lid notching after extensive electrolysis

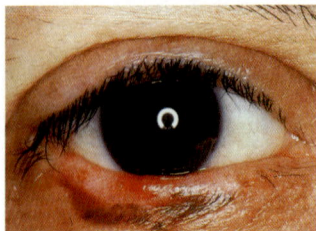

Figure 12: Madarosis and pigmentation after cryo

INVOLUTIONAL ENTROPION

Is the most common variety encountered.
It affects only the lower lids and is associated with aging.

Pathophysiology

It is due to:
- Laxity of the tarsal ligaments
- Weakness of retractors.
- Overriding and preseptal on pretarsal orbicularis.

Medical Treatment

- Patients with blephrits and meibomitis should by treated.
- Patients with dry eyes should by treated by artificial tears.

Surgical Treatment

1. Three suture technique.
2. Direct anatomic surgical approach.
3. Weis procedure.
4. Weis procedure with lateral tarsal strip.

Three Suture Technique

- It is best suited for poor risk patients at the bed side or in the office.
- The lid should not be too lax.
  A. Suture technique, sagittal view of 5-0 vicryl sutures passed through the retractor complex.
  B. The suture is brought out just anterior to the inferior tarsal border through orbicularis muscle to emerge 3 to – 4 mm below the lower lid cilia. This brings the retractors back to their normal anatomic position.

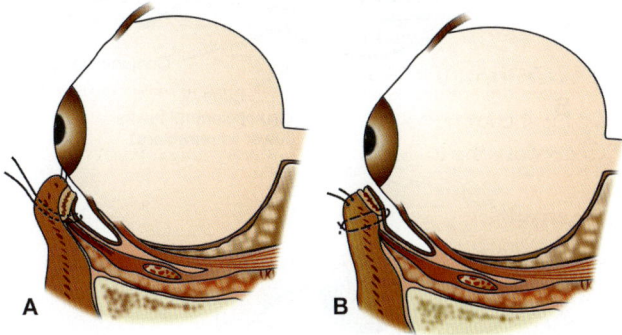

Figures 13A and B: Suture techniques (sagittal view)

Direct Anatomic—Surgical Approach

This approach seeks to correct the three main causative.

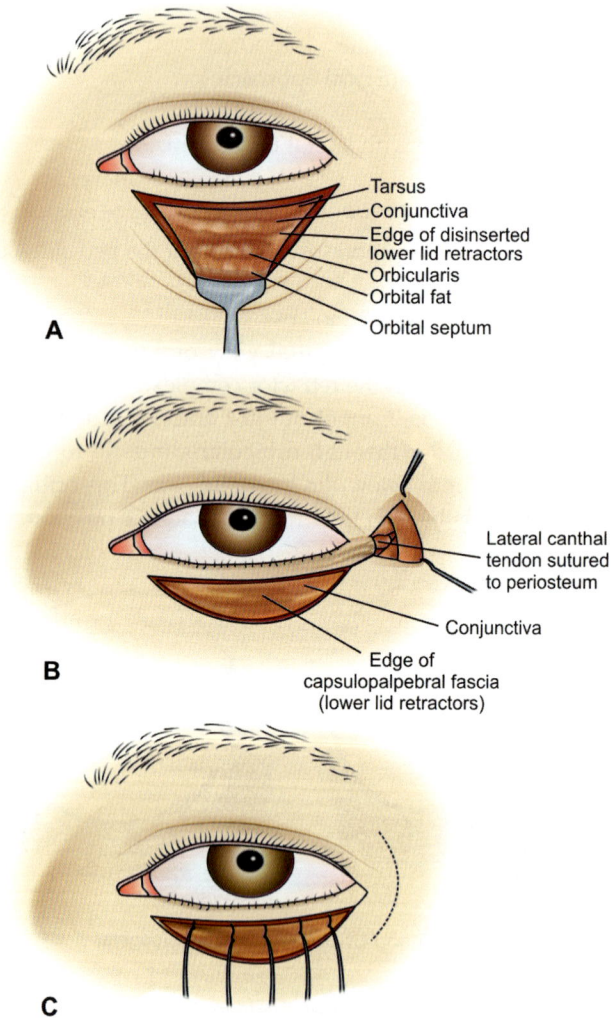

Figures 14A to C: Causative factors for surgical approach

Factors
- Overriding of orbicularis.
- Weakness of retractors.
- Horizontal lid laxity.

Direct anatomic approach:

A. A subciliary incision exposing the tarsal plate, dehisced edge of the lower eyelid retractors, preaponeurotic. fat, orbital fat, and orbicularis muscle.

B. A lateral tarsal strip is fashioned and sutured to: Periosteum of the inner aspect of the frontal process of the zygoma.

C. The edge of the lower eyelid retractor is advanced and sutured to the inferior tarsal border or to the cut edge of the pertarsal prbicularis with **6-0** silk.

Weis Procedure

A. Three double—armed 5-0 vicryl sutures are placed along the lower eyelid, through conjunctiva and retractors, anterior to the tarsal plate, exiting through the orbicularis and skin at the level of the lashes.

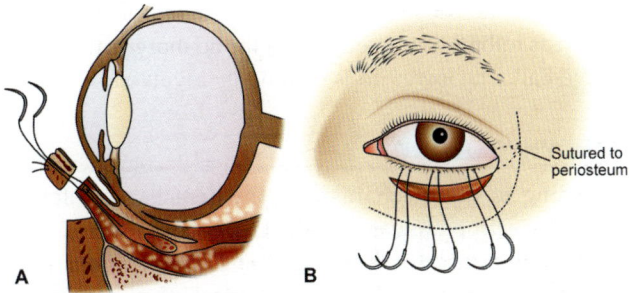

Sutured to periosteum

Figures 15A and B: Weis procedure

B. The tarsal edge of the horizontally shortened lid is sutured to periosteum. The **5-0** vicryl sutures have already been preplaced through conjunctiva and retractors, exiting anterior to the trasal plate through orbicularis and skin.

Weis procedure with lateral tarsal strip:
Used in weakens of retractors combined with congenital lid laxity.

Lateral tarsal strip procedure:
- Horizontal canthotomy .
- Inferior cantholysis.
- Excision of a part of skin and orbicularis
- Excision of a part of lid margin—according to lid laxity.
- Peeling of conjunctiva to prevent postoperative inclusion cyst.
- Suturing of tarsal strip by double armed vicryl **5/0** to the periosteum of frontal process of the zygoma.
- Closure of skin by interrupted sutures.

Ectropion

INTRODUCTION

It is one of the most common malpositions of the eyelid, defined as rolling-out "eversion" of the lid margin away from the eye-ball. The lower lid is commonly involved.

PATHOPHYSIOLOGY

According to the mechanism of the defect "pathological factor" the ectropion was classified to different types.
1. When the anterior lamella is shortened either post-operatively, trauma (burns or injuries), or ulceration, the resultant cicatricial ectropion will take place.

2. Supporting of the lower eyelid in its normal position depending on the orbicularis oculi muscle tone and loss of this support will lead to paralytic ectropion as in case of facial nerve palsy.

3. Senile or involutional which is caused by a horizontal lid laxity as a result of lengthening of medial and lateral canthal tendons with ageing changes, it is the most common type of ectropion and has a continuous pathological process that is aggravated by conjunctivitis and epiphora.

4. When the eyelids are well supported by a big eye-ball relative to its orbital cavity in presence of blepharospasm well cause a spastic ectropion and on the other hand when eyelids are less supported by a less prominent inferior orbital rim will lead to a midfacial hypoplasia with resultant ectropion as in case of exophthalmos and children.

5. Mechanical ectropion is caused by eversion of the lower lid by a tumor or a mass.

6. Congenital ectropion is a rare condition due to shortage of skin as in congenital ichthyosis or blepharophimosis.

Note: The condition of ectropion "during sleep" due to floppy eyelid syndrome should be suspected by exclusion in which the skeleton of lids "tarsus is lengthened and become more lax.

CLINICAL SIGNS AND SYMPTOMS

History

Patients with ectropion will complain of tearing, burning sensation and redness of the involved eye, however the age of the patient is an important clue in which the congenital ectropion is an infancy condition , epiphora is a less complaint of the elderly , but more common with young patients due to adequate tears production. Involutional ectropion is the most common type with patients while paralytic ectropion is more apparent in elderly rather than youngs with 7th C.N. Palsy.

Examination

It should be directed towards recognition of the ectropion and its severity .

1. Severity of ectropion:
   - *Mild*   : The lower punctum is everted
   - *Moderate*   : The tarsal conjunctiva is exposed
   - *Severe*   : The lower fornix is exposed
2. Extent of ectropion: Medial or lateral or involving the entire lower eyelid.
3. Presence of any traumatic or surgical scar tissue.
4. Presence of a horizontal lid laxity. Which is demonstrated by:
   a. Eyelid snap test: Pull the eyelid inferiorly.
      - If the eyelid springs to its normal position without a blink it means no lid laxity.
      - If it remains away from the eye for a time; it means a lax lid. Then the degree of lid laxity will be determined by the. Number of blink required to bring the lid on contact to the eye.
   b. Eyelid distraction test: By pulling the eyelid away from the eye, the lower lid should not move more than 6 mm from the eye.
5. Signs of lower facial nerve palsy as brow ptosis, lid retraction with incomplete blink, lagophthalmos and absence of nasolabial fold.

6. Weakness of the preseptal orbicularis oculi is tested by closure of the eyelids.
7. Examination of corneal sensation is a must .

TREATMENT OF ECTROPION

The management of ectropion depends on the cause, extent and presence or absence of a horizontal lid laxity.

1. Involutional ectropion:
   a. With no horizontal lid laxity: Medial conjunctivoplasty (medial spindle operation)
      " Excision of a diamond of tarsoconjunctiva"
      • With mild horizontal laxity:-lazy-T procedure (medial conjunctovoplasty and full thickness lid excision)
      • With severe horizontal laxity;-medial canthal tendon plication.
   b. Entire lid Ectropion
      • If no excess skin; Horizontal lid shortening .
      • If with excess skin; horizontal lid shortening plus blepharoplasty.
      • Lateral tarsal strip procedure.
2. Treatment of cicatricial ectropion
   a. If mild   : Z-plasty
   b. If severe   : Skin grafts or flaps
3. Treatment of paralytic ectropion.
   a. Temporary method:
      • Conservative (Artificial tears and ointment).
      • Surgical (Tarrsoraphy).
   b. Permanent methods:

- With ectropion
    i. Medical canthoplasty.
    ii. Lateral canthoplasty.
4. Medial canthoplasty with lateral tarsal strip.
5. Encirclement (with prosthetic silicon sling).
   a. Without ectropion
      - Upper lid weight (gold).
      - Graded levator recession.
      - Brow lift to correct brow ptosis.
6. Treatment of mechanical ectropion "Removal of the cause"
7. Treatment of congenital ectropion
   Skin graft ± horizontal lid shortening as appropriate
8. Treatment of spastic ectropion:
   a. Treatment of biepharospasm (Botulinum toxin injeciton
   b. Snellen's sutures: in which three double-armed sutures
      are passed from the lower fonix through the periostium
      of the inferior orbital margin to emerge on the skin of
      cheek and tied over small pieces of rubber of removed
      after 2 weeks.

PROGNOSIS

It is usually good with preservation of corneal wetting and clarity. Surgery results in long-term cure in functional obstruction.

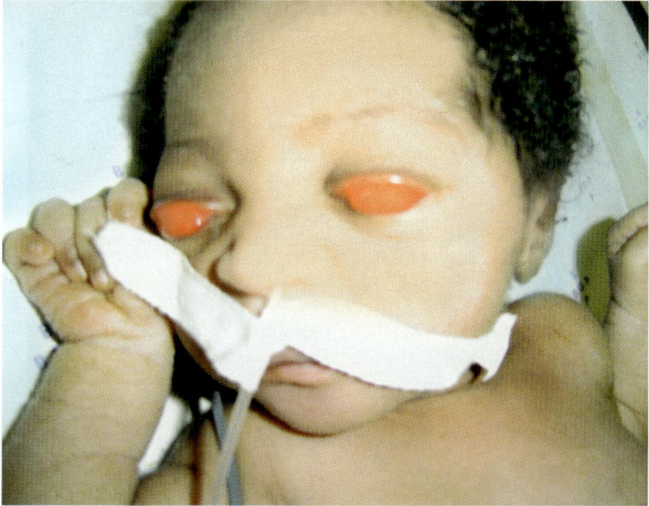

Figure 16: Congenital ectropion

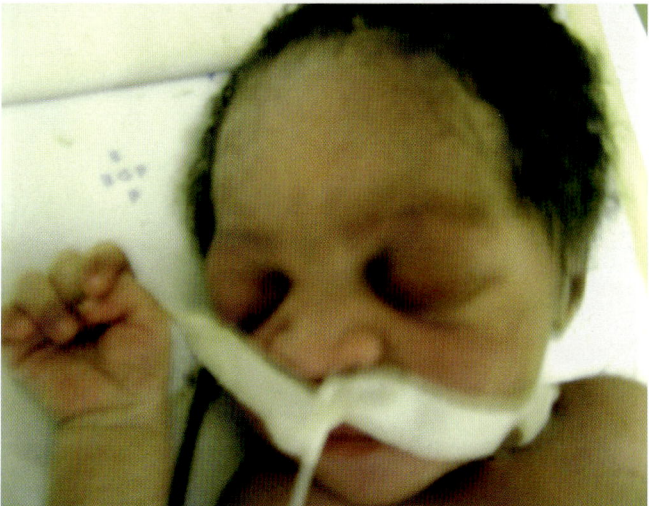

Figure 17: Congenital ectropion; immediate postoperative

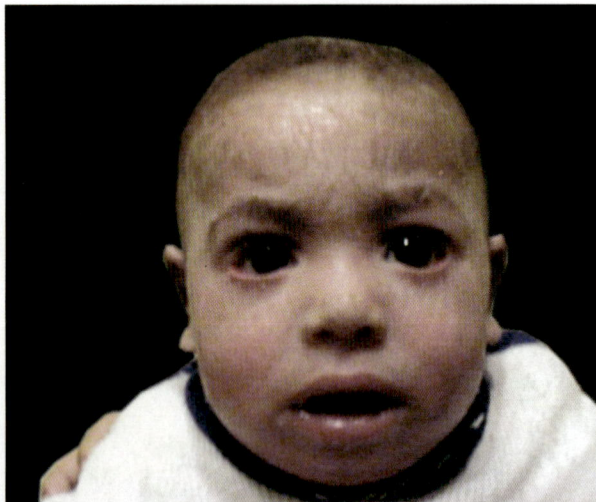

Figure 18: Congenital ectropion postoperative

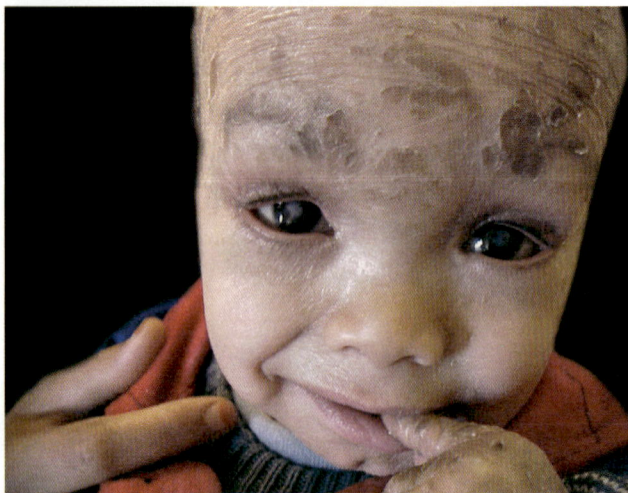

Figure 19: Congenital ectropion postoperative 1

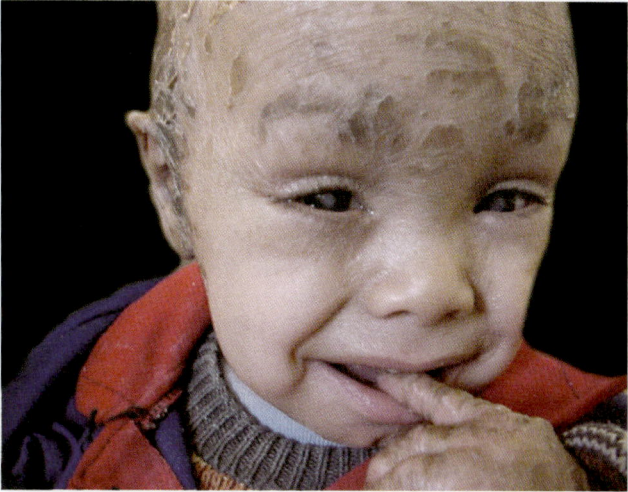

Figure 20: Congenital ectropion postoperative 2

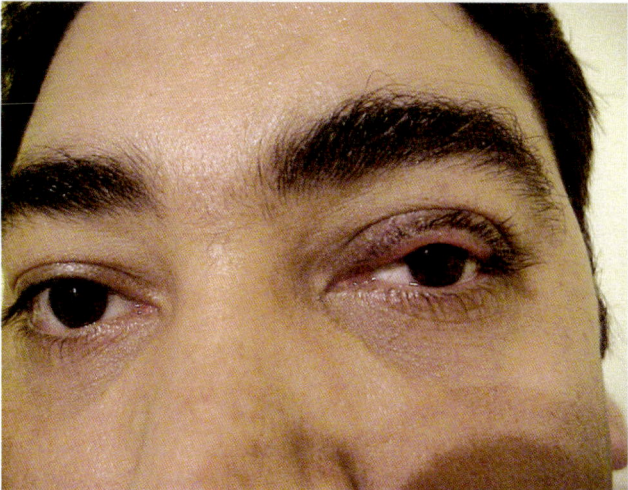

Figure 21: Floppy eyelid syndrome

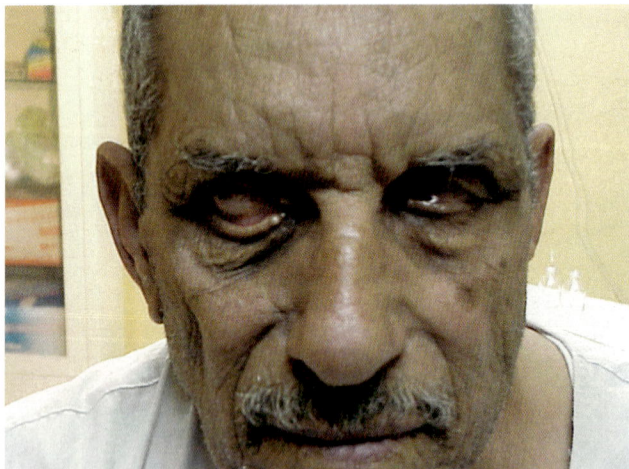

Figure 22: Ectropion preoperative

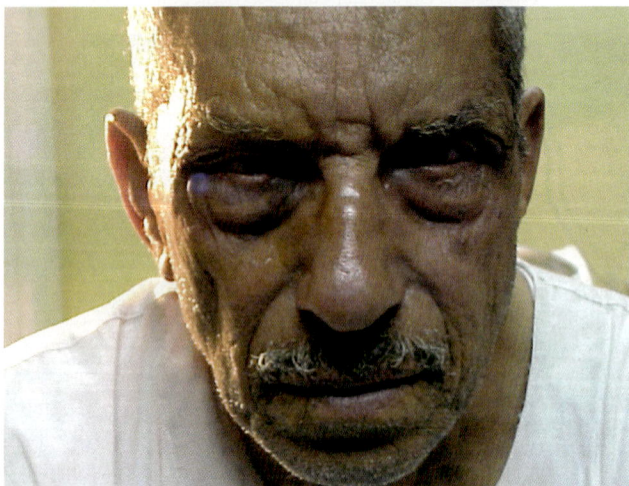

Figure 23: Ectropion postoperative

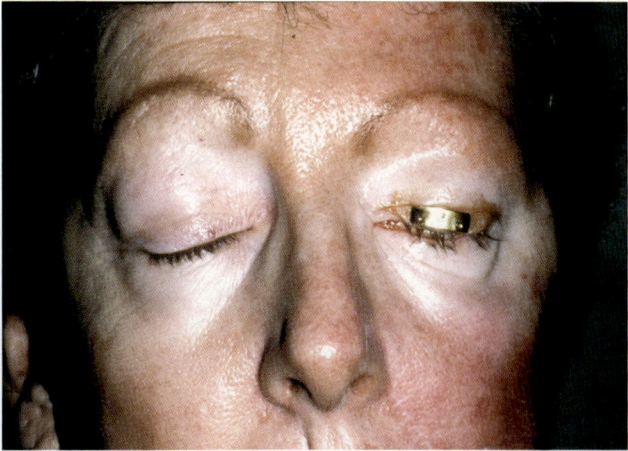

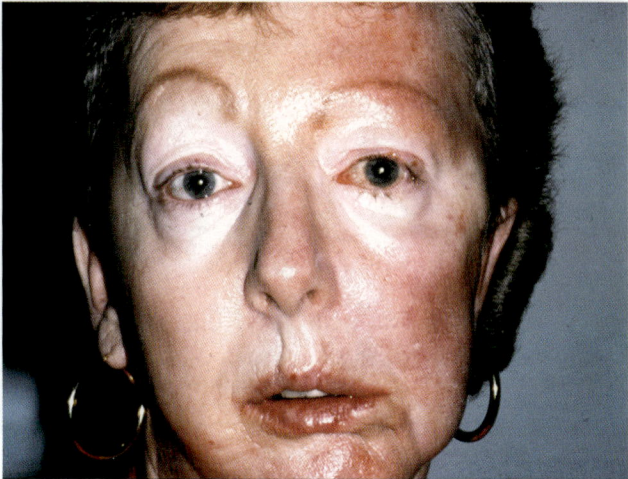

Figure 24: Gold weight implant preoperative

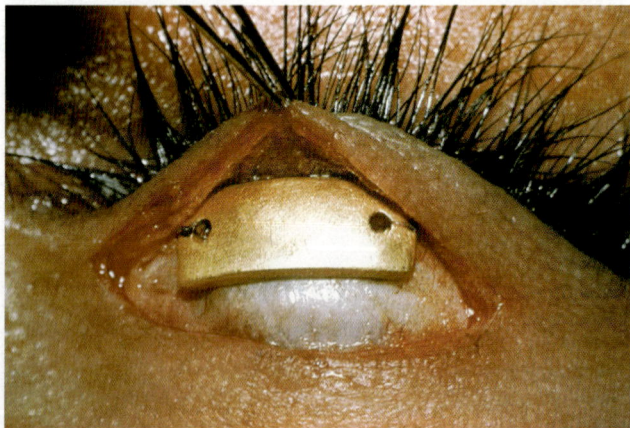

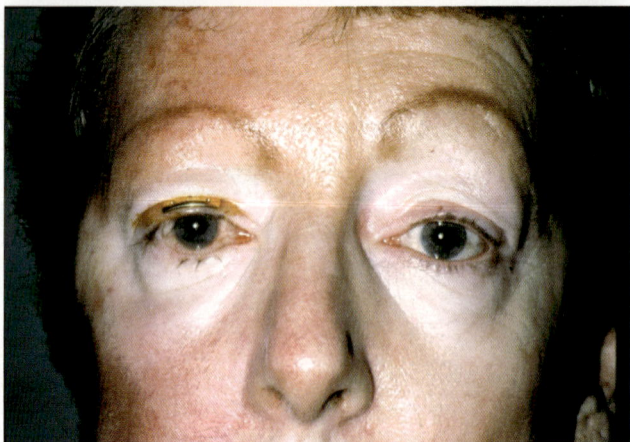

Figure 25: Gold weight implant trial & implantation

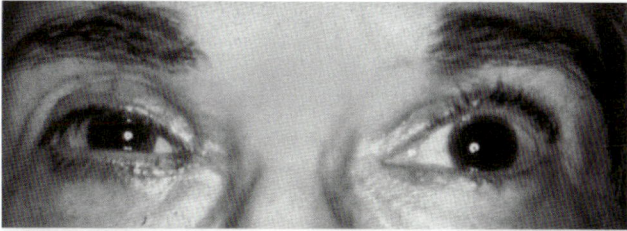

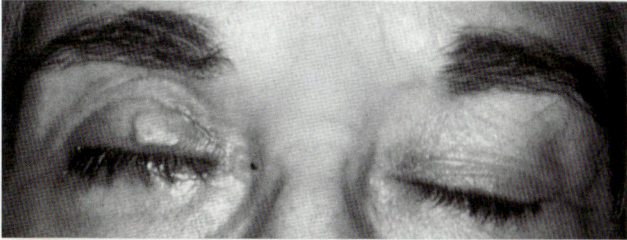

Figure 26: Gold weight implant postoperative

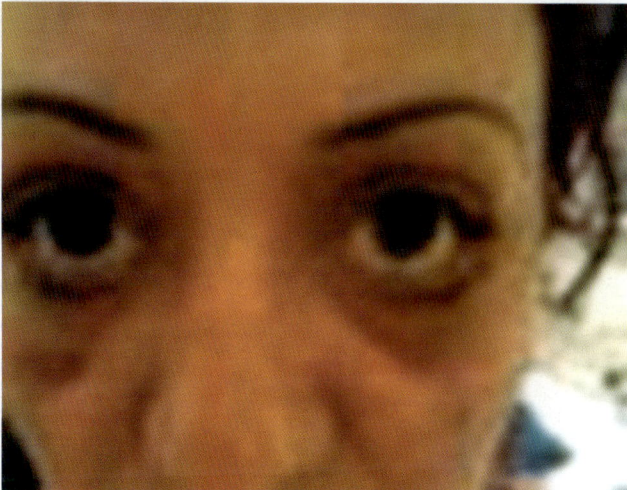

Figure 27: Post-blepharoplasty cicatricial ectropion preoperative

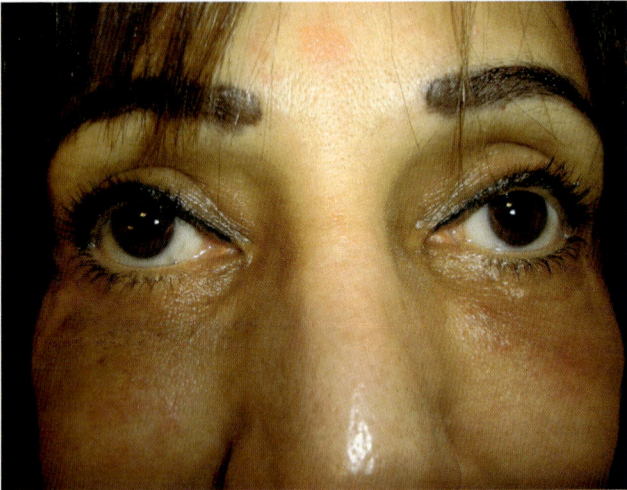

Figure 28: Post-blepharoplasty cicatricial ectropion postoperative

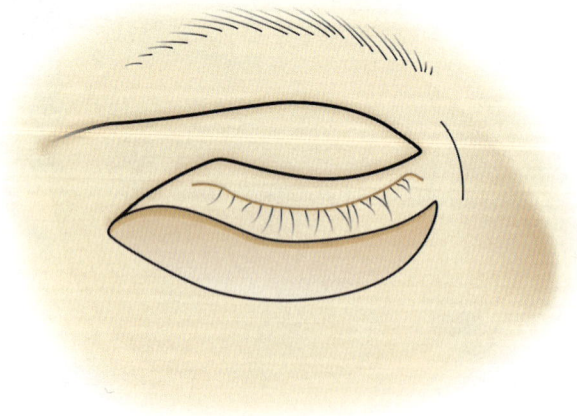

Figure 29: Transposition flap-1

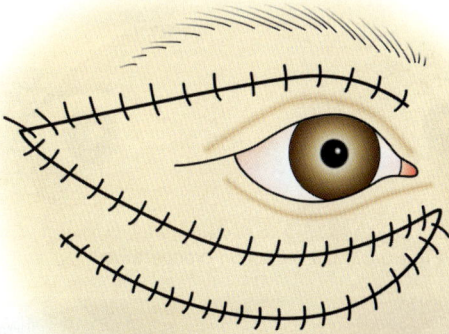

Figure 30: Transposition flap-2

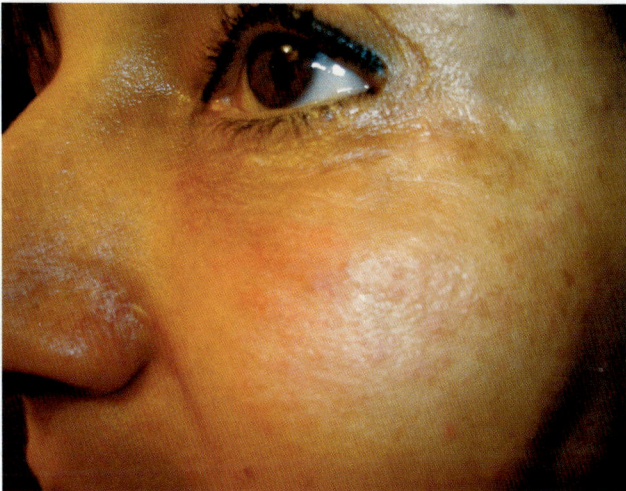

Figure 31: Transposition flap, magnified

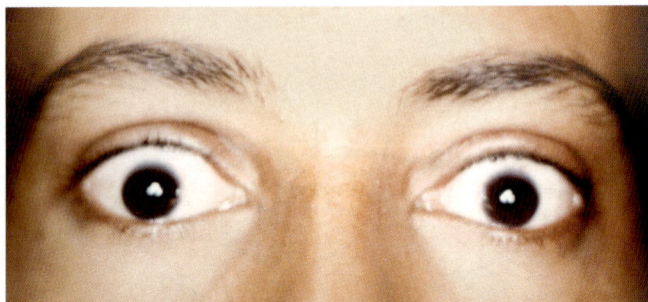

Figure 32: Lid retraction preoperative

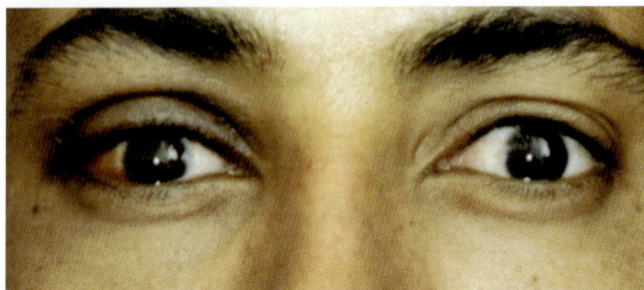

Figure 33: Lid retraction postoperative

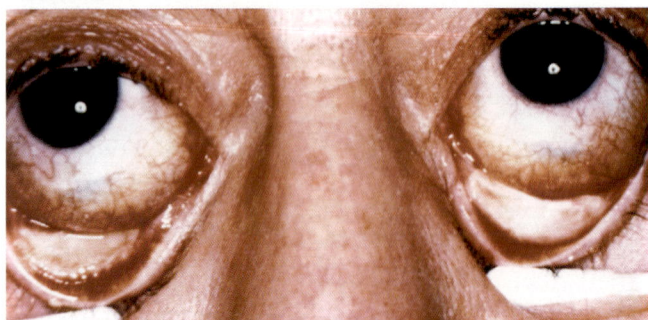

Figure 34: Hard palate graft

Diseases of
the Lids

4

Ashok Garg (India)

STYE (HORDEOLUM EXTERNUM)

Introduction

- Stye is an acute purulent infection (abcess) of Lash follicles and its associated gland of Zeiss or Moll.
- It is mainly Staphylococcal infection.
- Stye is generally seen in patients with staphylococcal blepharitis.

Clinical Signs and Symptoms (Figures 1 and 2)

- Stye presents as a painful inflamed swelling in lid margin pointing anteriorly through the skin.
- Symptoms are out of proportion to the diseae process.
- Redness and heat are present. After this a pus point develops at the root of the cilium and gets evacuated spontaneously.
- One lesion present can infect the surrounding follicles leading to a crop of lesions (Multiple minute abcesses).

Investigations

- Subjective ocular examination is sufficient to make the diagnosis and no specific investigations are indicated.

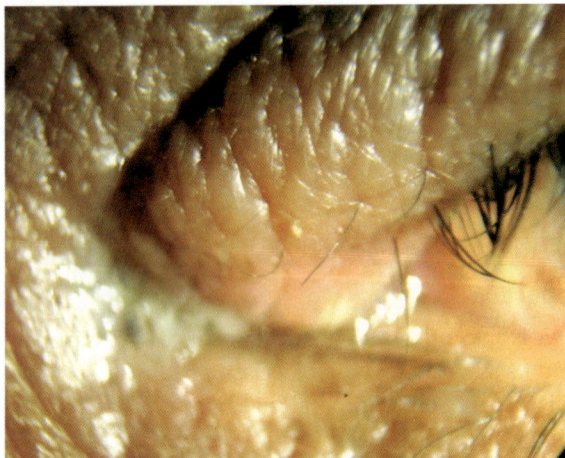

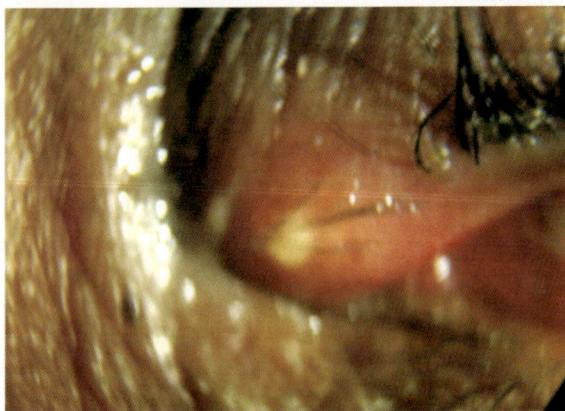

Figures 1 and 2: Hordeolum externum (Stye)

Differential Diagnosis

- International hordeolum
- Cyst of Zeiss and Moll.

Treatment

- Most styes either resolve spontaneously or evacuates anteriorly close to the eyelash roots.
- Resolution may be supported by removing the eyelash associated with the infected follicle followed by hot compresses helps in localization of the lesion and relief of symptoms.
- Application of local antibiotic ointment to the lid margin prevent the spread of the disease to the surrounding area.
- Systemic antibiotics and anti-inflammatory drugs are also advocated for reduction of infection and inflammation and relief of pain which in advanced stage is quite severe.
- Pus can also be evacuated once the lesion is localized and points on the surface under the cover of systemic broad spectrum antibiotics.
- Surgical incision is required only in case of large abcess under local anesthesia.
- Recurrence is prevented by the treatment of chronic blepharitis.

Prognosis

- Good

CHALAZION (MEIBOMIAN CYST)

Introduction

- Chalazion is a chronic inflammatory lipogranuloma of the tarsal glands.

- It is caused by infection of retained sebaceous material inside the neibomian gland due to obstruction of duct.
- Chalazion are common in patients with meibomian gland dysinfection.
- Chalazion is truly not a cyst as it's walls consist of granulomatous tissue and are not lined by epithelium.

Clinical Signs and Symptoms (Figures 3 to 6)

Clinically it starts slowly and without symptoms. In the beginning it is small and hard free from overlying skin.

- It is more common in upper lid and seen frequently in adults.
- Chalazion present as a painless, slowly enlarging roundish, firm lesion in the tarsal plate.
- Mostly the lesions remain stationary after growing to a certain size but sometimes spontaneous regression or secondary infection can take place.

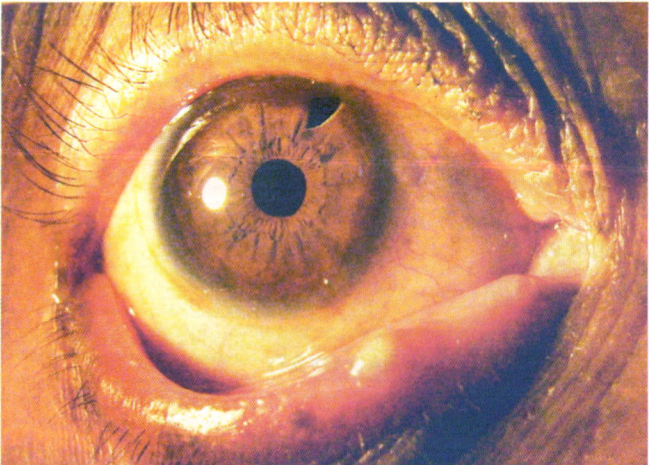

Figure 3: Marginal chalazion lower lid

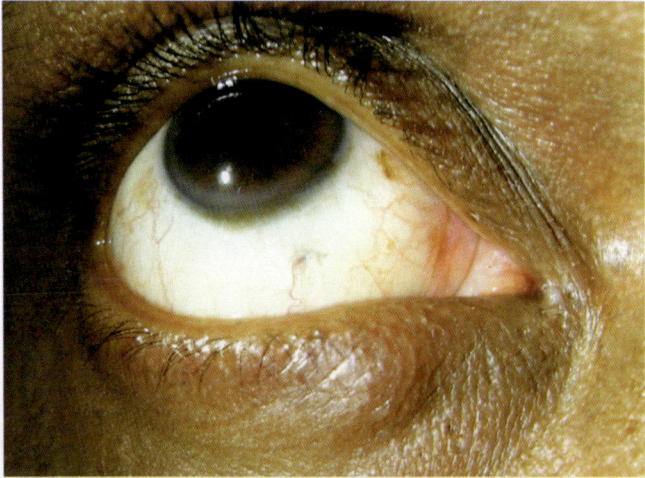

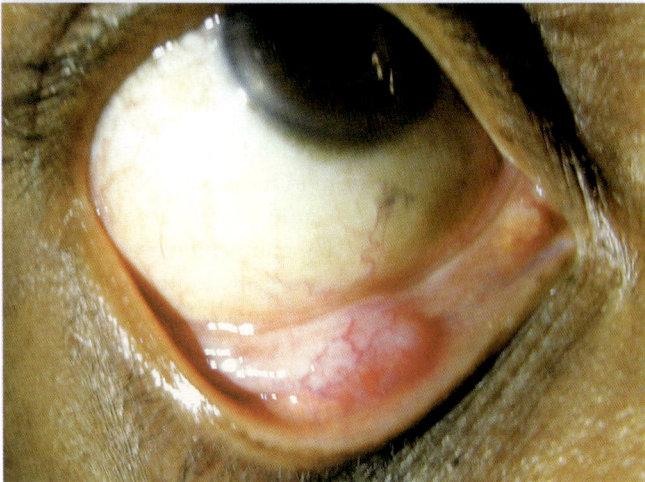

Figures 4 and 5: Chalazion lower lid

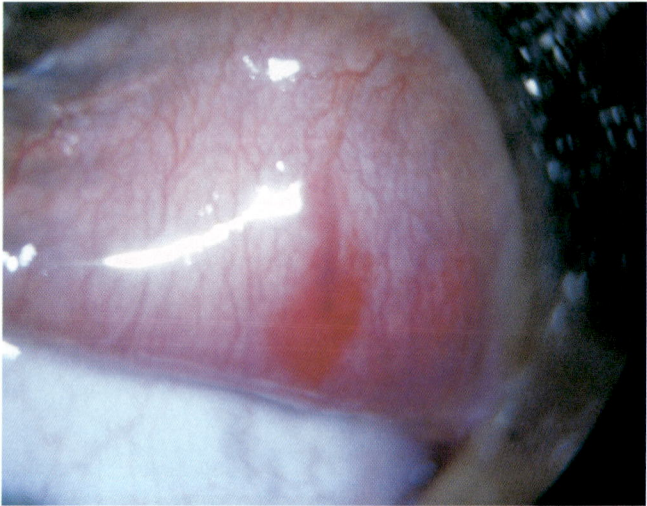

Figure 6: Incision and curettage for
chalazion upper lid (1st day postoperative)

- Sometimes Chalazion of upper lid presses on the cornea causing blurred vision from induced astigmatism.
- Pathologically, there is a unique inflammation of the meibomian glands producing granulation tissue. It affects the area around the acini and leads to fibrosis. There is infiltration of lymphocytes, plasma cells and epitheloid cells. In the center of the mass there is deposition of lipid producing a picture of lipogranuloma.
- There is a chronic low grade infection producing accumulation of sebaceous material in the acini which results in development of granulation tissue due to toxic irritation.

Investigations

- Subjective ocular examination is adequate to clinch diagnosis.
- Eversion of the eyelid may show the presence of an external conjunctival granuloma in the region of the cyst.

Differential Diagnosis

- Stye
- Cyst of Zeiss and Moll.

Treatment

- If chalazion is small and asymptomatic, it can be left alone.
- Medical management includes hot compresses and expressing out the material by massaging the lid.
- Intralesional injection of 1 mg triamcinolone is successful in mild to moderate cases.
- In majority of cases incision and curettage under local anesthesia is required.
- The lid is then everted with a special chalazion clamp.
- An incision is then made through the conjunctiva into the cyst, the contents are curetted and any associated external granulomatous tissue is excised with scissor. Evacuation of the granulation tissue is done with scoop.
- After proper evacuation, an antibiotic ointment is instilled and the eye is padded for about 6 hours. Systemic broad spectrum antibiotic and anti-inflammatory drugs are given.

Prognosis

- Generally prognosis is good.
- Recurrently occurring Chalazia should be closely watched and tissue must be examined for any malignancy.

BLEPHARITIS

Introduction

- Blepharitis is chronic inflammatory condition of the eyelid margin which leads to secondary changes in the conjunctiva and cornea.
- It is quite common but most of the time patient ignore it and goes undiagnosed.
- Etiology is varied one, but the most common causes are staphylococcal infection, seborrhea and meibomian gland dysfunction.

Clinical Signs and Symptoms (Figures 7 to 11)

- Itching in the eye specially at the lid margin is most common complaint of the patient.
- Red eye with watering and burning sensation may also be present.

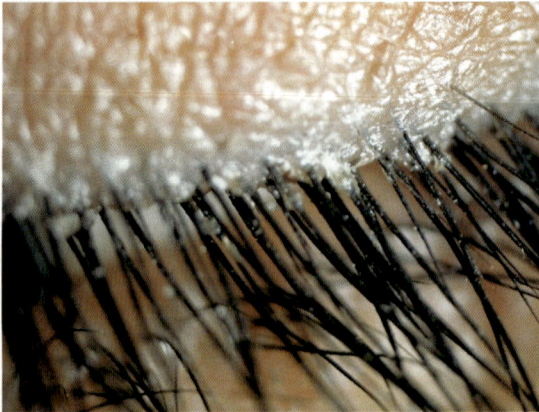

Figure 7: Seborrheic blephritis

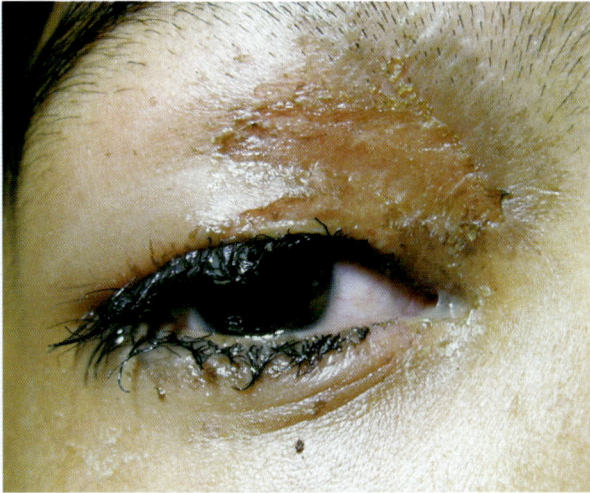

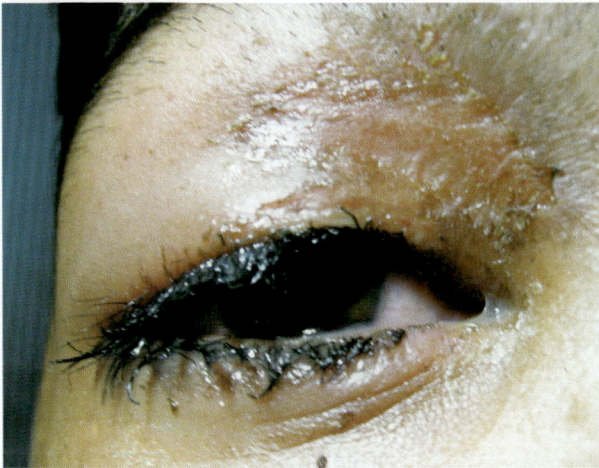

Figures 8 and 9: Blephritis (after thermal burns)

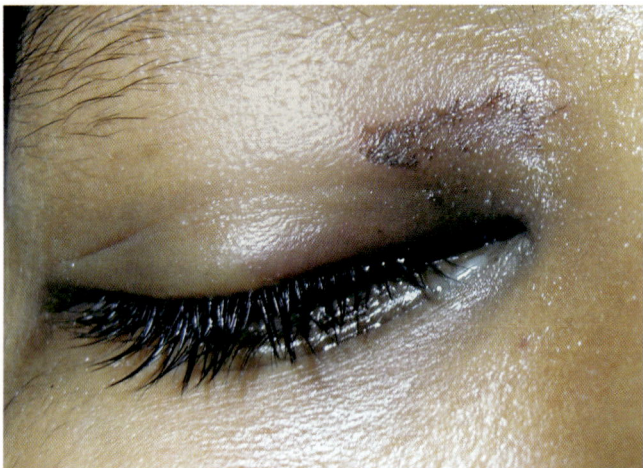

Figure 10: Blephritis (after injury)

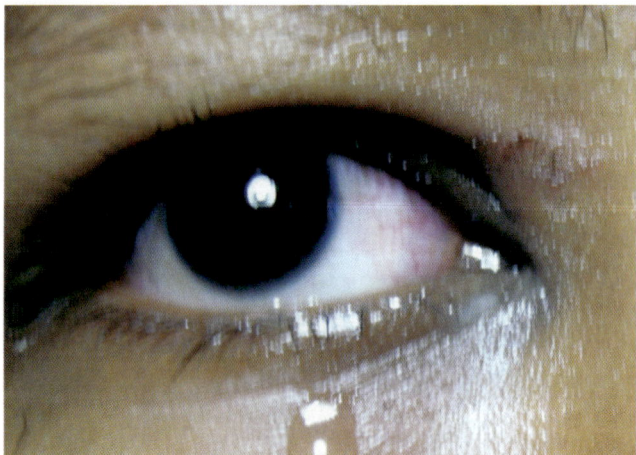

Figure 11: Blephritis

- This condition is more common in young females and is generally associated with dandruff of the scalp.
- Lid margin is thickened, edematous and may have dilated vessels. Gray or yellowish white scales are often observed along the lid margin, scraping of it may lead to tiny ulcers of fine points of bleeding.
- In chronic conditions cilia fall of (Madrosis) with fibrosis at the site. New misdirected cilia may grow (trichiasis).
- Infection can lead to recurrent stye and angular blepharitis – conjunctivitis.
- In some cases secondary changes are seen in the conjunctiva and cornea due to hypersensitivity to staphylococcal exotoxins. They may develop into chronic papillary conjunctivitis, punctuate epithelial erosions in the lower part of the cornea. Marginal corneal ulcers or Phlycten.
- In some cases cystic nodules are seen at the openings of meibomian gland ducts and a foamy discharge is floating over the tear miniscus.
- Tear film is disturbed causing dryness of the conjunctiva and cornea (sicca).
- This peculiar condition is known as triple 'S' Syndrome, a combination of Staphylococcal infection, seborrhea and sicca.

Investigations

- Subjective ocular examination is adequate to make the diagnosis.
- In cases of seborrheic blepharitis careful slit-lamp examination reveals minute oil globules at the orifices of the meibomian glands.

Treatment

Conservative long-term treatment is indicated as total eradication may not be possible.

Hot compresses are prescribed in melting solidified white deposits.

Hygeine of the lid margin with antiseptic soap with warm water atleast twice a day is important mechanical expression of excessive secretion from meibomian glands is advised.

- Local and systemic antibiotics are indicated to control the infection. Scales are softened by wetting with Boric acid and then mechanically removed by gentle scraping.
- Once the primary infection is under control, local steroids can be prescribed to treat secondary effects in the conjunctiva and cornea.
- Treatment with antibiotics and astringents should be continued for at least 2-3 weeks after visible cure.
- Simultaneous treatment of seborrheic dermatitis and dandruff with medicated shampoo is necessary.
- Improvement of general health with vitamins and antioxidants is essential to prevent relapses.
- In parasitic infection, mechanical removes of the organisms is most sufficient.

Prognosis

Generally prognosis is good however sustained medical treatment and compliance is required from the patient.

DERMATITIS

Introduction

- Skin of the eyelid is a very common site for inflammation even with very mild irritants as it is thinnest and most extensible in the body.

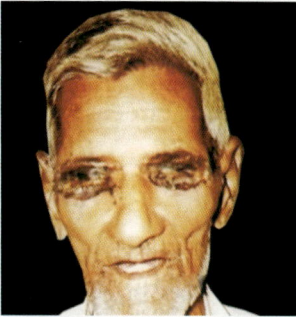

Figure 12: Drug induced dermatitis—Front profile

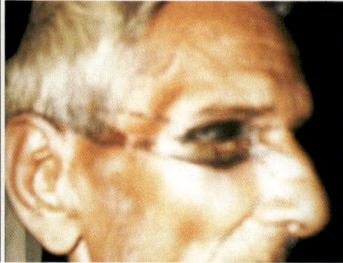

Figure 13: Drug induced dermatitis—Right profile

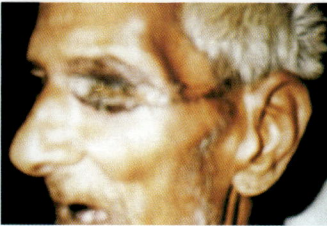

Figure 14: Drug induced dermatitis—Left profile

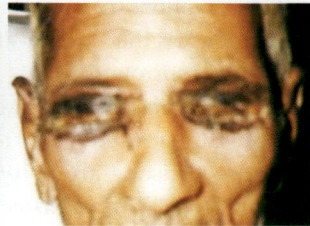

Figure 15: Drug induced dermatitis—Zoomed in

Clinical Signs and Symptoms (Figures 12 to 15)

- Acute dermatitis is characterized by erythema, vesiculation and crusting with burning sensation and itching.
- Chronic dermatitis is shown by thickening of the skin and itching with minimal erythema. Local drugs (Drops and Ointments) and cosmetics are the common irritants.
- In atopic dermatitis patient is sensitive to allergants to much greater degree than normal. They may have a past history of hay fever or asthma. chronic keratoconjunctivitis, keratoconus and lenticular opacities may be associated with atopy.

- Contact dermatitis involving the eyelids are common. It is caused by transmission of irritating substances to the lids by fingers. Failure to rinse the hands adequately following transfer of irritating chemicals in soaps or detergants is the most common cause.

Investigations

- Subjective ocular examination is required to make the diagnosis.

Treatment

- Conservations management involves patch testing in order to identify the irritant and then its removal from the patients surrounding.
- Acute dermatitis is best treated with cold compresses and non-fluorinated short-term corticosteroids like hydrocortisone are helpful. Long-term use of corticosteroids is contraindicated as it may aggravate the dermatitis.

Prognosis

Prognosis is good.

WARTS (VERRUCA VULGARIS)

Introduction

- Warts are small elevated lesions with a papillomatous surface.
- It is a virus infection caused by wart virus belonging to PAPOVA group.
- Sometimes it erupts as a crop of lesions which appear simultaneously.

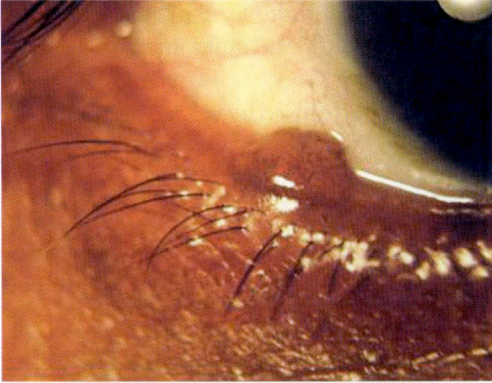

Figure 16: Verruca vulgaris lower lid

Clinical Signs and Symptoms (Figure 16)

It appears as elevated leision in the form of cyst either from upper and lower eyelid protruding anteriorly without any symptoms generally.

Investigation

Subjective ocular examination is generally recommended.

Treatment

Generally cryoapplication is recommended for the regression of wart.

Surgical excision is also indicated but it often leads to recurrence.

MOLLUSCUM CONTAGIOSUM

Introduction

- It is a caused by a viral infection and mostly affects children.

- The typical lesion is multiple, skin colored dome shaped nodule measuring from 1-3 mm sometimes umblicated are seen.
- It is due to infection caused by viruses belonging to a group of poxviruses.

Clinical Signs and Symptoms (Figure 17)

- Lesions when present close to the lid margin can produce follicular conjunctivitis due to liberation of the virus into the conjunctival sac.

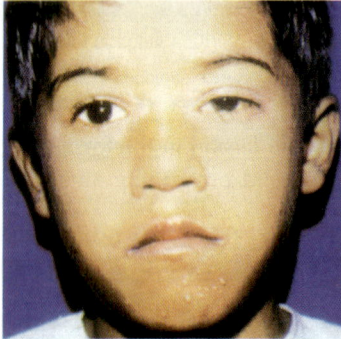

Figure 17: Molluscum contagiosum involving lids and face

Investigation

- Subjective ocular examination.
- Microscopically intracytoplasmic inclusion bodies can be seen which can displace and compress the nucleus to one side.

Treatment

Skin lesion treatment is recommended by expression or cauterization.

Prognosis

- Generally it is good.
- Immunocompromised patients including those of AIDS are prone to develop this virus infection.

TRICHIASIS

Introduction

- Trichiasis is an inward misdirection of the lashes. In this condition few cilia are misdirected backward and they rub against the cornea.
- Trichiasis is caused by trachoma, ulcerative blepharitis, ocular burns, membranous conjunctivitis, injury or operation on the lid margin. It can also be seen in congenital distichiasis.

Clinical Signs and Symptoms (Figures 18 and 19)

- Patient complain of foreign body sensation, irritation, lacrimation, photophobia and pain. The misdirected lashes may rub against the cornea or cause corneal erosions and vascularisation and in severe long standing cases corneal pannus may develop.

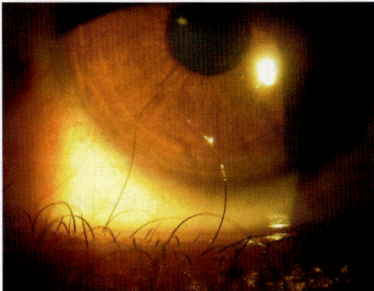

Figure 18: Trichiasis lower eye lid

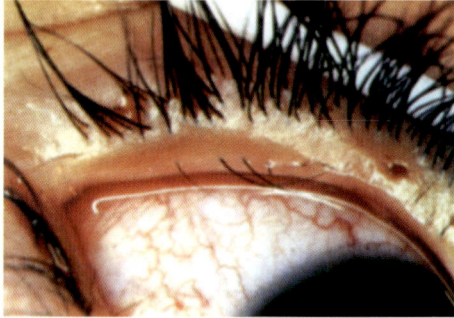

Figure 19: Trichiasis upper eye lid

Investigation

- Subjective ocular examination and slit-lamp examination clinch the diagnosis.

Differential Diagnosis

- Pseudotrichiasis secondary to entropion.

Treatment

- Epilation (Mechanical removal of cilia with forceps) is effective but recurrence with in 4-8 weeks is common with this method.
- Hair follicles can be destroyed by electrolysis. This procedure is not simple and frequent multiple treatments are required to obtain desired results. In this procedure passage of an electric current (3-5 milli amperes) is passed through a fine needle inserted into the root of the eyelash. Then eyelash is removed with the help of forcep. It is a painful procedure.
- Hair follicles can also be destroyed by passage of a current of 30 milli ampere for 10 seconds through a diathermy needle.

- Cryotherapy is safe and effective method for destroying the misdirected lashes. The cryoprobe with −20°C temperature is applied on to the root of the eyelash, **a** freeze-thaw-freeze technique is used. It destroys the hair follicles but leaves a depigmented area after healing.
- Trichiasis can also be corrected with argon laser but it is less effective than cryotherapy.
- Surgical correction may be required in patient with severe trichiasis.

Prognosis

- Generally prognosis is good if proper and adequate treatment is given.

Eyelid Retraction

Tamer Gawdat, Essam El Toukhy (Egypt)

5

INTRODUCTION

Lid retraction is a disorder of eyelid malposition whether the upper lid, the lower lid, or both. The condition is characterized by the appearance of a band of white sclera between the limbus and the eyelid margin or margins, when the eye is in the primary position. The most common cause of upper and lower eyelid retraction is thyroid ophthalmopathy.

ETIOLOGY AND PATHOPHYSIOLOGY OF EYELID CHANGES IN TED

Upper Eyelid Retraction

- Over action of levator muscle.
- Increased sympathetic tone to Muller's muscle.
- Proptosis.
- Fibrosis and contracture of levator aponeurosis.
- Adhesions of the levator to orbital septum and skin.
- Over contraction of superior rectus muscle (SRM)

Lower Eyelid Retraction Causes

- Contraction of inferior rectus muscle (IRM)
- Proptosis
- Secondary to inferior rectus muscle recession.

GRADING

Measuring of Upper Lid Retraction

- 1.5 mm must be added to distance between lid margin and 12.00 o'clock limbus.
- Mild = 1-2 mm
- Moderate = 2-5 mm
- Severe = >5 mm

Measuring of Lower Lid Retraction

- Mild = 1-2 mm
- Moderate = 3 mm
- Severe = > 3 mm

DIFFERENTIAL DIAGNOSIS

- TED
- Familial
- Marcus Gunn jaw winking phenomenon
- Contralateral ptosis
- Parinaud's syndrome
- Hydrocephalus
- High myopia
- Facial nerve palsy
- Postoperative following overcorrection of ptosis.

MANAGEMENT

Medical

Topical Sympatholytics (Adrenergic Blocker) (Guanethidine)

Side effects
- Miosis

- Conjunctival injection
- Punctate keratitis
- Discomfort

Botulinum A Toxin (Local Injection)

Side effects
- Temporary effect
- Ptosis
- SRM paresis → diplopia

Lubricants, Patching, Moist Chamber

Used to avoid corneal changes.

Surgical

Failure of conservative measures to control corneal changes (Functional and cosmetic).

N.B. Euthyroid state for 6-12 months with a prolonged control of local ophthalmopathy
- Tarsorrhaphy
- Eyelid lengthening procedure (post-lamella).

Tarsorrhaphy

Temporary for globe protection for 10-14 days.

Levator Marginal Myotomy

For moderate or severe lid retraction to lengthen a fibrotic contracted Levator and Muller's muscles.

Technique:
- Cut 40-50 % of the horizontal width of levator.
- Cut the levator apn Adhesions to nearby tissue.

- Followed by deep-suture lid crease to prevent upward migration of levator postoperative.

Disadvantages:
- Postoperative ptosis.
- Exact titration is not possible.
- Further levator surgery is difficult (adhesion).

Advantages:
- No foreign material is used.
- No changes of lid contour

Levator Recession and Mullerectomy

Anterior approach:
- Familiar anatomical approach
- Allows simultaneous lacrimal gland suspension.
- Debulking of preaponeurotic fat.
- No corneal irritation due to conjunctival sutures.

Post-approach:
- Less direct anatomic exposure
- Experience
- Damage of lacrimal gland ductules
- Bleeding is more common
- In severe lid retraction
- Levator is recession with a spacer
- Sclera (Eye bank)
- Auricular cartilage
- Fascia lata
- Hard palate mucosa.

Blepharotomy

- Transcrease full thickness lid incision.
- Skin suturing only.

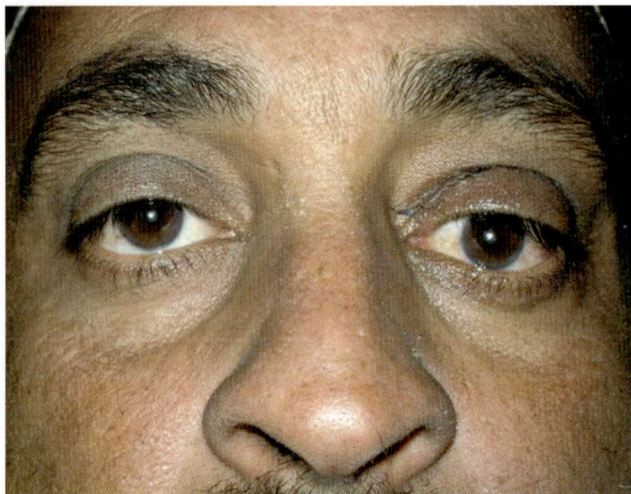

Figure 1: Left blepharotomy

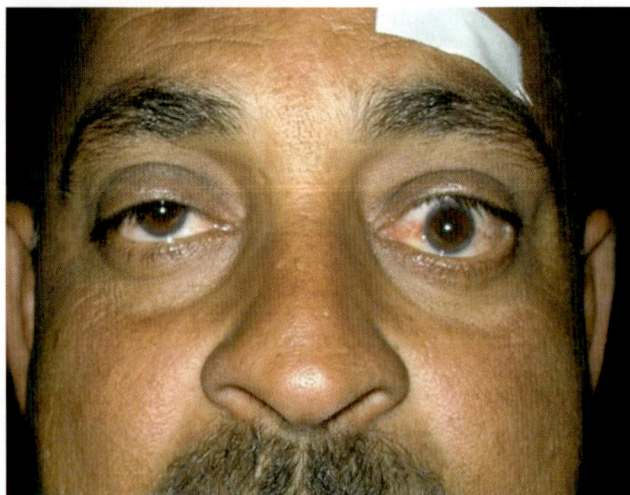

Figure 2: Left upper lid retraction

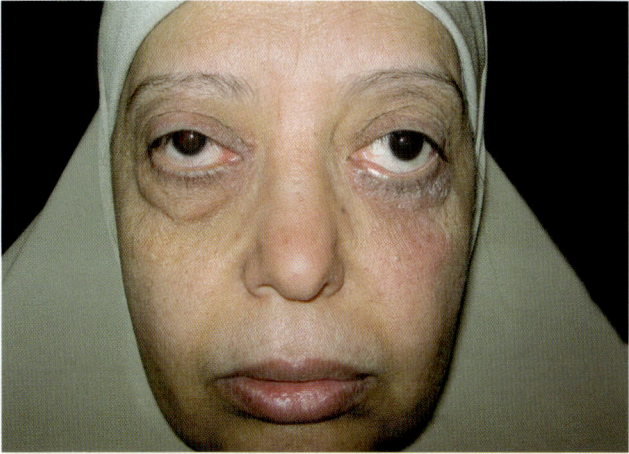

Figure 3: Lower lid retraction in myopia

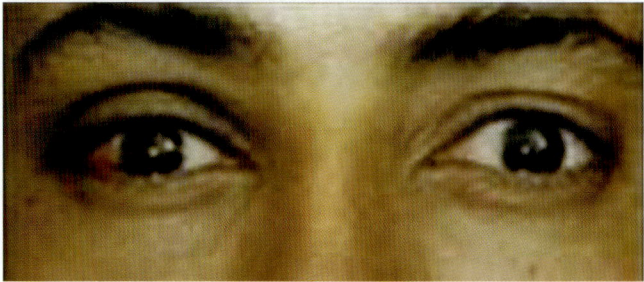

Figure 4: Postoperative—Levator recession and mullerectomy

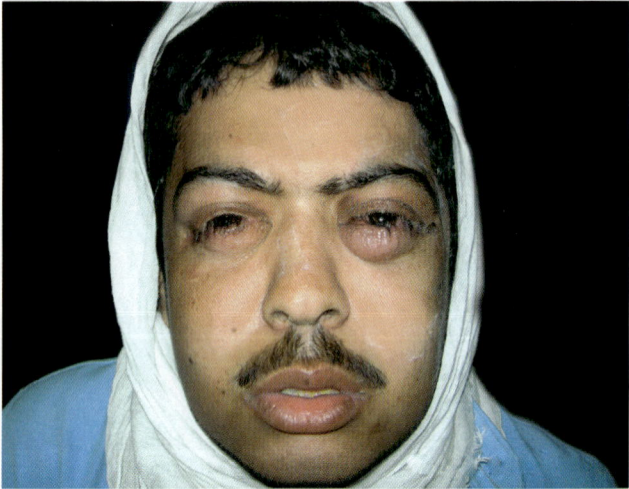

Figure 5: Postoperative—Left lower eyelid spacer (ear cartilage)

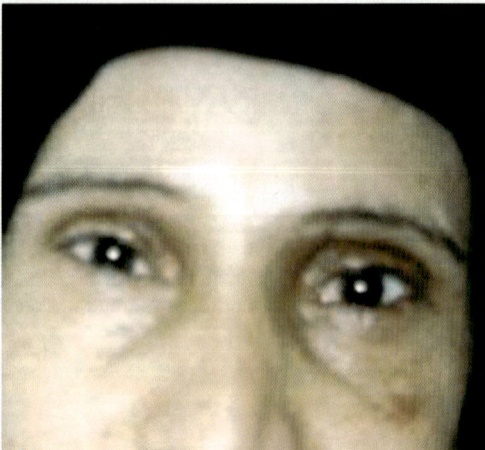

Figure 6: Postoperative—Levator recession and mullerectomy

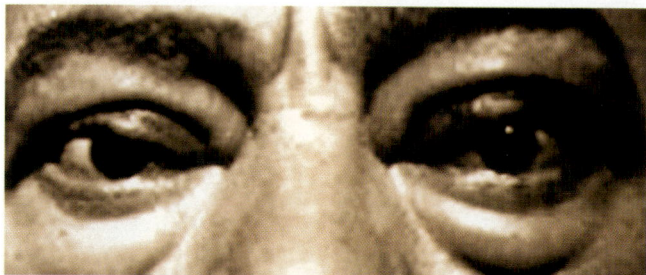

Figure 7: Postoperative—Levator recession and mullerectomy

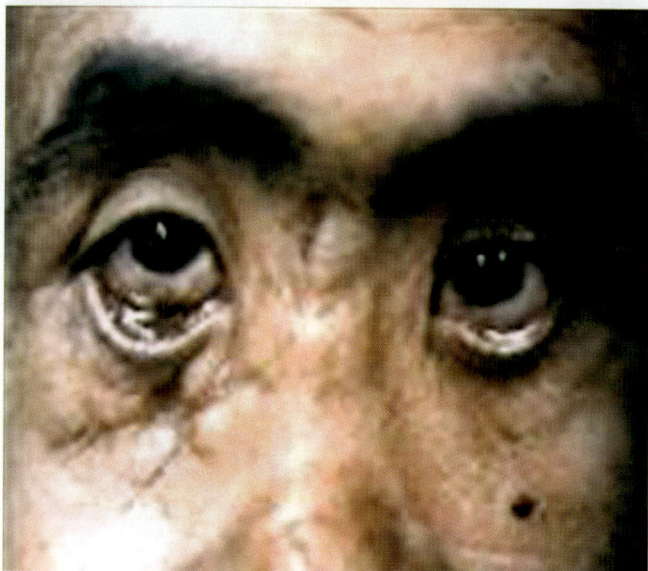

Figure 8: Post-traumatic lower lid retraction

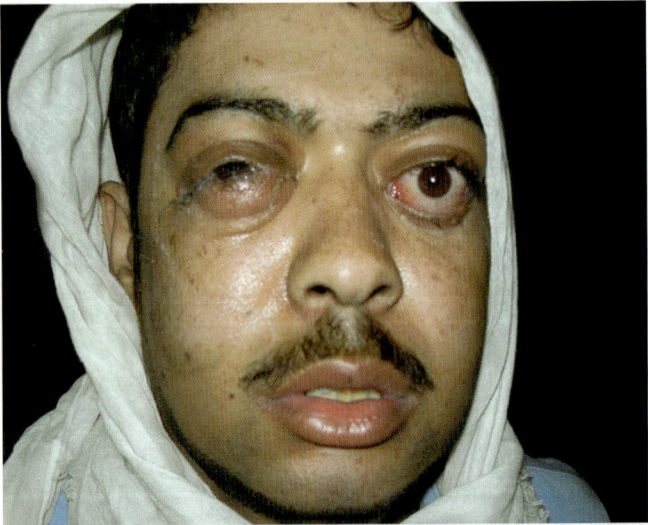

Figure 9: Preoperative left lower eyelid retraction

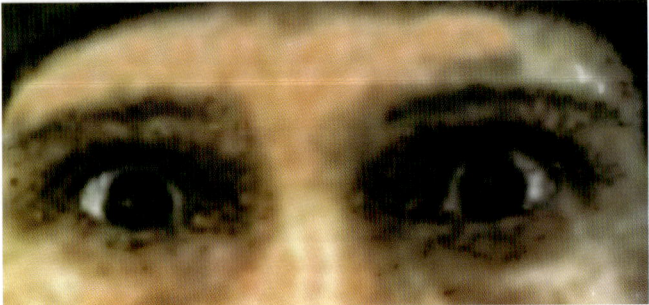

Figure 10: Preoperative upper lid retraction

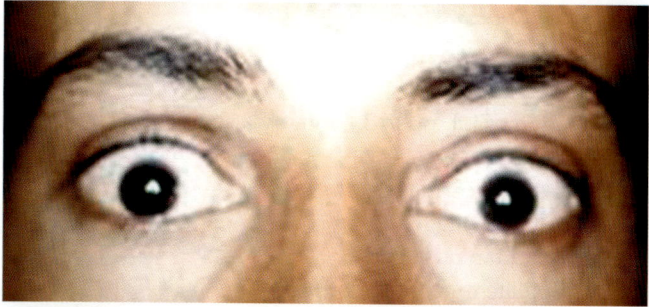

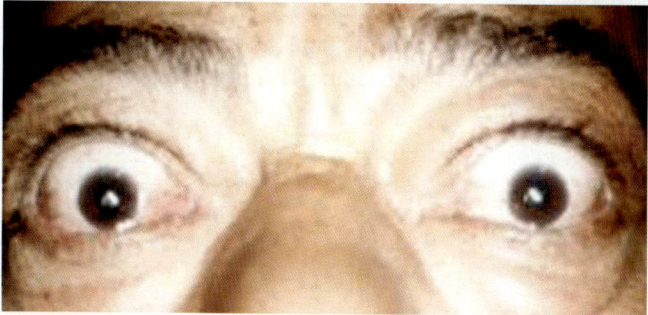

Figures 11 and 12: Preoperative upper lid retraction in TO

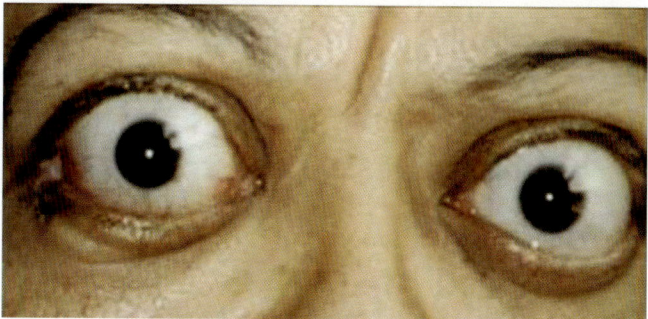

Figure 13: Upper and lower lid retraction in thyroid orbitopathy

Correction of Lower Lid Retraction

Posterior approach:

- Easier
- Elevation of L.L up to 3-4 mm by a spacer.
- Donor sclera
- Nasal septal cartilage
- Auricular cartilage
- Upper lid tarsus (Good)
- Hard palate mucosa (Good)

PROGNOSIS

God control of the thyroid status and proper choice of the surgical procedure are the important factors in prevention of recurrence.

Eyelid Injuries and Reconstruction— An Update

Quresh Maskati, Sunil Vasani (India)

INTRODUCTION

Most eyelid defects, full thickness or otherwise, come from cancers such as basal cell carcinoma or otherwise. In traumatic defects, the defect may be partial or full thickness and a simple inspection of the trauma site often reveals that slowly piecing the remnants together like a jigsaw puzzle will correct the defect. Most ophthalmic or oculoplastic surgeons must know the consistency and limitation of periorbital tissues to begin eyelid reconstruction. The same knowledge can also be applied for cosmetic surgery.

EYELID INJURIES

A careful history to evaluate the circumstances under which the injury was caused is mandatory. Some injuries are simple with only superficial lacerations of the lid while other facial trauma may involve injuries to the head and neck regions along with severe lid injury. The latter should be dealt with immediately as they may be life threatening. Hence, it is imperative to establish that the injury is localized only to the eyelid and surrounding adnexa before beginning management.

Classification

The authors prefer to classify eyelid injuries into:

1. Simple lacerations
2. Complex injuries
3. Full thickness margin defects a) with tissue loss b) without tissue loss
4. Damage to levator aponeurosis
5. Associated with eye/orbital injuries
6. Canalicular lacerations

ANATOMY REVIEW

The upper eyelid can be broadly broken up into:

a. Anterior lamella
b. Posterior lamella

The anterior lamella is broadly made up by skin (thinnest in the body) and orbicularis oculi muscle. The posterior lamella is broadly made up by the tarsal plate, conjunctiva, Muller's muscle and the levator aponeurosis in its posterior part.

An important surface anatomy landmark is the eyelid crease in the upper eyelid, which is formed by the attachment of a few fibers of the levator aponeurosis to the skin. A recession of the eyelid crease with ptosis and a good levator function may signify levator dehiscence.

Also important are the medial and central pads of fat that lie on and are important landmarks in finding the levator aponeurosis. The palpebral portion of the lacrimal gland replaces the lateral fat pad in the upper eyelid.

EXAMINATION

All examination should begin with a thorough search for any damage to the globe. In a conscious patient, visual acuity, intraocular pressure check, slit lamp bio microscopy and fundus examinations are mandatory. It is important to include assessment of ocular motility in the initial exam. Remember, even seemingly trivial eyelid injuries may be associated with underlying globe injuries. In patients with altered sensorium, a complete eye examination should be still carried out.

Assessment of Adnexal Injuries

In conscious patients complete and thorough evaluation of the eyelids and lacrimal system should be carried out. The levator muscle can be assessed by the eyelid crease, the margin reflex distance (MRD) and the levator function test. Medial lacerations may cause canalicular tears or canthal tendon disinsertion. The punctum may be displaced laterally.

Evaluation of the Orbit

Sometimes severe injuries may cause significant eyelid edema, which may hamper proper eye examination. Manipulation of the eyelids in these cases may exacerbate pre-existing globe damage. Such patients should be examined under anesthesia. Orbital injuries can be evaluated with CT scan with axial and coronal cuts to rule out associated orbital fractures and foreign bodies. CT scan may also help in assessing optic nerve compression or damage. A further MRI examination, after ruling out metallic foreign bodies in the orbit can be carried out if necessary for further optic nerve /muscle/adnexal studies.

If facial/nasal or head neck regions are affected, additional help from the concerned specialists should be sought.

MANAGEMENT

The aim of all management is to restore function, vision and cosmesis to as close to normal as possible. If the patient is intoxicated or unconscious and immediate surgery cannot be performed, tissues should be washed and repositioned as close to normal as possible. A light dressing with topical antibiotics can be given. Intravenous steroids and antibiotics or oral antibiotics should be administered. Intra-muscular tetanus toxoid injection should also be administered. The surgeon can safely wait 24-48 hours before attempting surgical intervention.

Anesthesia

Minor lacerations can be repaired in the outpatient department itself under local anesthesia. 2% lidocaine with epinephrine 1:100,000 can be infiltrated locally before closure. General anesthesia should be administered for complex or deeper injuries. However, sedation with monitored care along with local infiltration with or without a regional nerve block will suffice in most cases.

Surgical Tips

- Examine globe thoroughly for perforations and injuries – if necessary, explore.
- Wash all wounds with saline and a solution of 1gm cefazolin in 250 ml saline.
- Prepping can be done with diluted solution of povidone-iodine.
- Remove all foreign bodies after thorough exploration of all affected tissues.
- Check anterior and posterior lamella
- Look for lid laxity, indicative of canthal tendon injury

- Examine upper and lower canaliculi, lacrimal gland and levator muscle.
- To avoid lid notching, try to close wounds horizontally i.e. parallel to lid margin in the upper eyelid and vertically in the lower lid, i.e. perpendicular to lid margin **(Figures 1A and B).**

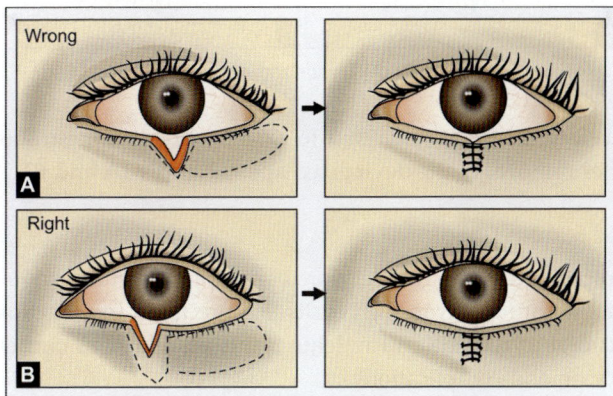

Figures 1A and B: (A) Incorrect closure with lid notch, (B) Correct closure

- Simple eyelid laceration can be closed directly with slight margin eversion. Care should be taken to avoid tension on wound edges. The authors prefer to close vertical lacerations in layers with 6/0 polyglactin and skin with 6/0 polypropylene. Horizontal lacerations spontaneously reapproximate themselves due to orbicularis sphincter action.

Disfigurement of the anterior lamella can cause complex lacerations. We try to undermine the edges to mobilize the tissue to aid anatomically perfect apposition. Debridement should be minimal. After debridement, a "V" shaped

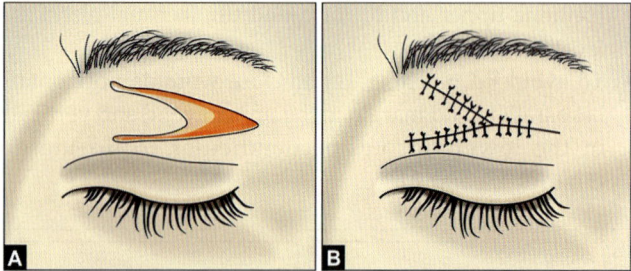

Figures 2A and B: (A) Devitalized apex, (B) Y-shaped flap

laceration can be converted to a "Y" shaped configuration after removal of the devitalized apex **(Figures 2A and B).**

Lid Margin Repair

Proper and immaculate closure of lid margin injuries should be sought for rewarding results. Failure to do so will cause lid disfigurement and notching and may lead to corneal drying and complications.

Evaluate lid tissue loss by trying to approximate the cut edges of the margins and see if closure can be achieved without tension. If this is possible, the marginal defect has to be closed in layers separately, i.e. the anterior and posterior lamellae **(Figures 3A and B).**

If there is tissue loss and the wound cannot be closed without tension, a lateral cantholysis or canthotomy **(Figure 4)** in mild cases and a Tenzel type rotational flap in moderate tissue loss can be carried out **(Figure 5).** For upper eyelid, the arc of the circle is below the lateral canthus and for lower it is above the canthus. For severe tissue or lid loss, Mustarde type flaps or lid sharing procedures can be used.

While attempting closure of small lid margin lacerations, the wound has to be modified to avoid formation of lid notch.

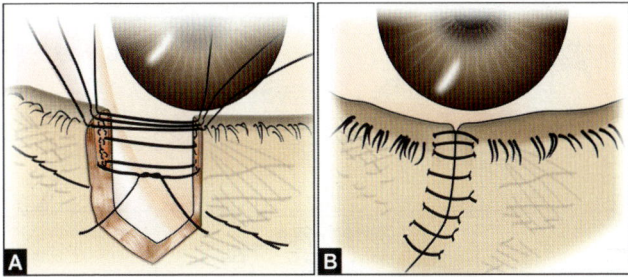

Figures 3A and B: (A) First silk suture through the tarsal plate is tied first. Second through the grey line. Third and fourth behind and in front of the lash lines, (B) Skin and muscles closed in layers

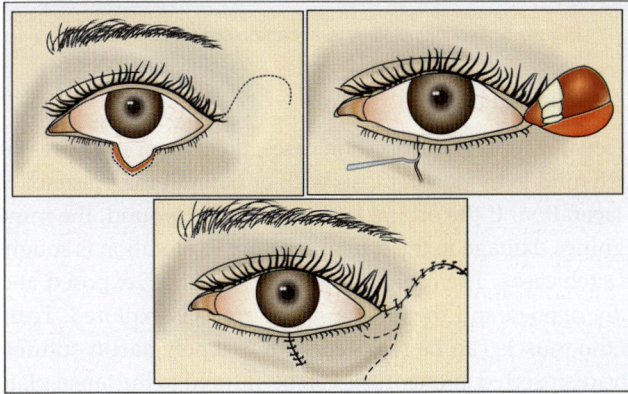

Figure 4: Tenzel rotation flap

The entire vertical portion of the tarsus has to be removed corresponding to the width of the deficit. The tarsal excision is carried out perpendicular to the lid margin. A "V" shaped defect is converted into a pentagon shaped defect before closure.

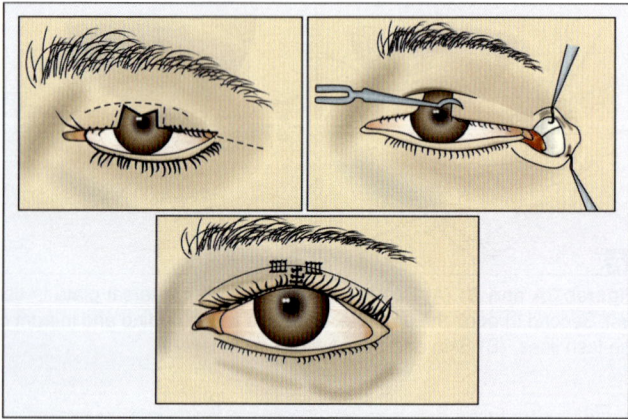

Figure 5: Technique for lateral canthotomy and lid closure

Levator Muscle Dehiscence

In levator muscle disinsertion cases, the patient may present with mild to moderate ptosis with or without the presence of a laceration. If the orbital fat is seen in the wound, the same signifies damage to the orbital septum. Exploration is sought in such cases. The orbital septum is identified, exposed and fully opened and the levator aponeurosis is explored. Tears in the muscle can be repaired with 6/0 polyglactin sutures. The disinserted aponeurosis can be sutured to the tarsal plate with 3 6/0 polypropylene sutures Care should be taken to preserve the lid contour. All prolapsed lacrimal gland tissue should be repositioned before closure. There should be no ectropion or lagophthalmos after closure is complete.

Canalicular Lacerations

- Commonly missed injuries.
- Look carefully for the severed edges.

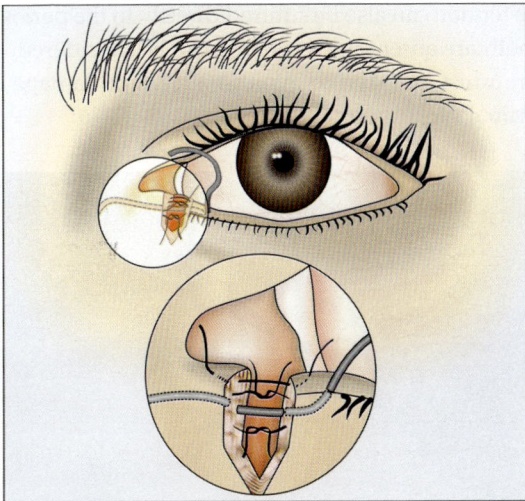

Figure 6: Canlicular repair with stent

- Irrigation from the ipsilateral punctum with fluoroscein stained saline or injection of air may help identify the cut edge of the punctum.
- Authors prefer to use bicanalicular stents, left in place for 6 months for repair **(Figure 6).**
- The surrounding lid margin and adventitia can be repaired as described earlier.
- In our opinion the pigtail probe should be avoided.
- Before repairing the canaliculi it is important to determine the presence of any canthal tendon avulsion **(Figure 7)**.
- Repair of the posterior horn of the medial canthal tendon is necessary to maintain the lacrimal pump function **(Figures 8 to 10)**.
- Approximation and suturing of the 2 cut edges of the tendon with 6/0 polypropylene is sufficient to maintain function.

- The tendon can also be sutured directly to the periosteum.
- If both are absent micro-plating can be considered.
- Care must be taken to avoid inadvertent damage to the lacrimal sac during repair.

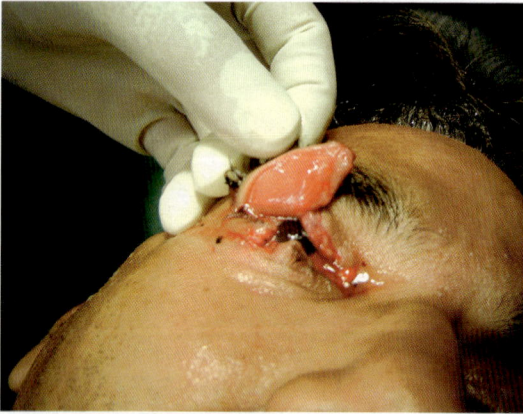

Figure 7: Eyelid avulsion preoperative

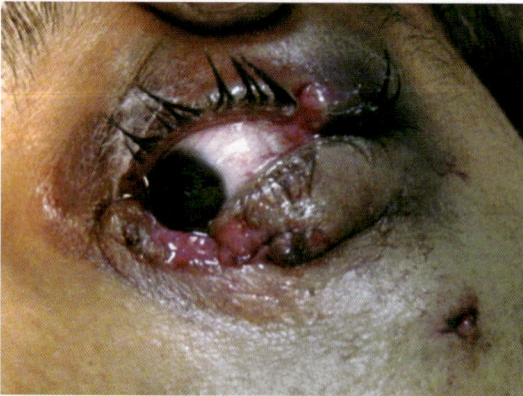

Figure 8: Eyelid injury with canalicular injury

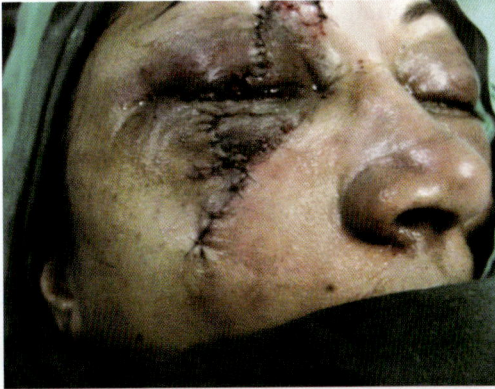

Figure 9: Eyelid injury with zygoma fracture 4

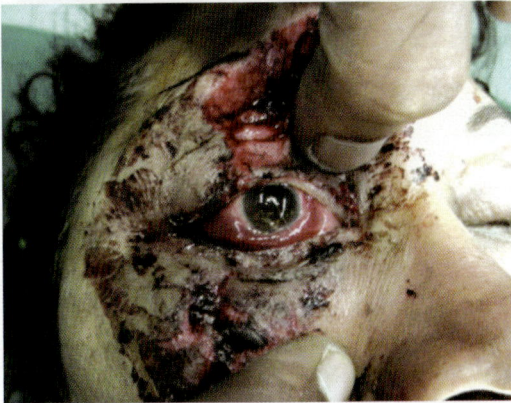

Figure 10: Eyelid injury with zygoma fracture 7

CONCLUSION

Though eyelid trauma has myriad manifestations, general surgical principles are to be followed in repair. Repair is to be attempted once the general condition of the patient permits;

meticulous cleaning of the injured area, maintenance of asepsis is essential. In most cases one can manage edge to edge apposition as the lids are fairly forgiving of minor tissue loss. However, in cases of major tissue loss or where there is concurrent injury to canaliculi or canthal tendons, plastic repair as outlined above will yield very satisfactory results in terms of function and cosmesis.

BIBLIOGRAPHY

1. Color Atlas of Ophthalmic Plastic Surgery: A.G.Tyers, J.R.O. Collins.
2. Oculoplastic Surgery: William P Chen.
3. Ophthalmic Plastic and Reconstructive Surgery: Frank A Nesi, Richard D Lisman, Mark Levine.

Congenital Nasolacrimal Duct Obstruction

7

Essam El Toukhy, Ibrahim Mosad (Egypt)

PATHOPHYSIOLOGY

A very common condition in which the extreme end of the nasolacrimal duct underneath the inferior turbinate fails to complete its canalization in the newborn period. Canalization of the nasolacrimal duct usually completed by eight month of gestation.

FREQUENCY

- Rate: 2-4% of newborn
- Race: no racial incidence
- Sex: no sexual difference.

CAUSES

Usually, these anomalies are sporadic, but genetics, prematurity, and maternal drug use can be possible influencing factors.

Ocular abnormalities are present in 20% of patients, and systemic abnormalities are present in almost 25% of patients with serious congenital nasolacrimal duct anomalies.

PRESENTATION

Amniotocele

This condition occurs in neonates as a distention in the lacrimal sac. Amniotic fluid enters the sac, is retained by a nonpatent nasolacrimal duct, and is trapped in the sac by the valve at the common caaliculus, the valve of Rosenmüller. Probing the nasolacrimal duct as an office procedure usually is curative.

Dacryocystitis (Acute Mucocele or Pyocele)

This condition exhibits acute distention and inflammation in the lacrimal sac region and may occur in the neonatal period. Probing is necessary in newborns with acute dacryocystitis to establish drainage as soon as possible. This procedure is performed with topical or local anesthesia only.

Tearing

Newborns who have congenital nasolacrimal duct obstruction may not develop acute dacryocystitis with a mucocele or pyocele of the sac in the early neonatal period but may simply have tearing with a chronic mucopurulent discharge, which usually manifests at 2 weeks. Topical antibiotics should be administered, and the parents must be instructed in the proper technique of lacrimal sac compression and massage. More than 90% of these cases clear and become asymptomatic with conservative management. Under normal circumstances, these children with mild-to-moderate symptoms of epiphora and lid crusting can be monitored for the first nine months life without serious sequela. It is rarely necessary to make probing mandatory at an early age before 6 month.

INVESTIGATIONS

- Fluorescein dye disappearance test—Grade as good, fair, or poor clearance
- Jones dye tests—Not as useful in practice with small children
- Imaging Studies:
- Intubation dacryocystography
- Scintillography

DIFFERENTIAL DIAGNOSIS

- Sinus mucocele
- Repeated conjunctivitis

TREATMENT

Medical Care

Congenital nasolacrimal duct obstructions resolves spontaneously in 90% of cases during the first year of life. Massage with digital pressure used as an aid to speeding up this natural resolution. Other than massage, topical antibiotics are useful for mucopurulent discharge, but the only treatment of efficacy for those patients who do not resolve spontaneously is surgery as follow.

Surgical Care

Probing

Probing cures 95% of congenital nasolacrimal obstructions. Prognosis for probing decreases with the increasing number of probings and the age of the patient. Rarely, it is successful after the third time or after 3 years.

Nasolacrimal Intubation

Success rates of 80-95% have been reported, in patients have only been probed twice or less and are younger than 2 years. Prognosis is poor for those patients with previous dacryocystitis and for those patients in which an obstruction is encountered during the procedure. Increasing duration of intubation was not associated with increasing chance of success but with a significantly higher risk of failure if longer than 18 months. The retention of silicone tubes for longer than 12 months was associated with a significantly lower success rate (67%).

Balloon Catheter Dilatation

Balloon catheter dilatation of nasolacrimal system with or without silicone tubing: This procedure has slightly better results than intubation alone.

Dacryocystorhinostomy with or without Intubation

This treatment indicated when a patent canalicular system is present with failed previous treatment.

Conjunctival Dacryocystorhinostomy

If the upper system is scarred or atretic then it can be bypassed using a prosthesis, such as a Lester-Jones tube. This procedure probably should be avoided until the child is older than 10 years because the prosthesis requires care from the patient and often has minor complications and revisions.

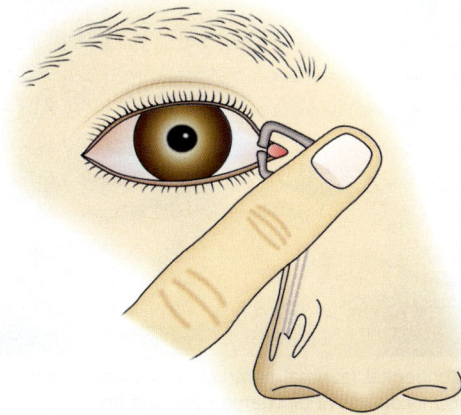

Figure 1: Massage technique for congenital nasolacrimal duct obstruction

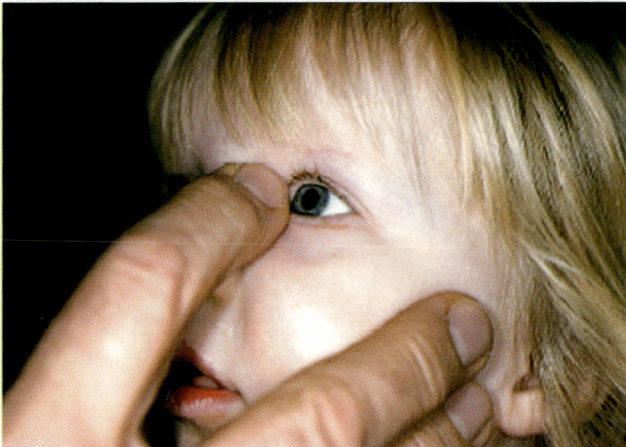

Figure 2: Massage technique for congenital nasolacrimal duct obstruction

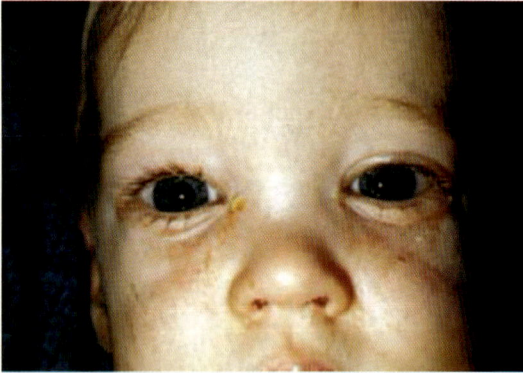

Figure 3: Congenital lacrimal obstruction presenting with persistent watering and mucopurulent discharge observed from the first month of life

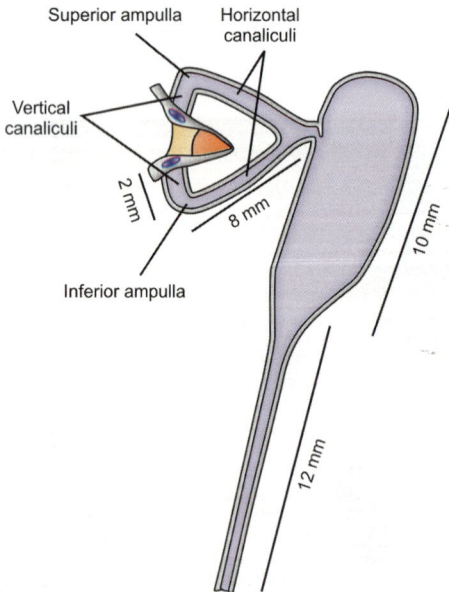

Figure 4: Important dimensions of the lacrimal drainage system

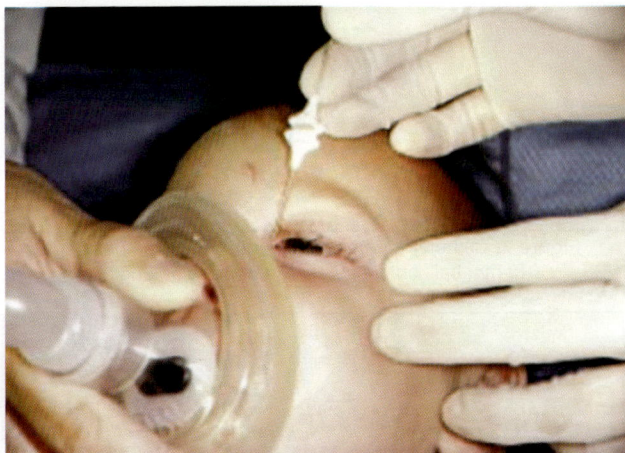

Figure 5: Probing of nasolacrimal duct under general anesthesia by mask

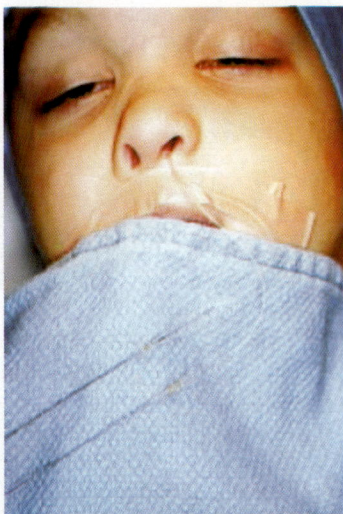

Figure 6: Both ends of the silicone tubing have been passed through canaliculus, sac, and duct, and have been retrieved from the nose

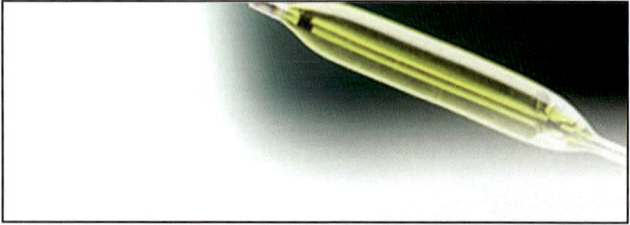

Figure 7: Catheter for patients older than 30 months of age
(3 mm balloon diameter, 15 mm balloon length)

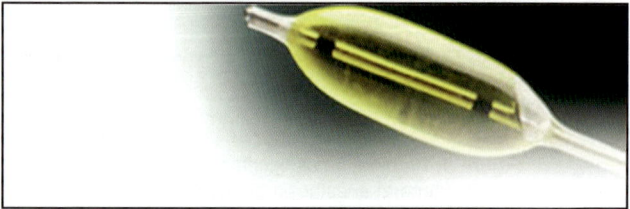

Figure 8: Balloon catheter for adults
(5 mm diameter, 8 mm balloon length)

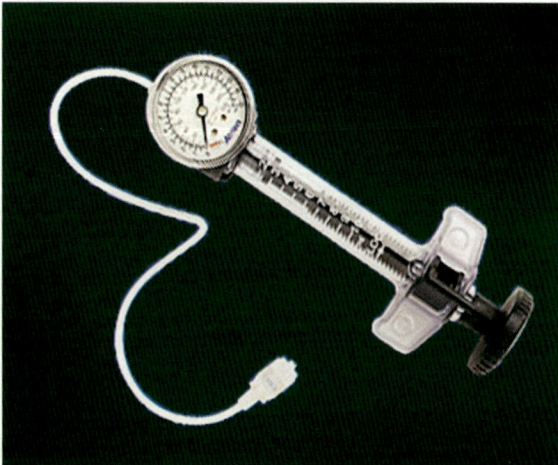

Figure 9: The balloon catheter inflation device

COMPLICATIONS AND PROGNOSIS

Bleeding

Serious bleeding is rare, occurring in only 1-2% of surgeries or postoperatively.

Surgical Failures

In these complicated conditions, a 10% rate of failure occurs.

Wound infections: These occur in 5-10% of patients, usually as wound abscesses on the fourth postoperative day.

Silicone or Polyethylene Tubing Complications

These complications occur in about 15% of cases and include the following: corneal abrasion, pyogenic granuloma, low-grade infection, chronic nasal irritation and congestion, epistaxis, sinusitis, and pharyngitis.

Bypass Tube Complications

These frequently occur in at least 40% of patients postoperatively and include tube loss or migration and tube obstruction.

Anesthesia Complications

In children, these complications are more frequent due to drugs, blood loss, malignant hyperthermia, and pseudocholinesterase deficiency.

Acquired Lacrimal Obstructions

8

Hatem A Tawfik, Norlaila Talib, Essam El Toukhy (Egypt)

INTRODUCTION

In an ideal situation, the amount of tear output should be equal to the amount to be eliminated. Unfortunately this is not always the case, and tearing is a frequent symptom in Ophthalmology clinics. Among the various causes of tearing, primary acquired nasolacrimal duct obstruction (PANDO) is the most frequently encountered cause.

PATHOPHYSIOLOGY

The exact cause of PANDO is not known. Diverticula of the lacrimal passages, descending infection from the eye, ascending infection from the nose, abuse of topical medications, and the use of carbon based cosmetics (Kohl) have all been listed as possible etiologies.

Pathological findings in PANDO include fibrous or fibrovascular obstruction of the surrounding cavernous body and the lumen of the nasolacrimal ducts. Other interesting pathological findings include squamous metaplasia in the stenotic area, in addition to loss of goblet cells. Dacryoliths may also be found in 10-20% of patients with acquired lacrimal obstructions. They are particularly common in the lacrimal sac. Their presence is of clinical importance because contrary to classical lacrimal teaching, which states that the presence of positive regurge of pus from the sac means no further investigations, syringing may still be of help if the cause of the obstruction is a lacrimal stone as it may be pushed through an otherwise healthy nasolacrimal duct causing relief of the situation. Furthermore, failure to observe and remove a dacryolith during lacrimal surgery may result in recurrence.

CLINICAL EVALUATION

History

Answers to be sought include whether the tearing is on daily basis or interrupted, whether the tears are watery or viscous, whether there has been a previous history of facial swelling (acute attack). History of abuse of topical medications or systemic chemotherapy is also important as these may serve as a cause of punctal or nasolacrimal duct obstruction.

A gritty, foreign body sensation, an itching eyelid, and the absence of daily epiphora usually alert the physician to a local ocular cause for epiphora not in the lacrimal drainage system

Clinical Evaluation

The *dye disappearance test (DDT)* is used to determine whether the outflow system is working or not. A drop or 2 of fluorescein are placed in the conjunctival sac in both eyes regardless of whether one or both eyes are asymptomatic. The eyes are evaluated a few minutes later **(Figure 1)**, to observe the amount of fluorescein stained tears in the conjunctival sac. A positive result is more easy to observe if obstruction is unilateral.

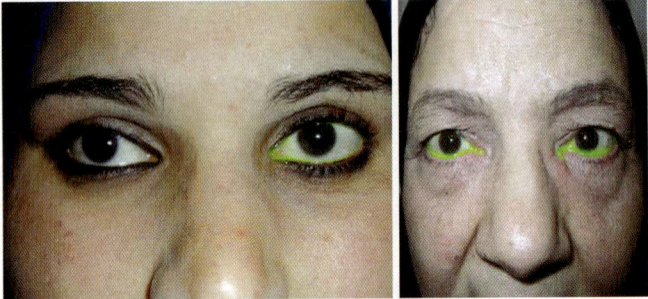

Figure 1: Unilateral and bilateral positive DDT

In *Lacrimal syringing,* a lacrimal cannula is introduced through the canaliculus; preferably the upper. If a *soft stop* is encountered, this indicated canalicular obstruction, and the cannula is withdrawn and the length of patent canaliculi is measured in millimeters. If no obstruction is encountered, normal saline is irrigated through the lacrimal canaliculi. If the fluid passes immediately into the nose, the lacrimal outflow system is patent. If the fluid initially regurges through the opposite canaliculus, then passes to the nose a couple of seconds later, then a partial obstruction should be suspected. If all fluid regurges through the opposite canaliculus then PANDO should be diagnosed. If fluid regurges through the same punctum, then a canalicular obstruction is present. **Figure 2** summarizes all the possible results of syringing.

Radiological Evaluation

Generally speaking, evaluation of the tearing patient is clinical not radiological. Several radiological tests are available like dacryocystography (DCG), scintillography, CT-DCG, and ultrasonography of lacrimal system may be needed in children

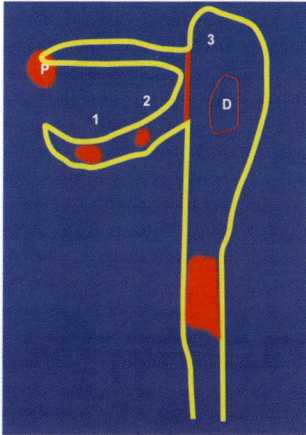

Figure 2: Possible sites of acquired lacrimal obstructions. 1,2: Distal and proximal canalicular obstruction, 3: Common canalicular obstruction, 4: Nasolacrimal duct obstruction, P: Punctal stensosis, D: Dacryolith in the lacrimal sac

or in uncooperative patients who refuse office syringing. A formal computed tomography, and nasal endoscopy may be needed if there is a history of associated sinus disease or if there is a suspicion of nasal or lacrimal system neoplasia.

DIFFERENTIAL DIAGNOSIS

The most important is to differentiate other causes of tearing from PANDO. This includes : dry eyes, functional tearing due to lacrimal pump failure and secondary nasolacrimal duct obstruction as in cases of nasal pathology or old fractures **(Figures 3 to 5)**.

TREATMENT

Dacryocystorhinostomy or DCR is the gold standard to treat PANDO. Three different approaches exist but they all have a common goal which is to create an alternative long-term pathway for the tears by creating an epithelial lined tract

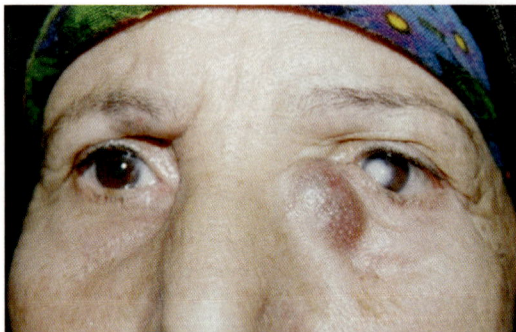

Figure 3: Mucocele of the lacrimal sac

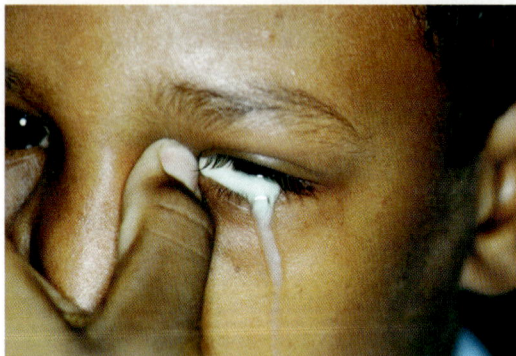

Figure 4: Positive resurge of pus from
the sac upon digital pressure

between the lacrimal sac and the nasal mucosa. These different approaches simply differ in the route used to create the fistula. The international standard is the external transcutaneous route introduced by TOTI way back in 1904 and is still by far the most frequently performed and the most successful lacrimal procedure worldwide. Endonasal techniques; either endoscopic or non-endoscopic have been in the rise in the past 20 years, but they still suffer from several drawbacks,

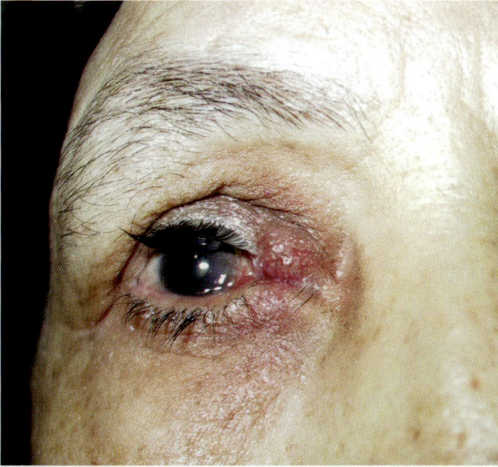

Figure 5: Canaliculitis of the upper and/or lower canaliculi should never be confused with a mucocoele, because the management is entirely different

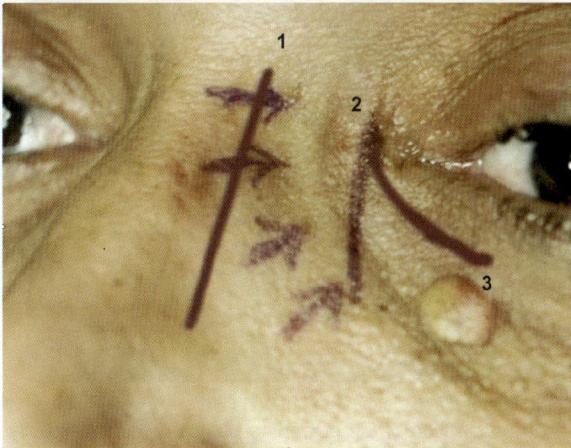

Figure 6: EXT-DCR, skin incision designs. Care should be taken to avoid injuring the angular vein (arrows)

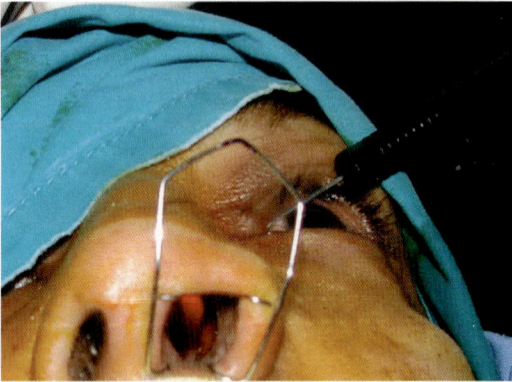

Figure 7: Endonasal non-endoscopic DCR. A 20-gauge vitrectomy light probe is gently introduced through the upper canaliculus top (to) visualize the surgical site without the aid of an endoscope

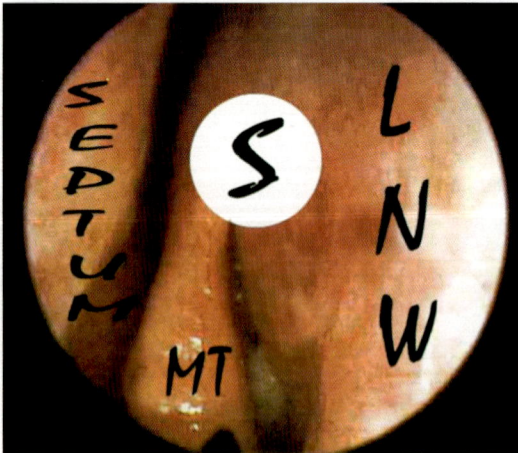

Figure 8: Endoscopic view of the left nasal cavity. The endoscope allows excellent visualization of the procedure but interferes significantly with the inlet and exit of surgical instruments especially in the presence of a deviated nasal septum, or a hypertrophied middle turbinate. LNW, lateral nasal wall. MT, middle turbinate. S, Intended surgical fistula site

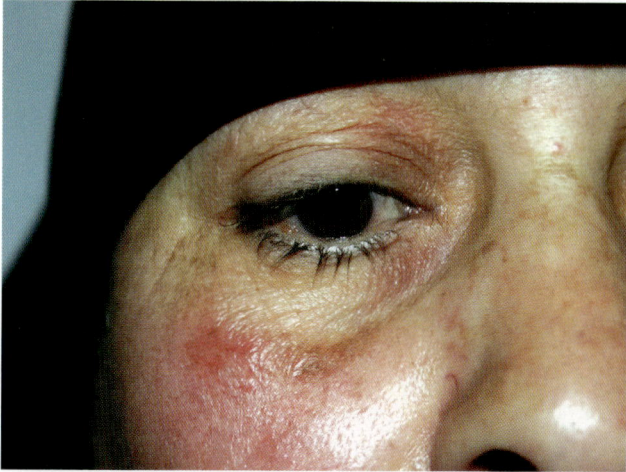

Figure 9: Complete disappearance of the DCR
scar one month after surgery

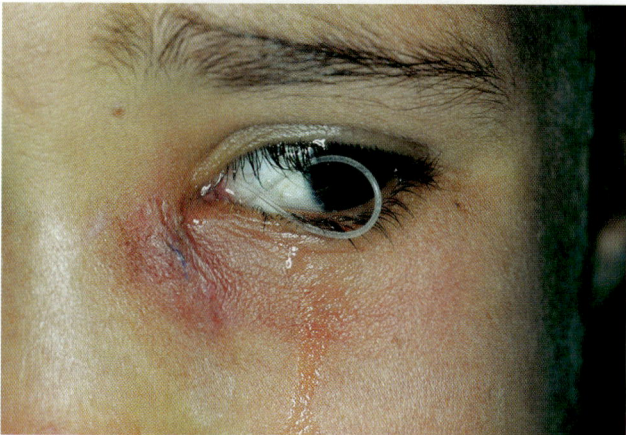

Figure 10: Prolapsed lacrimal tube after successful
EXT-DCR (Spaghetti sign)

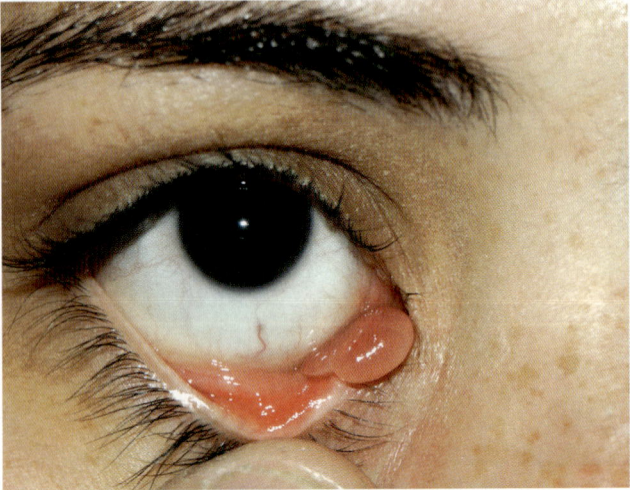

Figure 11: Pyogenic granuloma developing on top of a silastic stent

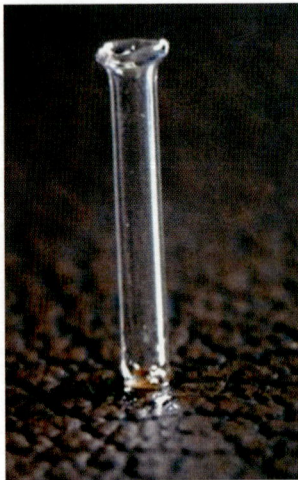

Figure 12: The Jones pyrex tube could be used as a bypass conduit of tears in case of complete punctal and canalicular stenosis

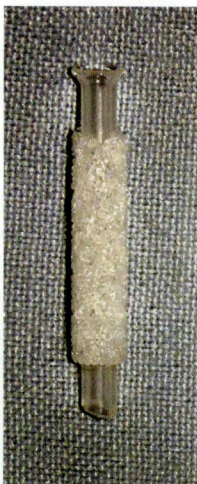

Figure 13: The Medpor coated glass tube is an alternative to the traditional Jones tube

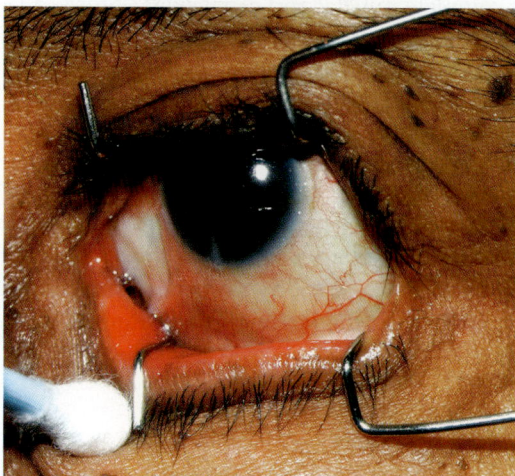

Figure 14: Scleral necrosis prompting removal of the Jones tube

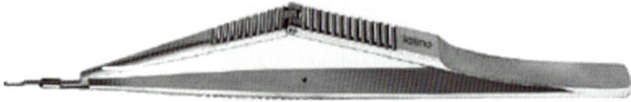

Figure 15: The Kelly glaucoma punch could be used to cut–open stenosed puncti

including the inability to create flaps that could be sutured to create primary intention healing, plus the poor access to the superior bone opposite the fundus of the sac which still places endonasal techniques as a second choice after the external route **(Figures 6 to 15)**.

Surgery in Special Situations

In case of isolated punctal stenosis, a DCR is not needed. Dilatation of the punctum plus stenting with a perforated plug, a monocanalicular tube or pigtail probing is enough. In case of complete punctal and canalicular fibrosis, a lacrimal bypass tube, the Jones pyrex tube, or one of its newer alternatives may be needed.

PROGNOSIS

External DCR has a success rate of over 90% in expert hands. Canalicular obstruction has a much lower rate of success even with successful intubation. If functional success (relief of symptoms) does not coincide with anatomic success (patency on syringing), then the lacrimal pump function should be reevaluated.

Lacrimal Injuries

9

Rania Abdel Salam, Essam El Toukhy (Egypt)

INTRODUCTION

Lacrimal injuries are usually not isolated. They are almost always associated with lid injuries or orbital or nasal fractures. Eyelid, orbital and adnexal injuries can be a part of multisystem trauma. The basic ABCs of the trauma management should be considered and once the patient is stable, it is possible to properly examine the eyelid with the upper lacrimal passages, orbital injuries as well as the associated globe or optic nerve affection. It should be remembered that upper lacrimal drainage system can be involved in chemical or thermal injuries

EVALUATION OF LACRIMAL INJURIES

History

The conditions of trauma can give an idea about the nature and the extent of injury. Being usually associated with lid or orbital injuries, high index of suspicion should exist to be able to detect lacrimal passage injuries. Lacrimal gland injury is usually rare and may be associated with orbital roof fractures or deep upper lid wound.

Review of medical history is essential as well as drug allergy history of tetanus immunization and problems encountered with anesthesia.

Examination

Routine systematic examination of the eyelid, globe and orbit should be performed. Canalicular injury is suspected when the injury lies medial to the punctum which is usually laterally displaced compared to the other side or the opposite one. Medial or lateral canthal injuries as well as tissue loss should be ruled out.

Lacrimal passage injuries associated with orbital or nasal fractures may be overlooked especially with the edema or ecchymosis. However, associated nasal bone fractures as well as traumatic telecanthus should raise the index of suspicion.

In case of late presentation of lacrimal drainage system injuries, systematic evaluation should be adopted. This includes, evaluation of the conjunctiva for presence of adhesions as well as assessment of the punctal position, direction and patency. Positive regurge test is a sure sign of nasolacrimal duct obstruction. Dye disappearance test show delay as compared to the other side. Probing may show strictures of the canaliculi or fibrosis of the lacrimal sac that usually felt as a soft stop. Irrigation test can show the extent of NLD obstruction. Nasal examination is very important is such cases as a deviated septum resulting from the original trauma may be the reason of the lacrimal passage problems.

Orbital CT whither conventional cuts or in three dimensions can show the fractures sites and their extent as well as associated nasal deformities.. Dacryocystography can show nasolacrimal duct obstructions site and extent.

PROPER LACRIMAL SYSTEM

Proper lacrimal system evaluation is necessary for choosing the treatment protocol.

Wounds Associated with Canalicular Injuries

They can result from direct trauma to medial canthal area or indirectly by avulsive forces caused by trauma to the orbit. They are common with dog bites and midface injuries. Early repair of the canalicular injury is much easier and more successful than late repair or conjunctivodacryocystorhino-stomy with Jone's tube.

Canalicular lesions may be missed. They should be suspected in injuries medial to the punctum that may be and may be laterally displacement. The diagnosis is confirmed by direct visualization of the cut edge or passing a probe into the canaliculus.

Repair of canalicular injuries is done under general anesthesia. A stent should be placed through the transected canaliculus. Bicanalicular silicone tube is commonly used however, some surgeons use monocanalicular tubes. In case of bicanalicular tube use, the severed canaliculus is intubated first. Both are retrieved from the nose. The marginal wound is then repaired and canthal tendon wound is also repaired before tying the silastic tube **(Figure 1)**. After the wound is approximated, the tube is secured by three square knots and left in place for 6 months **(Figures 2A and B).**

The medial cut end of the canaliculs could be identified under the microscope with high magnification. It can also be identified using injection of a fluorescein dye or viscoelastic material into the sac through the intact canaliculus. Pooling saline in the medial canthal area with injecting air into the intact canaliculus will point at the site of cut canaliculus where the air bubbles. If the wound is ragged freshening of the edges may be helpful. Retrograde intubation using Pigtail probes is better avoided as it can cause a false passage.

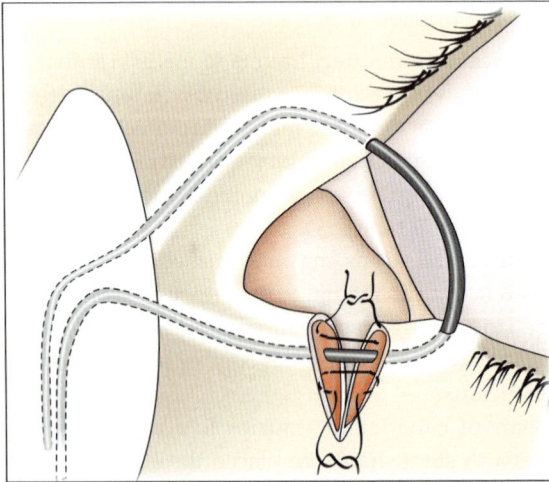

Figure 1: A diagram showing lower canalicular injury with a bicanalicular tube inserted first before the repair of the marginal wound

If the punctum is lacerated, the medial canaliculus could be marsupialized or opened to the conjunctival sac and the lid wound is repaired ignoring the injured punctum and canaliculus.

Lacrimal Sac and Nasolacrimal Duct Injuries

These lesions may be missed as these parts are included in a protective bony structure. A high index of suspicion should be present to anticipate these problems. They are usually associated with nasoethmoidal fractures, sometimes with blow out fractures of the orbit and types II and III Le Fort fractures.

A nasoethmoidal fracture usually results from a force delivered across the nasal bridge and it's very common in automobile accidents in which the face strikes the dashboard.

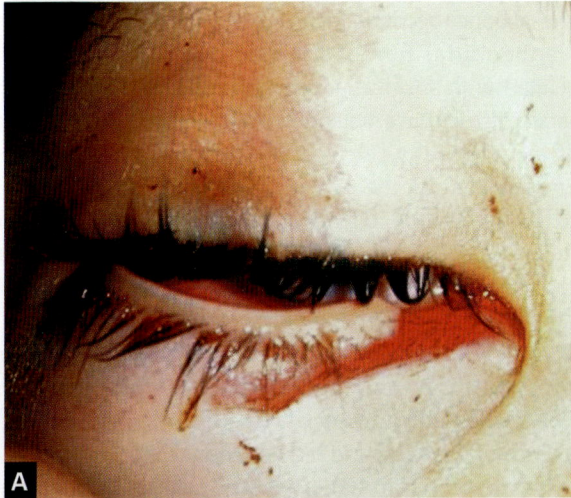

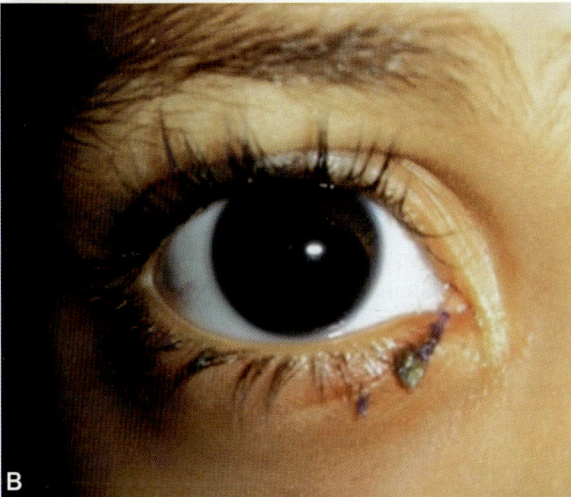

Figure 2: Left shows lower lid marginal wound involving the lower canaliculus. Right photo shows it after inserting the tube and repair of the wound

The nasal bones become fractured and displaced. The lacrimal and sphenoidal bones are usually crushed. They are associated with surgical emphysema. Traumatic telecanthus is usually present in association with lacrimal passage injury.

If the fracture is detected and repaired, irrigation of the lacrimal system by the end of the repair should be done. If there is a free system irrigation, nothing more is needed to be done. If there is some minor resistance exists, probing and bicanalicular silicone intubation where the tube is left for 3-6 months may be of use.

If these fractures are not detected and corrected, chronic dacryocystitis can occur and needs dacryocystorhinostomy (DCR). It is sometimes associated with excess bone formation in the area of the nasal and lacrimal bone that accentuates the possibly present traumatic telecanthus. This bone can be debulked while performing the DCR. The surgery can be associated with repair of the present telecanthus.

Old Traumatic Lacrimal Passage Injuries

Management of such injuries varies according to the site and extent of obstruction and addressed in a similar way as non traumatic cases. For example, destruction of the upper lacrimal system especially with chemical injuries and obliteration of the canaliculi usually necessitates conjunctivodacryocystorhinostomy (CDCR) with insertion of Lister Johns tube. Chronic dacryocystitis or complete NLD obstruction are treated by conventional DCR.

Congenital Ptosis: Evaluation and Management

AK Grover, Shaloo Bageja (India)

10

INTRODUCTION

Congenital ptosis is a common entity managed by the oculoplastic surgeons. It results from a developmental dystrophy of the levator muscle of unknown etiology. Management of the condition requires a thorough understanding of the surgical anatomy and a meticulous surgical technique based on a proper evaluation.

SURGICAL ANATOMY OF THE UPPER EYELID AND EYEBROW

The thorough understanding of the surgical anatomy of eyelid is necessary to give good functional and cosmetic results.

The layer of upper eyelid from anterior to posterior are skin, subcutaneous tissue, orbicularis muscle, submuscular tissue, orbital septum and preaponeurotic pad of fat, levator aponeurosis, muller muscle, tarsal plate and conjunctiva **(Figure 1)**.

Skin of the upper lid is thinnest in the body. The skin is attached loosely over the eyelid, but firmly over the brow, lid margins and canthi.

Orbicularis muscle is responsible for blinking and lid closure. It originates from medial palpebral ligament and the fibers spread in elliptical fashion. It is divided in to orbital and palpebral portion. The palpebral portion runs from medial canthal ligament to lateral palpebral raphe.

Submuscular layer is corrected with the submuscular layer of the brow and thus the infection can spread through this plane. Most of the blood vessels and nerve lie in this area.

Orbital septum and tarsal plate – form a continuous layer of fibrous tissues and is mainly responsible for the stability of the eyelid.

Levator muscle – is the main retractor of the upper eyelid. It originates above the optic foramina under the lesser wing of sphenoid. It moves forward under the orbital roof and above the superior rectus muscle. Near the equator of the globe it is transformed in to fibrous aponeurosis, which travels forwards and inferiorly and gets inserted into the upper 2/3rd of the anterior tarsus. The other attachments of the levator aponeurosis are to skin of the upper lid after penetrating the orbicularis muscle forming the lid crease. Its medial and lateral extensions are known as 'horns'. The lateral horn attaches to the orbital tubercle. by the canthal ligament. It is important to remember that the lateral horn separate the lacrimal gland into palpebral and orbital part. The medial horn forms the medial canthal ligament.

Muller muscle – is a thin sheet of non-striated muscle which arises near the junction of the levator and its aponeurosis from its under surface and attaches to the superior forward border of tarsus. The superior transverse ligament (Whitnall's ligament) arises from the under surface of the levator. It assists in suspension of the levator muscle.

Conjunctiva – is inner most layer of the lid. The palpebral conjunctiva is transparent, highly vascular and is strongly attached to tarsus of upper lid. It is continuous with the bulbar conjunctiva via superior fornix.

Frontalis muscle – originates from epicranial aponeurosis anterior to the coronal suture and inserts into skin and subcutaneous tissue of the eyebrow. It helps in elevation of upper lid by drawing the scalp, raises the eyebrow and form the crease on forehead.

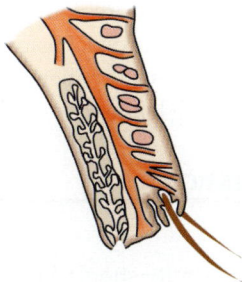

Figure 1: Showing surgical anatomy of the eyelid

CLASSIFICATION OF CONGENITAL PTOSIS

Congenital ptosis may be classified as:
- Congenital simple ptosis
- Complicated
  - With oculomotor abnormalities
  - With Blepharophimosis syndrome Synkinetic ptosis
- Marcus Gunn Jaw Winking
- Misdirected third nerve ptosis

CLINICAL EVALUATION

Pre-operative history and examination are vital because these decide the choice of surgery.

History

It is important to determine whether the condition is congenital or acquired. Relevant history should be elicited in all patients regarding the time of onset, any variation of the ptosis during the day, associations with any jaw movements or abnormal ocular movements and head posture. Photographic records of childhood often reveal important information.

A family history of similar conditions should be determined. Any history of previous surgery or trauma or use of steroid should be recorded. History of any reactions to previous anesthesia both by the patient and his relatives need to be asked. Any bleeding tendencies should also be recorded.

OCULAR EXAMINATION

Visual Acuity

Best corrected visual acuity should be checked to record the presence of amblyopia in the ptotic eye.

Palpebral Aperture

The measurement of the palpebral aperture is necessary as the difference between the two eyes gives the measurement of the ptosis in unilateral cases or the difference from the normal in the bilateral cases. Should be seen in up gaze, down gaze and primary gaze

Normal – 9-10 mm in primary gaze

However, judging the amount of ptosis by difference in the size of palpebral aperture has limitations due to possible alterations in the position of lower eyelid.

Margin Reflex Distance (Figure 2)

Hold the light source directly in front of the patient looking straight ahead. The distance between the center of the lid margin of the upper lid and the light reflex on the cornea would give the MRD 1. If the margin is above the light reflex

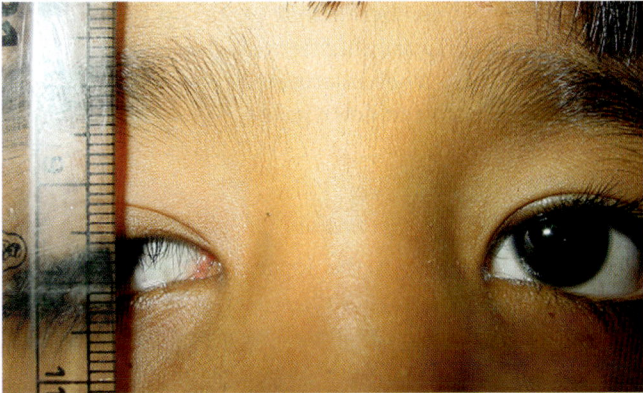

Figure 2: Measurement of margin reflex distance 1 (MRD1)

the MRD 1 is a +ve value. If the lid margin is below the corneal reflex in cases of very severe ptosis the MRD 1 would be a –ve value. The latter would be calculated by keeping the scale at the middle of upper lid margin and elevating the lid till the corneal light reflex is visible. The distance between the reflex and the marked original upper lid margin in –ve sign would be the MRD 1.

Margin reflex distance 1 (MRD 1) : Normal 4 - 5 mm

The mean measurement in Indian eyes is 4.1 ± 0.5.

Amount of ptosis

The difference in MRD 1 of the two sides in unilateral cases

or

the difference from normal in bilateral cases

gives the amount of ptosis.

Amount of ptosis may be classified as:

Mild ptosis	2 mm or less
Moderate ptosis	3 mm
Severe ptosis	4 mm or more

It must be remembered that ptotic lid in unilateral congenital ptosis is usually higher in down gaze due to failure of levator to relax. While in acquired ptosis it is invariably lower than normal lid in down gaze.

Levator Function

Berke's Method (Lid Excursion)

Measures the excursion of the upper lid from extreme down gaze to extreme up gaze with action of frontalis muscle blocked. The patient is positioned against a wall while the surgeon's hands press the forehead above the eyebrows ensuring that there is no downward or upward push. The patient is then asked to look at extreme downgaze and then in extreme upgaze and the readings are recorded in millimeters. The measurements need to be accurate. The levator action of the two eyes is compared. In our study in a North Indian population levator action in normal eyelids was 13.8+0.1mm. Crowell Beard reported normal eyelid excursion to be between 12-17 mm **(Figures 3A and B).**

The levator function is classified as:

8 mm or more	Good
5-7 mm	Fair
4 mm	Poor

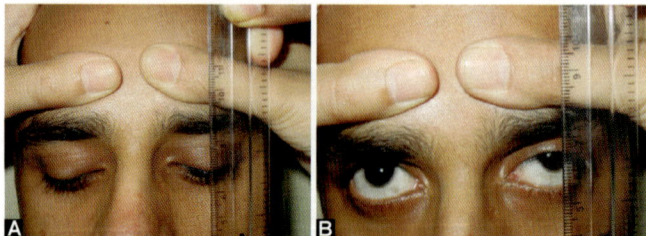

Figures 3A and B: Measurement of levator action by Berke's method

Putterman's Method

This is carried out by the measurement of distance between the middle of upper lid margin to the 6'o clock limbus in extreme up gaze. This is also known as the Margin limbal distance (MLD) **(Figure 4).**

Normal is about 9.0 mm

> The difference in MLD of two sides in unilateral cases
>
> or
>
> the difference with normal in bilateral cases multiplied by three would give the amount of levator resection required.

Assessment in Children

Measurement of levator function in small children is a difficult task as no formal evaluation is allowed by the child. The presence of lid fold and increase or decrease on its size on movement of the eyelid gives us a clue to the levator action. Presence of anomalous head posture like the child throwing his head back suggests a poor levator action.

Iliff Test

This is another indicator of levator action. It is applicable in first year of life. The upper eyelid of the child is everted as

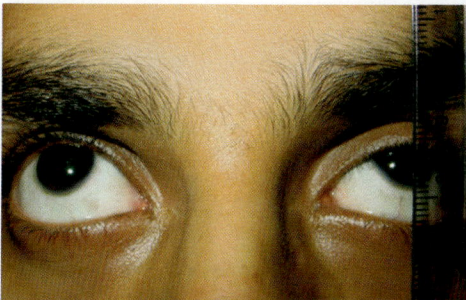

Figure 4: Measurement of margin limbal distance (MLD)

the child looks down. If the levator action is good lid reverts on its own.

Margin Crease Distance (MCD)

Measurement of the margin crease distance (MCD) is the next important step in examination. The height of the crease on the normal side should be measured and compared to the ptotic eyelid in the downgaze. In case of a very faint lid crease it can be made prominent by using a cotton tipped applicator below the lid margin. In patients, when more than one lid creases are present, the most prominent one should be considered **(Figure 5)**

MCD in Normal eyes is 5-7 mm.

The distance of the lid crease from the margin is measured as it helps in planning the surgical incision. Also presence of a distant lid fold in a case of moderate to severe ptosis with good levator action indicates a levator aponeurotic dehiscence.

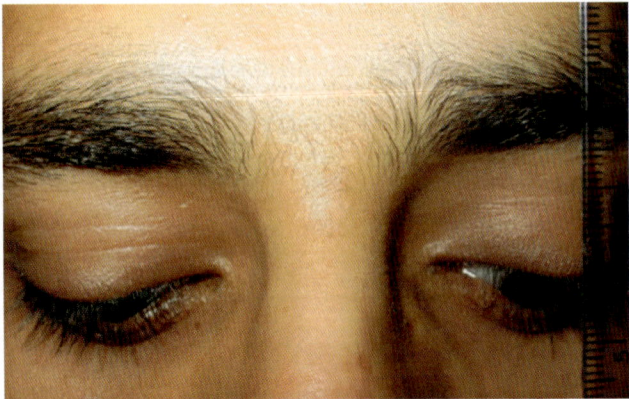

Figure 5: Measurement of margin crease distance (MCD)

Bell's Phenomenon

It is the upward rotation of eyeball on closure of the eye. This is referred to as Bell's positive.

Confirmation of presence of Bell's phenomenon is important before undertaking any surgical procedure to avoid risk of postoperative exposure keratopathy **(Figure 6).**

Corneal Sensation

The presence or absence of corneal functions should be noted using a cotton wisp **(Figure 7).**

Ocular Motility

The extraocular muscle functions especially the elevator muscles should be recorded. Any association of eye movements with change in degree of ptosis should be looked for **(Figure 8).**

Tensilon Test

This test is done in doubtful cases where an acquired ptosis due to Myasthnia gravis is suspected. In adults 1 mg of

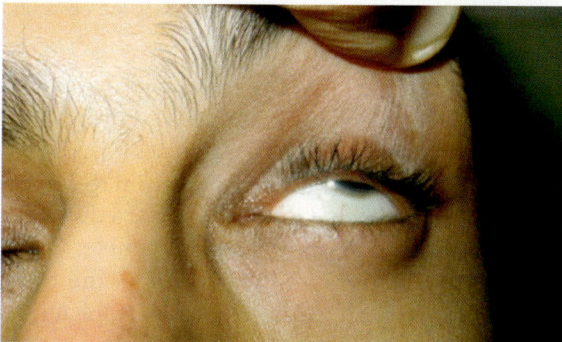

Figure 6: Assessing the Bell's phenomena

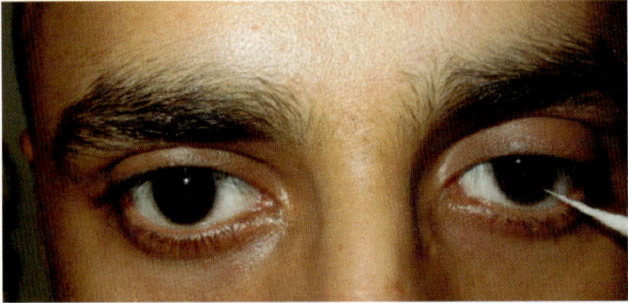

Figure 7: Assessing the corneal sensation

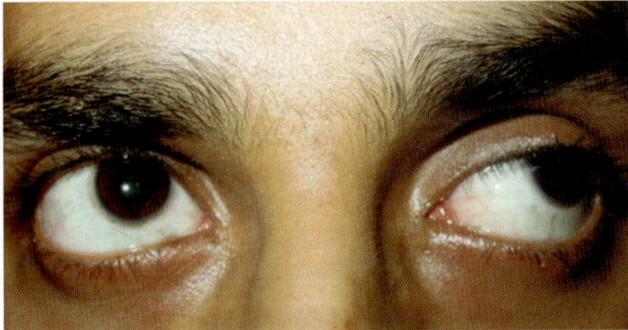

Figure 8: Assessing ocular motility especially the elevators

neostigmine is injected I/M. The ptosis improves in 5 to 15 minutes if Myasthnia gravis is the cause. Edrophonium is more faster and effective than neostigmine. It is loaded in a tuberculine syringe and 2 mg injected slowly in 15-30 seconds. The needle is left in situ and rest 8 mm is injected slowly if no untoward incident is observed within 1 minute. The effect occurs in 1 to 5 minutes if myasthenia is the cause. If cholinergic reaction occurs 0.5 mg of atropine sulphate is given intravenously.

Phenylephrine Test

Phenylephrine 10% drops are used to assess mild cases of ptosis as in Horner's syndrome. Positive phenylephrine test suggests that patient would respond well to Muller's muscle resection.

Associations

The presence of jaw winking oculomotor anomalies and blepharophimosis syndrome should be noted. The presence of any other associated ocular anomaly should also be recorded.

The presence of jaw winking is assessed by moving the jaw from side to side (chewing movements), opening and closing the mouth. Before considering for the surgery the possible causes for pseudoptosis should be excluded viz. hypothalmos, enophthalmos, epicanthus, overhanging skin etc.

It is advisable to wait till 3-4 years of age when the tissues are mature enough to withstand the surgical trauma and as better assessment and postoperative care is possible due to patient's co-operation. There should be no delay in surgical management in cases of severe ptosis where pupil is obstructed and the possibility of the development of amblyopia is high. In these cases a temporary procedure may be opted early on followed by definitive surgery later.

SURGICAL APPROACH

Surgical approach depends on:
1. Ptosis is unilateral or bilateral
2. Severity of ptosis
3. Levator action
4. Presence of abnormal ocular movements, jaw winking phenomena or blepharophimosis syndrome.

The choice of surgical procedure for congenital ptosis depends primarily on:

1. Amount of ptosis as determined on the basis of MRD.
2. Levator action.

Commonly Performed Surgeries (Table 1)

- Fasanella Servat operation
- Levator resection
- Brow suspension ptosis repair

Table 1: Indications for the choice of different surgical procedures

Ptosis	Levator action	Surgery
Mild	> 10 mm	Fasanella Servat or small levator resection
	< 10 mm	Levator resection
Moderate	Good	Levator resection
	Fair	Levator resection
	Poor (rare)	Whitnall's sling or Brow suspension
Severe	Fair	Levator resection or Brow suspension ptosis repair
	Poor	Brow suspension ptosis repair

Surgery for Bilateral Ptosis

In cases of bilateral ptosis, bilateral surgery is preferred to ensure a similar surgical intervention in the two eyes. However in cases where gross asymmetry exists between the two eyes the eye with a greater ptosis may be operated first and the other eye is operated after 6-8 wks when the final correction of the operated eye can be assessed.

SURGICAL TECHNIQUES

Modified Fasanella Servat Surgery

It is the excision of tarsoconjunctiva, muller's and levator. We use a simple modified technique that avoids the use of hemostat or any special clamp.

Xylocaine with adrenaline is used for local anesthesia in adults but general anesthesia is necessary for children.

Surgical Steps (Figures 9A to E)

Eyelid is everted and tarsal plate is exposed. Three sutures are passed close to the folded superior margin of the tarsal plate at the junction of middle, lateral and medial one third of the lid. Three corresponding sutures are placed close to the everted lid margin starting from conjunctival aspect near the superior fornix in positions corresponding to the first 3 sutures. Proposed incision is marked on the tarsal plate such that a uniform piece of tarsus, decreasing gradually towards the periphery is excised. This is necessary to avoid the central peaking. A groove is made on the marked line of incision and the incision is completed with the scissors. The first set of sutures help in lifting the tarsal plate for excision. The second set aids suturing by lifting and supporting conjunctival and tarsal edges during suturing. The tarsal plate not more than 3 mm in width is excised.

5-0 plain catgut is used for continuous suturing and the knot is buried within the wound. Postoperatively the patients are kept on antibiotics and antiinflammatory agents and cornea is observed for any sign of abrasion.

The preoperative and postoperative photographs of a patient taken up for Fasanella servat surgery in the primary, up and down gaze are shown in **Figures 10A to F.**

Complications of Fasanella Servat Surgery

1. Under or overcorrection—If the lid is too low then reoperate. If the lid is too high, in early postoperative traction might help otherwise reoperate.
2. Dry eye—Surgery should be avoided in patients with dry eye symptoms as the procedure removes some of the

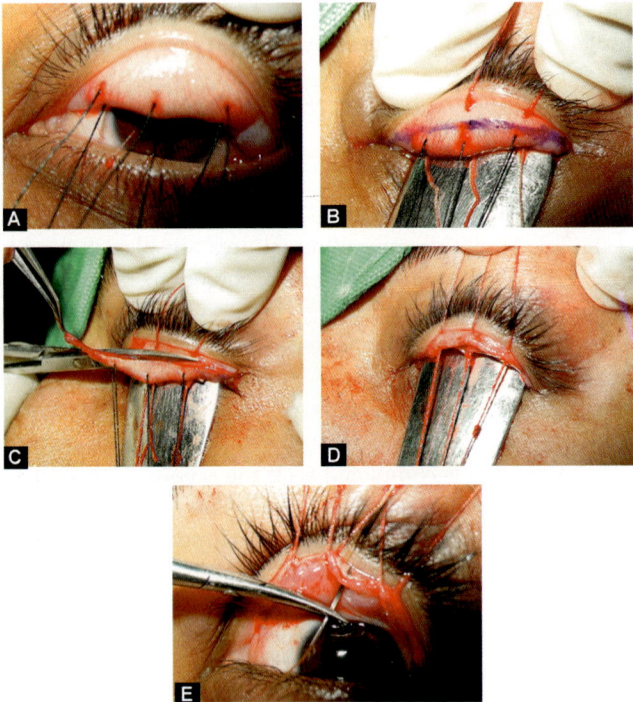

Figures 9A to E: Modified Fasanella Servat surgery. (A) Lid everted and sutures passed through the superior margin of the tarsal plate. (B) Marking along the proposed line of excision. Corresponding sutures passed close to everted lid margin. (C) A scissors is used to cut along the groove created by the knife. (D) Excision is completed. Conjunctival and tarsal edges are raised with the aid of the traction sutures, to assist in suturing. (E) Continuous sutures with 5'0 plain catgut, with knots buried within the wound

accessory lacrimal glands. The patient should be treated with lubricating drops and ointment.

3. Keratopathy—Results due to the suture or scar beneath the lid and abrades the cornea.

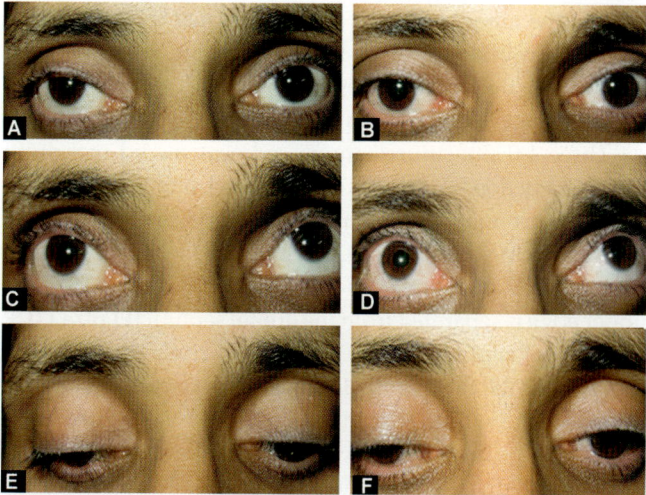

Figures 10A to E: (A and B) Preoperative and postoperative photograph following modified Fasanella Servat surgery. (C and D) Preoperative and postoperative photograph in upgaze. (E and F) Preoperative and postoperative photograph in downgaze

Levator Resection

This is the most commonly practiced surgery for ptosis correction. It may be performed by skin or conjunctival route but the former is preferred by most surgeons because it allows a good titration/assessment on the table and creates a good lid fold.

2% xylocaine with adrenaline is locally infiltrated. The injection is also used in cases being operated in general anesthesia to achieve hemostasis.

Surgical Steps

The proposed lid crease is marked to match the normal eye considering the margin crease distance of the normal eye as well as the amount of skin show measured in the primary position. In bilateral cases highest forming crease is used which is usually at the superior border of the tarsus or standard measurements can be used.

Three 4-0 silk sutures are passed near the lid margin to provide traction. A lid spatula is placed under the lid and incision through the skin and orbicularis made along the crease marking **(Figure 11A)**. The inferior skin and orbicularis are dissected away from the tarsal plate **(Figure 11B)**. The upper edge is separated from the orbital septum **(Figure 11C)**. The orbital septum is cut completely across exposing the preaponeurotic fat **(Figure 11D)**. Fat is retracted posteriorly exposing the whole tendinous aponeurosis **(Figure 11E)**. Three partial thickness traction 4-0 silk suture are passed through the distal end of the aponeurosis. The fibers of the aponeurosis are cut from their insertion in the inferior half of the anterior surface of the tarsus **(Figure 11F)**. The levator is freed from the adjoining structures. The lateral and the medial horn are cut **(Figure 11G)**. The direction of the cut should be vertical to avoid damage to the lacrimal gland laterally or the pulley of superior oblique muscle medially. Care should be taken that Whitnalls ligament is not damaged which is visualized as a whitish fascial condensation running across the junction of the muscular and aponeurotic part of the levator about 15 mm from the insertion. A double armed 5-0 vicryl is passed through the centre of the tarsal plate by a partial thickness bite. It is then passed through levator aponeurosis and intraoperative assessment is made **(Figure 11H)**. Two more double armed vicryl 5-0 sutures are passed through the tarsus about 2 mm from the upper border in the center and at the junction of central third with the medial and lateral thirds **(Figure 11I)**. These sutures are then placed in

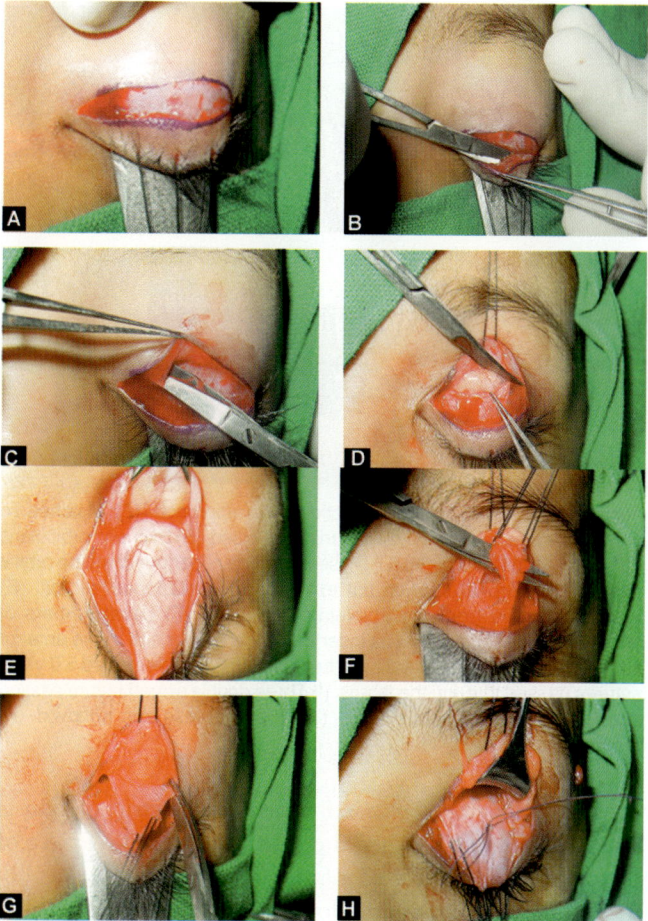

Figures 11A to H

the levator and intraoperative assessment made. The lid level and contours are evaluated. The eyelid is left at the position determined preoperatively based on the levator action.

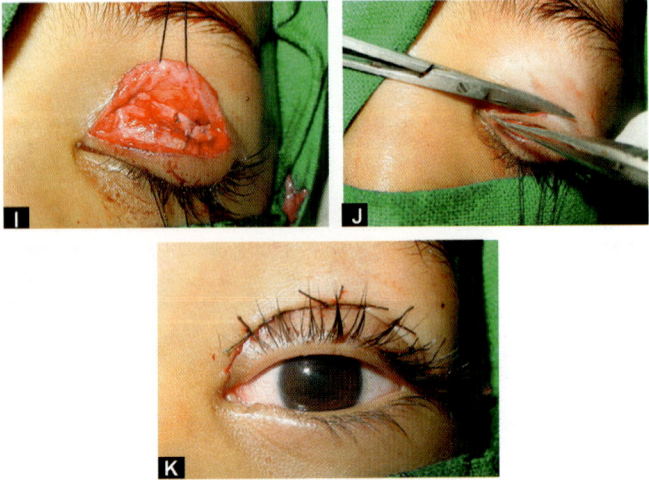

Figures 11A to K: Levator resection: Skin approach. (A) Matched lid crease is marked. Skin and orbicularis are incised. (B) Skin and orbicularis dissected from tarsal plate. (C) Dissection done superiorly from the orbital septum. (D) Orbital septum cut exposing the preaponeurotic fat. (E) Levator is freed from the adjoining structures. (F) Levator fibers of aponeurosis being cut from its insertion in the inferior half of the anterior surface of tarsus. (G) Lateral horn being cut. (H) Double armed 5'0 vicryl sutures passed through the tarsus. (I) Three double armed suture passed through the levator and tightened. (J) Strip of excess skin removed. (K) Skin sutures applied

Excess levator is excised. If required a strip of skin is removed from above the lid crease **(Figure 11J)**. A piece of orbicularis may be excised inferior to the lid crease to debulk the lid. Four to five lid fold forming sutures are placed. The sutures pass through skin edges taking a bite through the cut edge of levator **(Figure 11K)**. An inverse frost 6-0 silk suture is passed through the lower lid margin over a bolster

We use a modification of Berke's criteria based on our postoperative observations.

The position of the lid aimed at during the table assessment should be as follows:

Levator action	Recommended placement of lid
2-4 mm	1 mm above the limbus (when levator resection is chosen to be undertaken.
5-7 mm	1 mm below the limbus
8 mm or more	2 mm below the limbus

- Patients are prescribed oral antibiotics and antiinflammatory agents.

Preoperative and postoperative photographs are demonstrated in **Figures 12A to F.**

Complications of Levator Surgery

1. *Undercorrection:* Multiple factors may be responsible for undercorrection **(Figure 13)**, It may either be due to inadequate resection of levator or due to a thin friable or fibrotic levator muscle associated with poor levator action where even a large levator resection may prove inadequate. In these cases even where a good correction is achieved in early postoperative period, there may be a late development of drooping in a few months time. **The surgeon should wait for a couple of months before considering for re-surgery.**

2. *Overcorrection:* Overcorrection may be due to too large a resection of the levator or due to advancement of the levator too far down on the tarsus **(Figure 14).**

   Massage and traction on the lashes can be tried in the early postoperative phase. But in late phase tarsotomy, levator recession or recession with a spacer such as scleral graft is required depending on the amount of overcorrection.

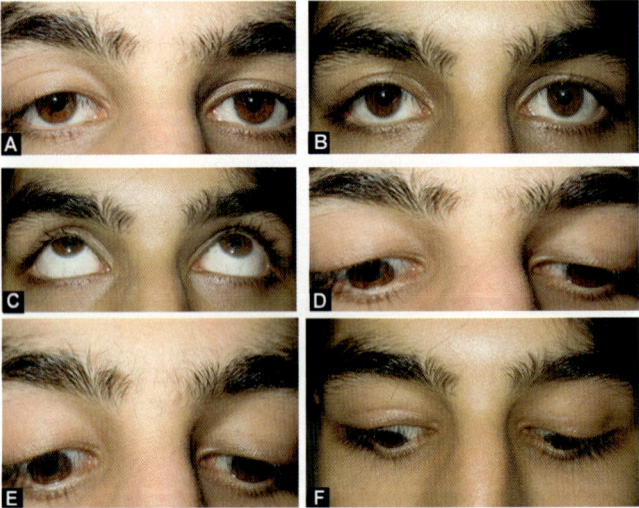

Figures 12A to F: (A) Preoperative simple ptosis. (B) Postoperative following levator resection. Note the symmetrical lid crease and contour. (C and D) Preoperative and postoperative: Upward gaze, (E and F) Preoperative and postoperative: Downward gaze

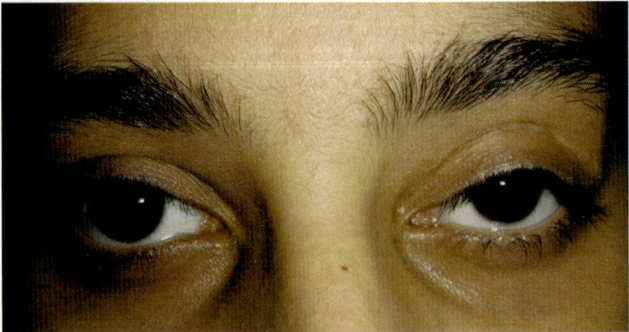

Figure 13: Showing residual ptosis following levator resection

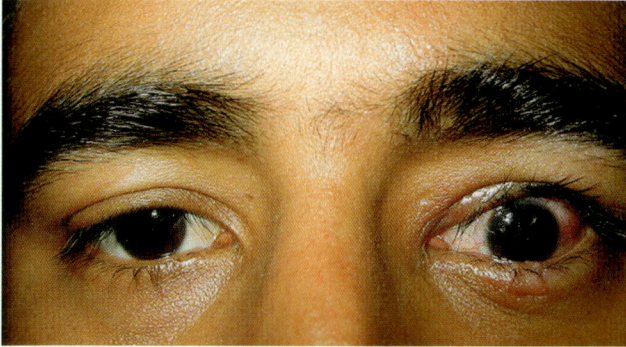

Figure 14: Showing overcorrection following surgery

3. *Lagophthalmos:* Lagophthalmos is usually severer in the early postoperative period and diminishes with the passage of time **(Figure 15).**
4. *Entropion:* Entropion occurs due to surgical shortening of the tarso-conjunctival layer as compared to anterior skin muscle lamina **(Figure 16).**
5. *Ectropion:* Massage can be tried in early phase otherwise surgical correction is carried out by advancement of skin and muscle flap.

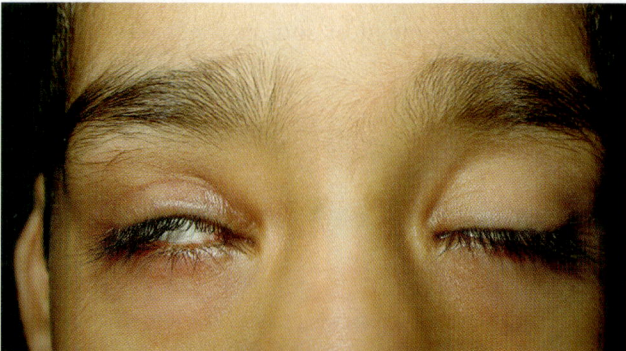

Figure 15: Showing mild lagophthalmos

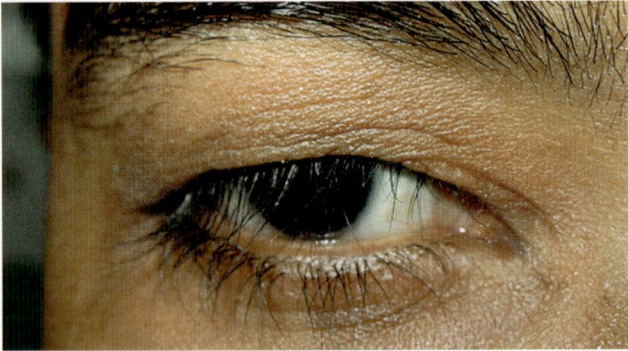

Figure 16: Showing excess skin with entropion

6. *Lid fold:* Lid fold may be placed asymmetrically due to appropriate position of the skin incision. The correction may require recreations of the lid crease **(Figures 17A and B).**

7. *Lid lag:* This is an inevitable association of levator resection as the levator resection raises the lid to a higher position, but does not alter the tone of the muscle **(Figure 18).**

8. *Notching of the lid margin:* Notching of the lid margin may occur due to irregular resection of the tarsus or due to improper placement of sutures for levator resection **(Figure 19)**.

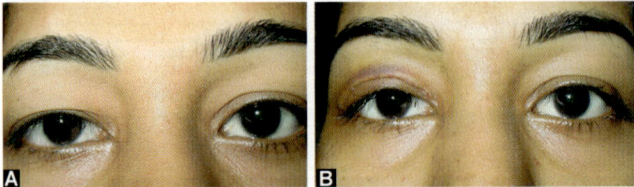

Figures 17A and B: (A) Showing excess skin with poor lid fold. (B) Postoperative skin removal with lid fold creation

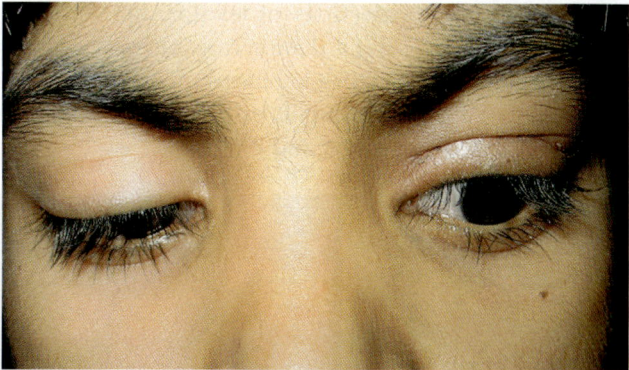

Figure 18: Showing lid lag which is an inevitable association of levator surgery

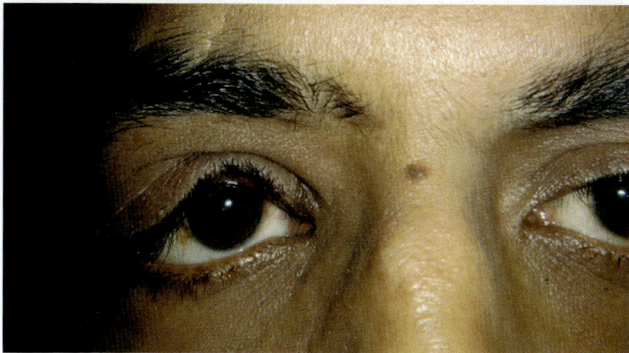

Figure 19: Showing lid notching

9. *Exposure keratitis:* Keratopathy can occur after any type of ptosis surgery as it is accompanied by lagophthalmos. The milder forms usually respond to tear substitute drugs and taping of eyelids **(Figures 20A and B).**

10. *Conjunctival prolapse* **(Figure 21)***:* This is usually due to separation of fibers of levator attaches to the superior

fornix in large resections of levator. Reposition of prolapsed conjunctiva is done in early phase. If this fails, it can be corrected by passing the suture from prolapsed conjunctiva through the lid or by excision of excess conjunctiva **(Figures 22A and B).**

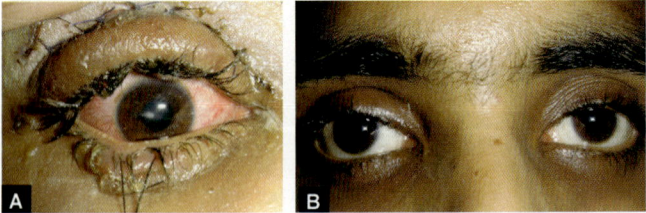

Figures 20A and B: (A) Showing exposure keratitis following levator surgery. (B) Exposure keratitis responded to tear substitutes and lid taping

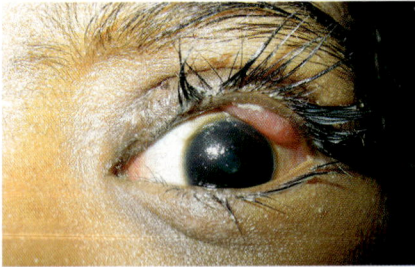

Figure 21: Showing fornix prolapse

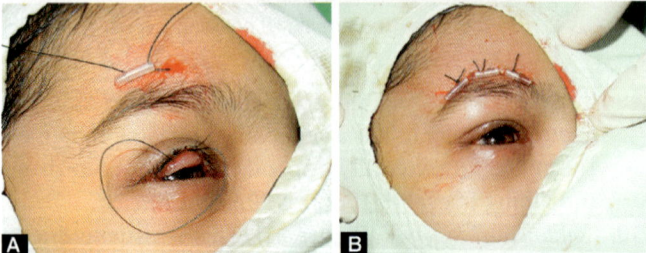

Figures 22A and B: Double armed 4'0 silk suture is passed through prolapsed fornix

Brow Suspension Repair

This surgery is the procedure of choice in simple congenital ptosis with a poor levator action. A number of materials like non absorbable sutures, muscle strips, banked or fresh fascia lata strips, extended Poly Tetra Fluoro Ethylene (ePTFE) have been used for suspension. We prefer Poly tetra fluoro ethylene (ePTFE) sutures for temporary thread sling procedure and fresh autogenous fascia lata for permanent brow suspension.

Temporary Sling

Thread sling is carried out in very young children with severe ptosis where prevention of amblyopia and uncovering the pupil is the main aim. We use CV 0 ePTFE (Goretex) sutures by modified Crawford technique for brow suspension. The suture sling procedures have a relatively higher recurrence rate of 20-30% or may show formation of suture granuloma. Definitive surgery may be performed at a later date when a fascia lata sling is carried out.

Fascia Lata Sling

It is considered in children above four years of age having severe congenital simple ptosis with poor levator action We prefer fresh autogenous fascia for suspension. Even in cases of unilateral severe ptosis a bilateral procedure is preferred because a unilateral surgery causes marked asymmetry in down gaze. Results of bilateral surgery are more acceptable.

All cases are done under general anesthesia. Infiltration with 2% xylocaine and adrenaline is done in the region of the proposed incision in the thigh, eyelid and the eyebrow region.

Harvesting of Fascia Lata

A line joining the lateral condyle of femur to the anterior superior iliac spine is marked. A lower thigh incision about 2 inches above the lateral condyle on the marked line is site of incision. However due to lower thigh scar we often use the upper thigh for past 2 yrs which is about one inch in size. The skin incision is deepened through the fat till the glistening fascia is visible. The fascia is then cleared of the overlying tissue for a length of four inches upwards from the incision. A 12 mm incision is then given at the lower end of the exposed fascia lata. Dissection is carried out beneath the fascia lata separating it from the underlying vastus lateralis muscle along the whole length of the previous dissection. Two linear incisions are given 12 mm apart on the fascia along the length of dissection using a long scissors. The superior end of the fascia is made free by making horizontal cut using a long bladed scissors while the assistants retract the skin and the subcutaneous tissue. The subcutaneous tissue is closed using 4–0 chromic catgut and the skin is closed using 4–0 silk sutures. We now have an autologous fascia lata four inches long and 12 mm wide. It is kept in a bowl containing Ringer lactate and 1 cc of gentamycin **(Figures 23A to D)**.

The fat is trimmed from the fascia lata strip **(Figure 23E)**.

The fascia lata strip is kept on a wooden board, stretched and fixed. It is divided into four pieces each of about 3 mm width by a scalpel blade **(Figure 23F)**.

Fascia Lata Sling Suspension

Three traction sutures are passed along the lid border. Four incisions are made 2-4 mm above the margin.The placement of these determines the position of lid fold. The two central incisions are on either side of the center of the lid while the other two are at the junction of middle and lateral thirds and middle and medial thirds of the lid. A lid crease incision is also given.

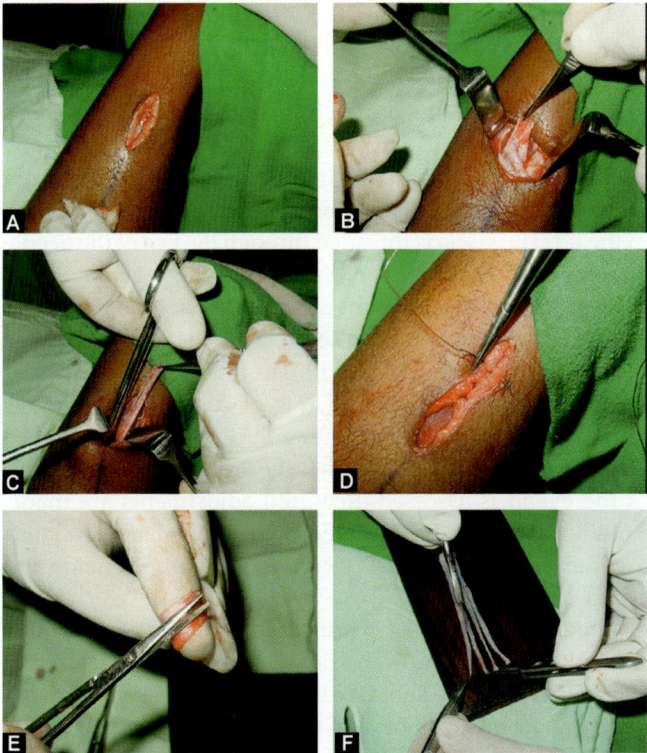

Figures 23A to D: Harvesting fascia lata. (A) Incision marked. 2 inches above the lateral condyle. (B) Fascia lata is exposed. (C) 12 mm fascia lata strip being removed. (D) Subcutaneous tissue closed with 4'0 catgut. (E) Trimming of the strip, fat removed. (F) Strip placed on a wooden board and divided into 4 strips of 3 mm width each

The eyebrow incisions are marked next. They are made at a line perpendicular to the intersection of two lateral eyelid incisions and the two medial incisions while the eyelid is placed in the desired normal position. A third incision is made in the middle of the first two but 4-6 mm higher than the first two incisions.

The eyelid incisions are made down to the tarsus and the brow incisions are made upto the frontalis. Blunt dissection is carried out to make pockets for the fascial knots. The two ends of a strip are then passed from the outer eyelid incisions to the central eyelid incision using a Wright's fascia lata needle. The needle is passed in the submuscular plane from the lateral brow incision to emerge from the lateral incision in the lid. The fascia is threaded through the eye of the needle and is pulled through. The Wright's needle is again passed from the lateral incision to the second eyelid incision threaded with fascia and drawn up. The procedure is repeated on the medial side **(Figures 24A and B)**. The fascial strips are pulled up and a single tie is made so as to place the eyelid margins as high as possible without lifting the eyelid from the globe **(Figures 24C and D)**. After a single tie the position and contour of the eyelid is assessed. Required adjustments are made. Presence of good lid crease is ensured at this stage. The knots are then secured using 5-0 vicryl. A second tie is made and secured **(Figure 24E)**.

One end of fascial strip from each brow incision is pulled through the central brow incision. Knots are tied and secured **(Figure 24F)**. All the knots are buried in the pockets prepared for them. The excess of skin created by shortening of the posterior lamina is judged and excised by removing a spindle of skin from above the eyelid crease. Eyelid incisions require no closure. The brow incisions are closed with 5-0 silk and the eyelid crease incision by 6-0 silk.

Patients are prescribed oral antibiotics and antiinflammatory agents. An appropriate selection and meticulous execution of surgical technique hold the key to obtain excellent functional and cosmetic results in patients with ptosis.

The preoperative and postoperative photographs of patient with severe ptosis corrected by bilateral fascia lata sling are shown in **Figures 25A to H**.

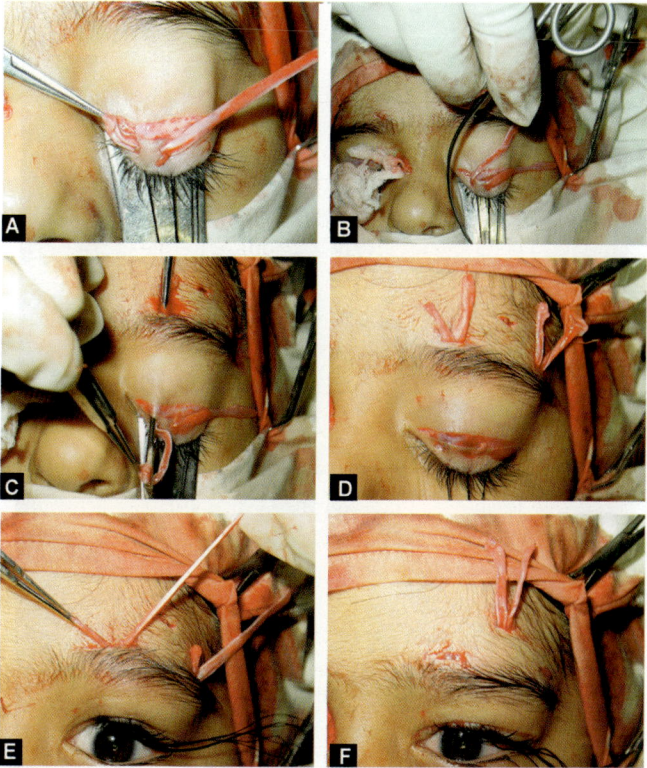

Figures 24A to F: Fascia lata sling surgery by modified Crawford double triangle technique. (A and B) Fascia lata needle is passed through submuscular plane on medial side and strip pulled. (C) Needle passed from brow incision to medial lid incision. (D) Fascial strips pulled from both medial and lateral brow incisions. (E) Knot tightened and secured to get proper lid position. (F) One end of fascial strip passed through central brow incision and tightened

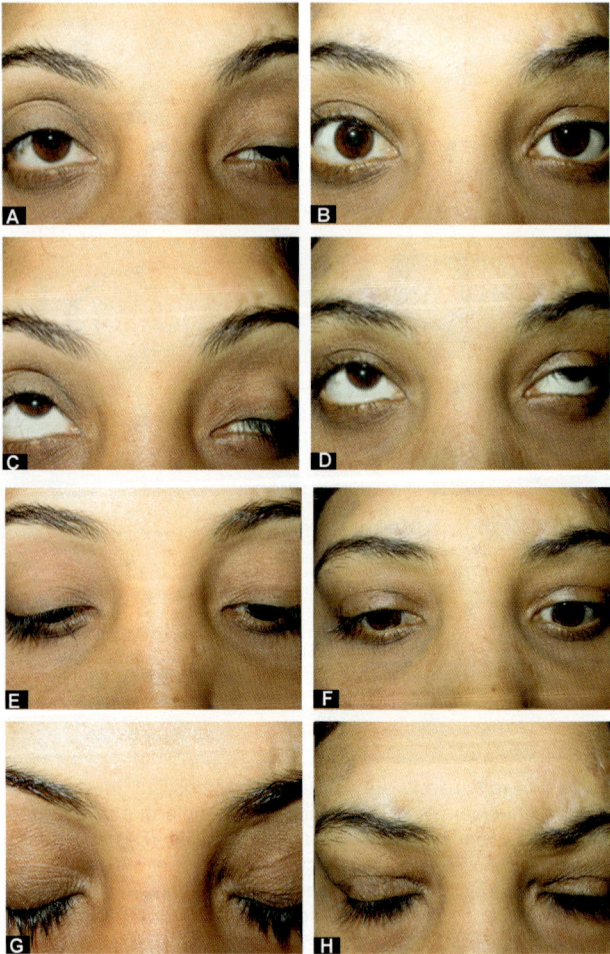

Figures 25A to H: (A and B) Preoperative and postoperative: primary gaze following fascia lata sling surgery. (C and D) Preoperative and postoperative: Upward gaze. (E and F) Preoperative and postoperative: Downward gaze. (G and H) Preoperative and postoperative: On lid showing minimal lagophthalmos

Complications of Frontalis Sling

Though the sling surgery is much simpler than levator surgery, but it is accompanied by some complications.

Unavoidable Complications

1. *Lid Lag:* Lid lag is more prominent in uniocular cases, thus the bilateral sling is preferred to maintain the synchronicity between the two eyelids. The patient can be taught to bend his head down instead of turning the eyes down **(Figure 26).**

2. *Lagophthalmos:* Normally the patient has little difficulty with lid closure as the eyeball rolls upward sufficiently to protect the cornea though the sclera may remain exposed **(Figure 27).**

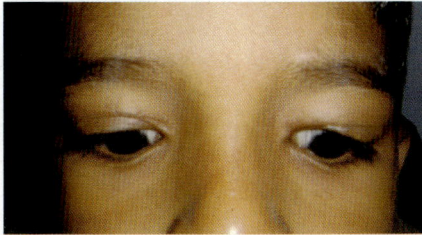

Figure 26: Showing lagophthalmos, inevitable complication of fascia lata sling

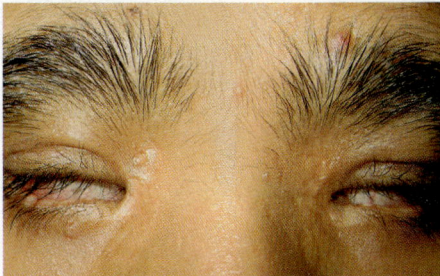

Figure 27: Showing lid lag following sling surgery

The frequent use of lubricants and ointment at night time is prescribed for longer duration.

Avoidable Complications

1. *Undercorrection:* Usually due to failure to raise the lid sufficiently high or due to placement of lid at a lower position due to improper judgement under GA **(Figure 28).**
2. *Overcorrection:* Overcorrection is not a common complication. It results due to excessive tightening of the sling. The management is difficult and requires the loosening of subcuticular tissue sufficiently to allow drooping down of lid.
3. *Notching or tenting:* Usually occurs due to high position of one of the fascial strips. This can be corrected intraoperatively by loosening of the strip so that lid curve is maintained.
4. *Recurrence:* It is possible due to release of suture ends or rupture.
5. *Ectropion:* Ectropion may occur due to too much tightening of the strip.

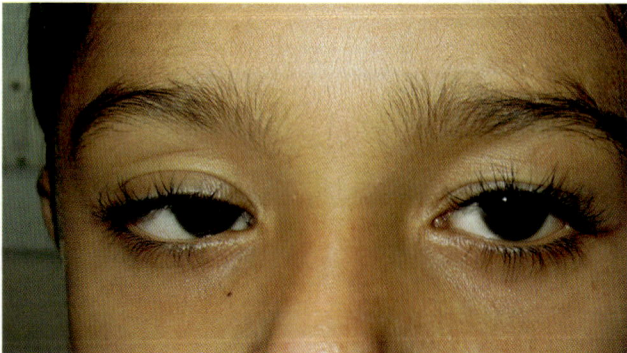

Figure 28: Showing undercorrection

6. *Exposure keratitis:* Requires use of lubricants and patching at night.
7. *Granuloma formation:* This is commoner with synthetic material **(Figure 29)**
8. *Infection:* Infection either early or later may occur. This is commoner with synthetic material. Infection is rare with use of autogenous fascia lata **(Figure 30).**

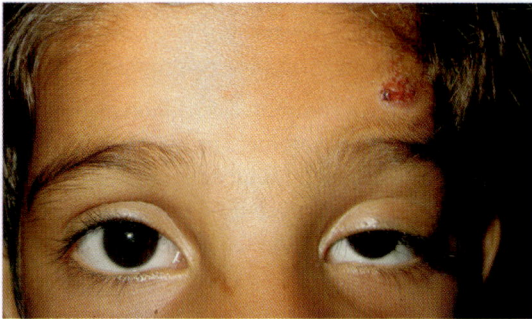

Figure 29: Showing suture granuloma with synthetic material

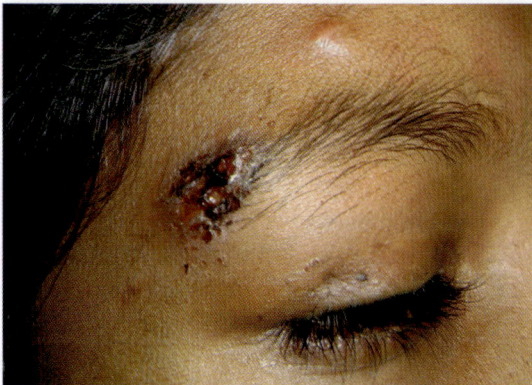

Figure 30: Infection following sling surgery, more common with synthetic material

MANAGEMENT OF COMPLICATED PTOSIS

Ptosis with Oculomotor Abnormalities

It is necessary to correct the ocular motility problem before correction of ptosis because the restriction of the superior rectus and accompanying hypotropia makes the assessment of ptosis difficult. Secondly, the hypotropic eye with poor Bell's penomenon is extremely vulnerable to exposure keratopathy due to postoperative lagophthalmos.

Congenital Ptosis with Superior Rectus Weakness

Superior weakness is a common association as both muscles develop from the same myotome. The hypotropia is corrected by an inferior rectus recession at times combined with superior rectus resection as the first procedure. Ptosis correction is then carried out using the procedure indicated by evaluation.

Ptosis Associated with Double Elevator Palsy

Knapps procedure may be done for ptosis associated with double elevator palsy. The lateral and medial rectus tendons are transposed to the sides of superior rectus insertion. This does not cause significant limitation of adduction or abduction. Ptosis is corrected 3 months later.

Blepharophimosis Syndrome

The blepharophimosis syndrome comprises of ptosis, epicanthus inversus, telecanthus, horizontal shortening of palpebral aperture, flattened supraorbital ridges, arching of the eyebrow and lateral ectropion of the lower eyelid.
• Mustarde's double "Z" plasty or Y-V plasty with transnasal wiring is done as a primary procedure. This gives a good surgical result both in terms of correction of telecanthus as

well as deep placement of the medial canthus. The results are long lasting.

- Brow suspension is carried out 6 months after the first procedure for correction of ptosis.

Double Z Plasty or Y to V Plasty with Transnasal Wiring

Lateral canthotomy and canthoplasty may be carried out before the skin incision is made.

The markings for double Z plasty are made as shown in **Figure 31**. The first mark is made just medial to the medial canthus (A). The proposed canthal site (B) is marked such that intermedial canthal distance is half that of interpupillary distance. The two marks are joined. All the other lines drawn are 2 mm smaller than the line AB. Two lines are drawn from A parallel to upper and lower lid margins. From the centre point of AB(C), a line is drawn medially at 60° both above and below (CD). Another line is drawn outwards at an angle of 45° from the point of D (DE).

The markings for Y-V plasty are shown in **Figure 32A.** The incision are made through the skin down the to the orbicularis. The flaps are undermind **(Figure 32B).** The site of proposed canthus is cleared of all tissue upto the periosteum and the medial palpebral ligament is exposed. The periosteum is incised medial to the insertion of MPL and is reflected along with the lacrimal sac.

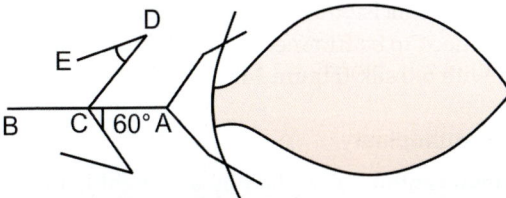

Figure 31: Z-plasty

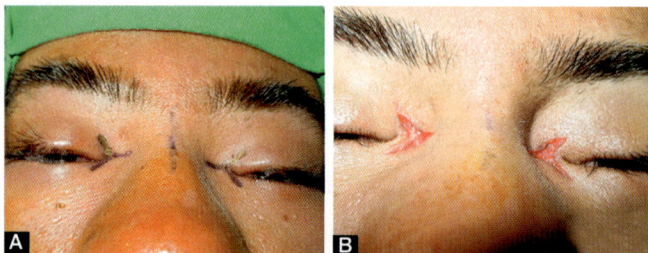

Figures 32A and B: (A) Markings of Y-V plasty. (B) Incision given and flap undermined

A large bony opening 12-15 mm high and 10-12 mm wide is made as for dacryocystorhinostomy but located more posterior and superior. The edges of the bony opening are smoothened. A similar procedure is performed on the opposite side.

Medial palpebral ligament (MPL) of one side is wired with 24 G stainless steel wire close to its attachment to the tarsus and the two ends of the wire are passed to the opposite side through the bony opening with the aid of an aneurysm needle or a Wright's fascia lata needle. The wire is threaded into the opposite MPL by a similar double bite. The two ends are tightened and a single twist given to the wires **(Figure 33)**. The position of the medial canthus is assessed from the front, above and the sides. Once the desired position is obtained the wire is twisted several times and cut. The ends of the wire are pushed into the bony opening. After achieving the hemostasis the incision is closed in several layers. The skin flaps may need to be trimmed before they are tranposed and sutured with 6-0 silk **(Figure 34)**.

Lateral Canthoplasty

Thee lateral canthus is crushed by a straight hemostat for a few seconds. A lateral canthotomy is performed. The bulbar

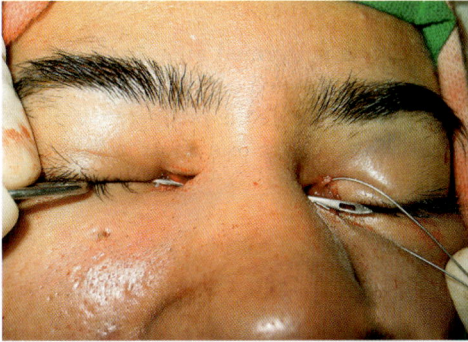

Figure 33: Transnasal wiring

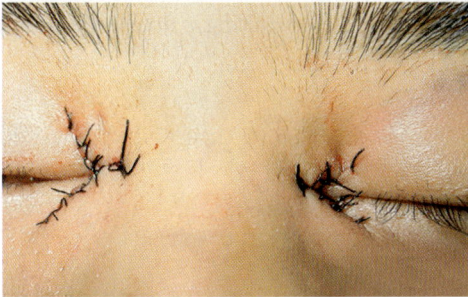

Figure 34: Skin sutured

conjunctiva at the lateral canthus is undermined. The apex of the conjunctiva is sutured to the proposed new position of the canthus which is short of the end of the skin incision. The skin edges distal to the new lateral canthus are apposed with 6-0 silk sutures. The similar procedure is repeated on other side.

The bandage is removed after 24 hrs and sutures are removed between 5-7 days.

Stage II

The second stage is performed after 6 months. A bilateral fascia lata sling is performed.

Figures 35A to C shows the preoperative photograph of a patient with Blepharophimosis syndrome after stage 1 and 2 procedure.

Marcus Gunn Ptosis

Ptosis associated with lid retraction on opening the jaw or its movement to the opposite side is classical marcus gunn phenomenon. An inverse Marcus Gunn phenomenon is also known.

Management depends on the cosmetic significance of the jaw winking. Where jaw winking is not significant the choice

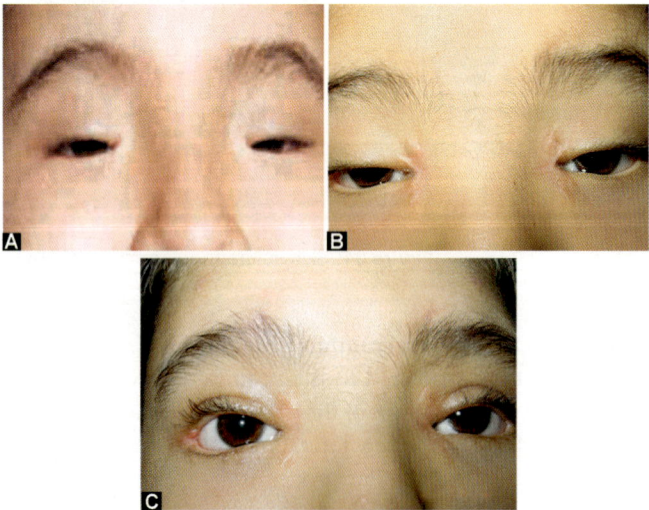

Figures 35A to C: (A) A patient with blepharophimosis syndrome. (B) Postoperative photograph following Y-V plasty and transnasal wiring. (C) Postoperative photograph following fascia lata sling surgery

of procedure depends on the amount of ptosis and the levator action, as in any case of congenital simple ptosis. A larger levator resection is necessary and undercorrection is common. In case with significant jaw winking bilateral levator excision with a fascia lata sling surgery is the procedure of choice **(Figures 36A to D).**

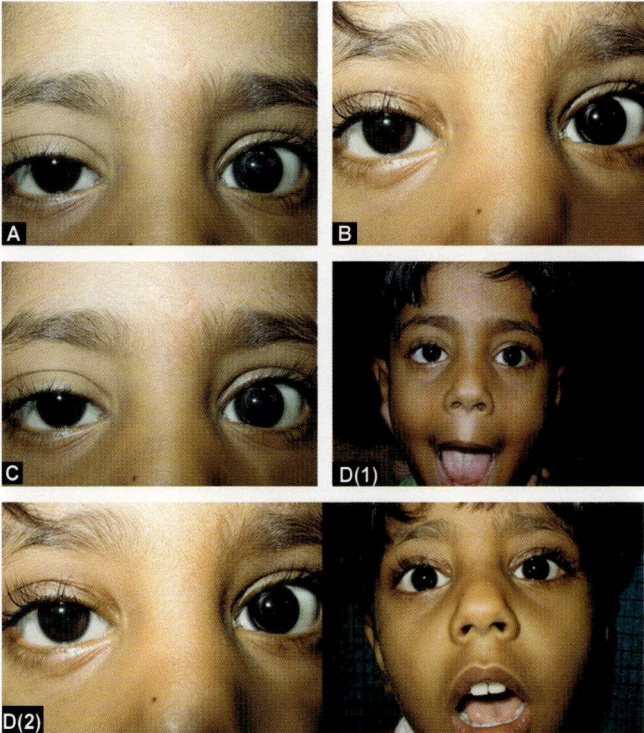

Figures 36A to D: (A) A patient with moderate ptosis with Marcus Gunn phenomenon. (B) Postoperative photograph following bilateral levator excision with fascia lata sling surgery. (C) Marcus Gunn phenomenon elicited on opening of mouth. (D) Postoperative photograph. Marcus Gunn phenomena is eliminated

Misdirected Third Nerve Ptosis

- In cases of misdirected third nerve ptosis where treatment is indicated levator excision with bilateral fascia lata sling is the procedure of choice.
- Ptosis associated with third nerve palsy is difficult to manage because of poor Bell's phenomenon. A crutch glass may be prescribed or a conservative sling surgery may be performed.

BIBLIOGRAPHY

1. Beard C. Ptosis, 3rd edition. St. Louis : CV Mosby Company 1981.
2. Berke RN. Types of operation for congenital and acquired ptosis – In Trauotman R, Converse J, Smith B (Editors): In Plastic and reconstructive surgery of the eye and adenexa. Washington DC Butterworths 1962.
3. Betharia SM, Grover AK, Kalra BR. Br J Ophthalmol. 1983;67:58-60.
4. Crawford JS. "Congenital Blepharoptosis" in Bryon C Smith - Ophthalmic Plastic and reconstructive surgery. Vol. 1, CV Mosby Company, 1987:631-53.
5. Crawford JS. Congenital Blepharoptosis in Byron C. Smith Ophthalmic plastic and reconstructive surgery, Vol. 1, CV Mosby Company 1987:631-53.
6. Grover AK, Gupta AK. Proceedings of the Golden Jubilee Conference of All India Ophthalmological Society, New Delhi 1992:54-56.
7. Grover AK, K Uma Chaturvedi, Sanjal Mittal. Presented at 53 AIOS Annual Conference at Bombay 1995.
8. Grover AK, Mittal Sanjay. A Clinico-pathological study of levator muscle for Congenital Ptosis. Thesis is submitted to Delhi University.
9. Gunn RM. Trans Ophthal Soc UK 1983;3:283.
10. Mustarde JC. Epicanthus and telecanthus. Int Ophthalmol Cli 4:1964.
11. Putterman. Basis oculoplastic surgery in Peyman GA: Principles and practice of ophthalmology, Vol. 3. Philadiphia: WB Saunders Company 1980:2246-33.
12. Smith B, McCord CD, Baylis H. Am J Ophthalmol 1969;68:92.

Frontalis Muscle Flap Advancement for Correction of Blepharoptosis with Poor Levator Function

11

Essam El Toukhy, Ibrahim Mosad, Lobna Khazbak (Egypt)

INTRODUCTION

Ptosis or dropping of the upper eyelid, is the most common lid malposition encountered in clinical practice in both adults and children population and is the most surgically correctable lid disorder.

The upper lid position is a function of the delicate balance between the lid retractors including levator muscle, Muller's muscle, and frontalis muscle, and the lid protractors including the orbital pat and palpebral part of the orbicularis oculi muscle. Normally the upper lid covers the upper 1-2 mm of the cornea in the primary position, providing no obstacle to image formation on the retina. It follows the globe on looking down with no lag. It provides complete coverage of the eye on lid closure. Finally, it rises up for up to 20 mm in extreme up-gaze.

Changing the activity of the levator, Muller's muscles, bring all of these movements about. The frontalis muscles are called into action only in extreme up-gaze. The orbicularis muscle in mainly used in forceful lid closure although its palpebral part shares in the blinking mechanisms.

Both upper eyelids are symmetrical. The brain considers both lid retractor as yoke muscle. They receive equal innervations form single subdivision of the oculomotor nucleus in the midbrain. Changes in the position of one lid will lead to affection of the position of the other in a similar fashion to the secondary changes occurring in extraocular muscle when its yoke muscle is weak, paralyzed or overacting.

A successful ptosis surgery provide a lid that is at or just below the limbus in the primary position and moves freely with the globe in up and down gaze. This result can be obtained only in mild to moderate degrees of ptosis when levator muscle can be attempted successfully.

However, when the levator function is poor (less than 4 mm), Frontalis muscle surgery has long been accepted as the best technique for managing the blepharoptosis. In these cases if levator muscle surgery is attempted, then In order to position the lid at an acceptable level, at least 25 mm or more of the levator muscle should be resected. This would entail cutting of both levator horns as well as the advancement of Whitnall's ligament and its suturing to the anterior surface of the tarsus.

The results are usually less than acceptable with a lid that is so shortened to be practically immobile or frozen. Lagophthalmos is invitable and corneal exposure is considered the major postoperative complication and occurs in over 75% of patients. In unilateral cases, marked asymmetry between both lids is noted. Most surgeons conclude that good results are seldom achieved with this procedure in poor levator function cases and recommend frontalis muscle surgery instead.

THE MECHANISM OF LID ELEVATION AFTER BROW SUSPENSION

The upper eyelid is suspended from the brow so the patient opens the eye by the brow and closes the eye by orbicularis contraction. The transmission of frontalis muscle activity to upper lid is achieved by the insertion of a biologically acceptable non-stretchable rod- shaped connection between the two. The mechanism of lid elevation after brow suspension is totally different from the mechanism when the levator muscle is lifting the lid. Normally, the elevating force vector of the levator muscle on the upper lid is superio -posterior. This is due to the pulley effect of Whitnall's ligament, which diverts the antero- posterior contractile fore of the levator muscle to a more superio-posterior direction.

In frontalis muscle suspension where the sling material is passed at a more superficial level from he brow to the anterior eyelid layers, the brow transmits a superior, and frequently, an antero- superior elevating force to the upper eyelid. This superior vector tends to pull the upper lid away from the globe and presents an even greater problem in patients with prominent brows or deep set eyes. The line of pull also tends to obliterate, rather than form, a lid crease.

This antro-superior elevating force could be directed posteriorly by placing the suspensory material behind the septum. Several problems arise from posterior placing of the sling. Depending on its nature, it might adhere to the septum and leave the upper lid at a frozen level. There is increase in the incidence of lagophthalmos and exposure keratopathy. If infection occurs it may result in an orbital space infection.

The ideal material used in frontalis sling should be chemically inert, noncarcinogenic capable of resisting mechanical stress, sterilizable, yet not physically modified by tissue fluids, dose not excite an inflammatory of foreign body reaction, not induces a state of allergy or hypersensitivity.

Several sling materials have been used; as fascia lata (autogenous or preserved); synthetic materials as silicone rods, sutures and meshes.

The frontalis muscle flap advancement is a technique of direct transfer of the force of the frontalis muscle to the eyelid without the insertion of fascia, suture or a graft between the muscle and the tarsus. Frontalis suspension by frontalis muscle flap is a well-accepted method of treating severe bleharoptosis. Being from the same patient, there is no risk of rejection or severe body reaction as may occur with homogenous or alloplastic materials. There is no risk disease transmission. A Frontalis flap grows with the child's growth and does not lead to cheese-wiring as synthetic materials. The frontalis muscle is well-developed before fascia lata maturation. Therefore, this procedure can be performed earlier, if indicated, in cases of infantile ptosis. Additional advantages of this technique include its technical simplicity, lack of remote scar as the donor site is in the primary surgical field, minimal ptosis on upgaze, less lid lag on downgaze, preservation of eyelid contour and less tendency for the lid to pull away from the eye. In contrast to traditional frontalis slings, only one 2 cm brow incision is required.

The mechanism of frontalis suspension surgery is to transfer the upward traction produced by the frontalis muscle to the eyelid. Most techniques described the transfer of this traction by the way of the insertion of a suture material or graft between the frontalis muscle and the tarsus. It seems that the relocation of the frontalis muscle insertion to the eyelid would be the ideal way to elevate the eyelid by direct frontalis muscle action. This direct linkage of the frontalis muscle to the eyelid has been documented by postoperative magnetic resonance imaging scan.

The frontalis muscle flap lifts the eyelid thorough natural contraction of the muscle, directly transferring the upward traction of the frontalis to the eyelid. The frontalis muscle itself is the ideal suspensory material for ptosis repair, especially in patient with poor levator function or previously failed levator resection surgery, yet its use largely has been overlooked.

ANATOMY OF THE OCCIPITOFRONTALIS

Occipitofrontalis covers the dome of the skull from the highest nuchal lines to the eyebrows. It is a broad musculofibrous layer consisting of four thin, quadrilateral parts—two occipital and two frontal connected by the epicranial aponeurosis. Each occipital part (occiptalis) arises by tendinous fibers from the lateral two-third of the highest nuchal line of the occipital bone and the mastoid part of the temporal bone, and ends in the aponeurosis. Each frontal part (frontalis) is adherent to the superficial fascia, particularly of the eyebrows.It is broader than the occipital part and has fibers that are longer and paler.

Although frontalis has no bony attachments of its own, the medial fibers are continuos with those of procerus muscle, the intermediate fibers blend with corrugator supercilii and orbicularis oculi muscles. And the lateral fibers also blend with orbicularis over the zygomatic process of the frontal bone. The frontalis muscle is closely adherent to the skin and subcutaneous tissues at the eyebrow region but is mobile on the underlying periosteum due to loose areolar connections between the frontalis and the periosteum of the supraorbital rim. From theses attachment the fibers ascend to join aponeurosis in front of the coronal suture. The medial margins of the frontal bellies are joined together for some distance above the root of the nose, but between the occipital bellies there is a considerable, though variable, gap occupied by an extension of the epicranial aponeurosis. Contraction of the frontalis muscle elevates the eyebrows strongly and the eyelids weakly.

The blood supply of the frontalis muscle is via the supraorbital, the supratrochlear and the superficial temporal arteries. Sensory branches of the supraorbital nerve course upwards over the frontalis muscle. The frontal or temporal branch of the facial nerve passes approximately 1.5 cm at the lateral brow to enter the undersurface of the frontalis muscle no higher than 2 cm above the eyebrow.

EVALUATION OF THE PATIENT

This procedure can be conducted on patients with ptosis and eyelid excursion measured as poor or less than 4 mm. The etiology of ptosis can be congenital or acquired.

Patients should subjected to full ophthalmological examination.

Slit lamp examination, fundus examination and refraction must be done. Best corrected visual acuity and presence or absence of amblyopia must be noted. Extraocular muscle functions must be evaluated for any associated abnormalities. Patients should be tested for jaw winking, Bell's phenomenon and abnormal head posture. Orbicularis muscle function must be assessed by noting eyelid closure. Measurement of the eyelid crease to determine the site of lid incision must be done.

The forehead must be examined to detect any abnormality as well. This surgery has an effect similar to a brow lift in that it affects forehead wrinkles and therefore is best indicated for patients with bilateral ptosis or unilateral ptosis with a smooth forehead preoperatively.

The amount of ptosis is measured using the margin reflex distance 1 (MRD 1), which is the distance from the light reflex to the center of the upper lid margin in primary position. Measurement of the vertical interpalpebral fissure height is also recorded. Measurement of levator muscle function by measuring the excursion of the upper eyelid from down gaze to upgaze with the frontalis muscle fixed is done. Cases with 5 mm or more of function should undergo levator muscle surgery. The procedure can be done on primary cases as well as cases with recurrent ptosis following previous levator muscle surgery or frontalis sling procedures.

SURGICAL TECHNIQUE

The frontalis muscle is exposed through a horizontal brow incision that begins 5 mm lateral to the supraorbital notch and extends laterally 2 cm on the upper border of the eyebrow parallel to the hair line. It is necessary to limit the lateral extent of the incision so the frontal branch of the facial nerve is not injured. A subcutaneous plane is then dissected downwards bluntly to free the frontalis from the brow till the orbicularis is seen, providing adequate length to be used in the flap formation. The anterior surface of the frontalis muscle is exposed by blunt dissection superiorly so that a superiorly based frontalis muscle flap can be designed. The frontalis muscle is incised along its attachment to the brow. Care is take to avoid injury to supra orbital nerve and vessels as they emerge from the notch.

Blunt dissection releases the under surface of the frontalis from the periosteum of the frontal bone, creating a flap 1 to 2 cm in length. Two vertical incision are made through the frontalis muscle parallel to the muscle fibers at the extremes of the eye brow incision to form a tongue of the frontalis muscle 7 to 12 mm in width to be advanced onto the tarsus. The dissection is performed so that the vertical height of the frontalis flap is 1 to 2 cm depending of the degree of ptosis and the power of the frontalis muscle.

An eyelid crease incision is made deep to the plane beneath the orbicularis oculi muscle to expose the tarsus downward. The dissection is continued superiorly to form a tunnel underneath the orbicularis muscle and then turns superficially to the subcutaneous plane by cutting the muscle layer transversely at the level of the inferior eyebrow margin. The inferior portion of the frontalis flap is then brought down through the tunnel above the septum and below the orbicularis and advanced onto the anterior surface of the tarsus.

The isolated flap is then fixated to the upper third of the tarsus with two – interrupted mattress sutures of 6-0 polypropylene.

In cases of bilateral ptosis the eyelid margin position is set at or 1 mm above the limbus on both sides, because the lid will lower approximately 2 to 3 mm when orbicularis function returns and gravity forces the eyebrow down in the upright position.

In unilateral cases, the lid should be set 2 to 3 mm above the level of the non-ptotic lid. Because of a tendency to undercorrection, we recommend suturing the side of the flap to the original frontalis muscle helping to maintain the level of the lid higher as needed. This modification reduces the incidence of late undercorrection that is reported with this technique, suspected to be due to gradual stretching of the flap.

The lid crease incision and eyebrow incision are sutured by 6-0 polypropylene in older children and adults, or 6-0 chromic cat gut in younger children. Polypropylene skin sutures are removed after 5 days, and ophthalmic antibiotic ointment is applied at bedtime for 2 weeks or until lagophthalmos resolve.

Our technique for frontalis muscle advancement differs from previously described technique, which likely explains our successful use of this procedure. Part of the frontalis muscle insertion is transferred directly to the eyelid in our surgical technique. We make the frontalis flap rectangular and base it superiorly, in contrast to the earlier reports of a superolaterally placed L – shaped flap. This distributes the pull of the frontalis muscle on the tarsal plate.

Our results suggest that a flap width of 7 mm in younger children and 12 mm in older ones provides adequate elevation if properly centered over the tarsus. Also, the tenting deformity described earlier, was not seen, likely because we make the flap in a rectangular fashion and undermine the flap as high as necessary to prevent overcorrection by a tight flap.

It should be emphasized that the length of the flap is adjusted according to the degree of ptosis and the power of the muscle. The more pronounced the ptosis, the shorter the flap must be to elevate the lid adequately. In this aspect the flap acts like a harness, the shorter it is, the closer the insertion (tarsus) is to the origin (brow), i.e. the higher and taughter is the lid. Accordingly, based on this experience, we believe that adjustment of the lid height can be done using recession or resection of the flap in cases of under or over correction post-operatively. The advanced flap can be shortened directly in cases of residual ptosis. Also, it is not necessary to advance a thick, bulky flap, a thin flap will cause less eyelid fullness and still elevates the lid well.

Lastly, we now perform the entire procedure through a lid crease incision, there by minimizing brow scarring.

COMPLICATIONS

Residual ptosis of +2.00 mm or less occurs in about 10% of cases. These can be redone with our modified technique and corrected as explained earlier.

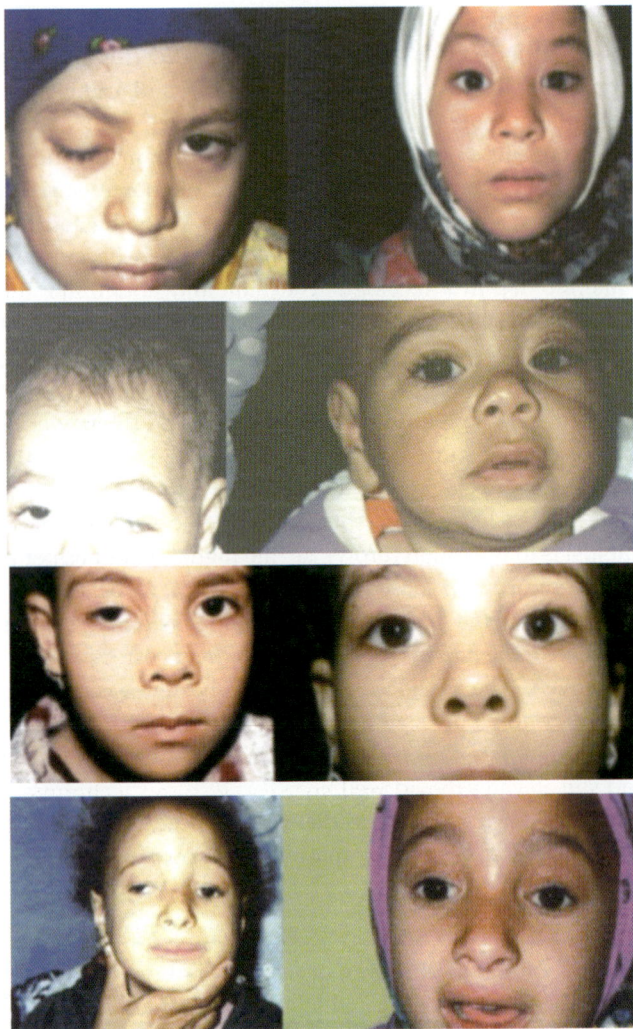

Figures 1A to D: Preoperative and postoperative photos of some patients showing improvement in lid height and the absence of scars at the incision sites. Notice the symmetry between both lids and the good closure

Entropion can occur due to lower insertion of the flap in the middle third of the tarsus. It should be immediately repaired by reinsertion of the flap in the upper part of the tarsus.

Late suture infection can be managed by removal of the suture, drainage of the pus and administration of systemic antibiotic. The flap is usually not affected nor its attachment to the tarsus. Suture infection and/or granuloma formation is a well-recognized complication of frontalis sling procedures. However, its treatment may necessitate removal of the sling and recurrence of ptosis.

Lagophthalmos is usually temporary in the first few weeks till edema resolves. It disappeares with the full recovery of orbicularis function and the patient can close his eyes by orbicularis contraction. Lubricants are prescribed until the lagophthalmos resolves.

Lid lag on down gaze and corneal exposure during sleep are potential complications of the procedure. In our cases, lid lag on down gaze occurred in almost all cases. It is an inherent side effect of all frontalis muscle surgery and should be well-explained to the patients or their parents. However, it is usually accepted as the price for correction of the ptotic lid in primary position and in upgaze.

Asymmetry between the lids of more than 1 mm can occur in patients with unilateral surgery. For any technique of frontalis surgery to be successful, the patient should be stimulated to use the frontalis muscle to lift the ptotic lid.

Therefore, severe unilateral ptosis corrected only with a unilateral frontalis surgery causes "a functional undercorrection" of the ptosis. The reason for this undercorrection is that the normal lid level on the contralateral side allows the patient to see well, and therefore, the patient is not stimulated to use the frontalis muscle. This is similar to the patient with jaw–winking phenomenon who learned to see well with either the contralateral eye in unilateral jaw–winking or with jaw movments in bilateral cases. This signifies the importance of documenting the trial to lift the lid preoperatively by the patient with frontalis contraction. The full correction of ptosis in the primary position can be noticed when the patient contractes the frontalis voluntarily especially in unilateral cases. A trial of occlusion of the sound eye can document the functional undercorrection and differentiate it from true anatomical undercorrection. Occlusion therapy (as in amblyopia cases) and excercises to develop and maintain binocular vision can help reducing this phenomenon.

Cases of over-correction rarely occurs. The postoperative lid height attained at 6 weeks visit is usually stable and maintained thereafter.

In conclusion, frontalis muscle flap advancement is a valuable technique in the management of severe ptosis with poor levator function in children and adults. Our modified technique helps to prevent postoperative under correction by preventing overstretch of the flap.

Upper Lid Blepharoplasty 12

Lucas Henrique Barbosa dos Santos,
Belquiz A Nassaralla (Brazil)

INTRODUCTION

Blepharoplasty is the surgical removal of the excessive eyelid tissues (skin, orbicularis muscle, and orbital fat), which can be for functional or aesthetic purposes. It is a useful procedure, not only isolated but also in conjunction with other procedures, such as ptosis repair, eyebrow suspension, among others.

Nowadays, there are an increasing number of patients seeking this type of surgery. The youngest patients typically go to the oculoplastic surgeon to improve their appearance, to raise their selfesteem or to be more competitive in the job market. On the other hand, the oldest individuals seek the surgeon with hope to improve their complaint of ocular fatigue and/or obstruction of the temporal visual field. Both conditions caused by the excessive skin on the upper lid. These are certainly functional reasons for the blepharoplasty.

Before removing any amount of skin or fat from the lids, it is of utmost importance to do a careful preoperative evaluation.

PREOPERATIVE EVALUATION

Careful medical history must be taken, including questions concerning the motives that drive the patient to undergo a blepharoplasty surgery. Some patients relate emotional reasons for the surgery, hoping that even a slight shift on their appearance could reverse some ongoing problem on their lives, such as marital troubles or better job opportunities. It is of good sense to lower the expectations, or in more complicated cases, to postpone the surgery or even rule out such patients.

Patients should be asked about pre-existing conditions such as systemic hypertension, diabetes, blood discrasias, current drugs in use (salicilates, anti-inflammatory, or anti-coagulating drugs), or smoking. Laboratory work should include complete hemogram, coagulogram and blood fast-glycemia. Also, if the patient is over 60 years old, a cardiac assessment should be performed by a cardiologist.

Ophthalmologic evaluation includes: visual acuity, extrinsical ocular motility and biomicroscopy, in order to rule out amblyopia, low vision, and strabismus. Biomiscroscopy must be thoroughly assessed. It can show Bell's phenomenon, cornea disorders such as puntacte keratitis, and lacrimal film disorders such as dry eye. Such conditions can get worse if too much skin is removed.

Ectoscopy is performed to assess the eyebrow position, the amount of redundant lid skin, the existence of fat bags (pockets) or the presence of lid ptosis. This will show if the blepharoplasty should be performed solo or along with other procedure such as brow correction or removal of fat bags. Careful measurements of the marginal reflex distance and the elevator muscle function determine if the patient also needs a ptosis repair. One can take advantage on this step, and give the patient a mirror to discuss along with him/her about the surgery.

Both physician and patient should get to an agreement about the right amount of skin that is to be taken. During this talk, the doctor can take some time to explain how the anesthesia is done (local only or with sedation), how long the surgery should take and how long should the patient recover in the clinic before going home. Also, the post-surgical care to be done at home should be discussed (local ice bag, anti-inflammatory drugs, local ointment, resting).

Photography is of extreme importance before any plastic surgery to document the patient's baseline. Full frontal face and close pictures should be taken, in order to compare the postoperative outcome.

The patient must be given the chance to ask any questions he/she may have regarding the procedure. Some doctors may think of it as "wasted time", but this is very important to strengthen the patient/doctor relationship, thus increasing the satisfaction with the results.

SURGICAL PROCEDURE

Anesthesia can be done either before or after the marking of the redundant lid skin. Some doctors understand that the volume of anesthetic can make the marking more difficult, losing the reference of the correct amount of skin to be taken.

Eyelid surgery is usually performed under local anesthesia, which numbs the area around the eyes, along with oral or intravenous sedatives. It requires approximately 5.00 cc of local infiltrative anesthesia per lid, using 2% Xylocaine with 1:100,000 epinephrine. We prefer to use intravenous sedation, because it makes the patient relaxed during the procedure. We should wait at least ten minutes for the epinephrine to make a good vasoconstriction, thus reducing the need for electrocautery during surgery. Mild compression of the lids can be done to help spreading the solution.

The inferior extent of the upper lid resection is demarcated over the natural skin crease with a marking pen, at least 8 to 10 mm superior to the lid margin **(Figure 1A)**. Next, we draw a line that goes just from above the lacrimal punctum, passing through the previously marked line, extending to the lateral cantus, following the natural existing crow's feet or laugh lines, if there is extra tissue in this area. If not, this marking may extend laterally 10 to 20 degrees to the horizontal line. We then pinch the redundant lid skin with an Addison forceps, always conservatively, and mark on the top of it **(Figure 1B)**. We repeat the process laterally and medially, and then we draw a line joining the 3 existing marks to complete the inferior and superior extents of the marking lines **(Figure 1C)**.

After placing a corneal protector, we proceed to the skin resection. The incision can be made with a 15 blade, radiofrequency, or CO_2 LASER, usually starting medially in the lower line, extending laterally. We follow the same procedure in the upper line. A slight portion of preseptal orbicullaris muscle should also be resected. This will help to form the lid crease **(Figure 1D)**. Meticulous hemostasis is obtained using an electrocoagulator, or the laser beam in a defocused mode. If excess orbital fat exists, we should open the orbital septum with delicate scissors. The orbital fat will protrude with a gentle pressure of the ocular globe. After prolapsing, the fat should be clamped with a hemostat and the distal part to the instrument should be resected either with scissors or a blade **(Figure 1E)**. Electrocautery is then applied over the entire extent of the cut surface within the hemostat, and after being sure that there is no bleeding, the hemostat can be released. The fat removed can be placed over gauze, for better comparison of the volume taken on each side. There is no need to suture the septum. A continuous or separated

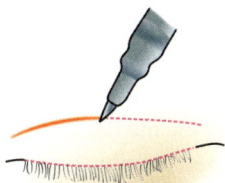

A: Marking the incision sites, following the natural lines and creases of the upper eyelid

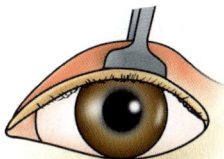

B: Pinching the redundant skin

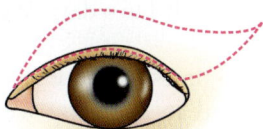

C: Inferior and superior extents of the marking lines

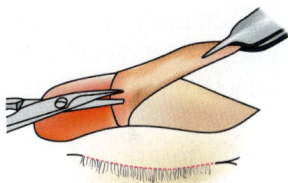

D: Removing excess skin

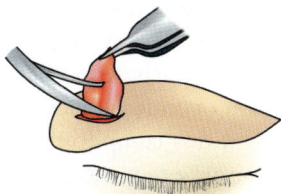

E: Removing protruding fat pockets

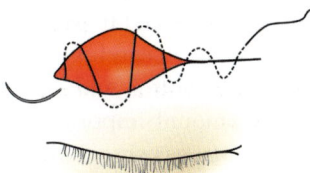

F: Suturing incision

Figures 1A to F: Upper lid blepharoplasty technique

skin suture with 6.0 nylon or 6.0 prolene is used to approximate the margins of the wound **(Figure 1F).** It is advisable to deepen the suture in three or four points taking skin, muscle and septum to create a lid crease. Sometimes it can be necessary to take extra skin in the medial third of the superior margin, especially in older people. For that, a Burrow's triangle can be resected.

POSTOPERATIVE CARE

Ice packs are used over the closed eyes to minimize edema and postoperative hemorrhages, extending its use for 48 hours. The sutures can be removed from 4 to 6 days. We use to remove them as soon as possible.

An antibiotic ointment is used 3 times a day for 15 days, in order to prevent infection and to keep the wound moistened, avoiding crusts around it. Oral anti-inflammatory drugs are prescribed for 7 days, and moderate rest is advised.

COMPLICATIONS

The most serious complication of blepharoplasty is visual loss which may be caused by an orbital hemorrhage. The surgeon should be skilled to perform a lateral canthotomy or should this occur. A careful attention to hemostasis, good blood pressure control, and discontinuation of anticoagulants are of paramount importance to prevent this complication. If hemorrhage is observed, the wound can be reopened and an incision on the septum performed, in order to alleviate the intraorbital pressure.

Damage to the extraocular muscles can cause strabismus. Excessive fat removal can cause an aesthetically displeasing, hollow appearance to the orbit. If too much skin is taken, that can lead to insufficient lid closure and lagophthalmos, followed by keratopathy. Other infrequent complications described are hypertrophic scaring, cheloid, ptosis, optic atrophy and even blindness.

Careful preoperative examination, as well as a thorough understanding of the eyelid anatomy and surgical techniques are essential to prevent unwished complications and to achieve natural and pleasant results.

BIBLIOGRAPHY

1. Bosniak S. Cosmetic Blepharoplasty, Upper Lid Blepharoplasty, 1992;37-53.
2. Matayoshi S, Forno E, Moura E. Manual de Cirurgia Plástica Ocular 2004:149-65.
3. Reeh M, Beyer C, Shannon G. Practical Ophthalmic Plastic and Reconstructive Surgery 1976:133-40.

Pterygium Excision

13

Belquiz A. Nassaralla, João J. Nassaralla (Brazil)

INTRODUCTION

Pterygium is a fibrovascular growth of the conjunctiva over the ocular surface extending over the nasal sclera onto the cornea and may eventually obstruct vision, necessitating surgical removal **(Figure 1).**

Surgical excision of a pterygium is usually indicated if the visual axis is threatened, in case of considerable irritation, if there is restricted ocular motility and for cosmesis.

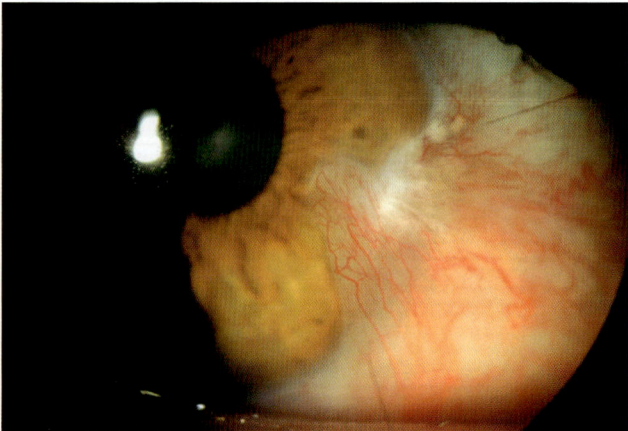

Figure 1: Primary pterygium

CAUSES

Risk factors for pterygium include the following:

- Increased exposure to ultraviolet light, including living in subtropical and tropical climates.
- Engaging in occupations that require outdoor activities.
- A genetic predisposition to the development of pterygia appears to exist in certain families.
- A predilection exists for males to develop this condition in significantly higher numbers than females, although this finding may represent an increased exposure to ultraviolet light in this portion of the population.

DIFFERENTIAL DIAGNOSIS

- *Pseudopterygium:* is a fibrovascular scar arising in the bulbar conjunctiva that extends onto the cornea. Pseudopterygia are the result of previous ocular surface inflammation from such varied causes as chemical or thermal burns, trauma, surgery, cicatrizing conjunctivitis, or marginal corneal disease.
- *Pingueculae:* is a small elevated, yellowish mass confined to the limbus and bulbar conjunctiva in the intrapalpebral fissure and may occasionally become inflamed. Surgical excision is rarely indicated, but if done, the lesion tends not to recur.
- *Tumors:* the most common acquired limbal masses in order of their frequency are papilloma, squamous cell conjunctival carcinoma, conjunctival melanoma, and pagetoid or sebaceous carcinoma. Because of their appearance, most of these lesions are easily distinguished form a pterygium.

PATHOGENESIS

The occurrence of pterygia is strongly correlated with UV exposure, although dryness, inflammation, and exposure to wind and dust or other irritants may also be factors. UV-B is mutagenic for the p53 tumor suppressor gene in limbal basal stem cells. Without apoptosis, transforming growth factor-beta is overproduced and leads to collagenase up-regulation, cellular migration, and angiogenesis. The ensuing pathologic changes consist of elastoid degeneration of collagen and the appearance of subepithelial fibrovascular tissue. The cornea shows destruction of Bowman's layer by fibrovascular ingrowth, frequently with mild inflammatory changes. The epithelium may be normal, thick, or thin, and it occasionally shows dysplasia.

A pterygium is nearly always preceded and accompanied by pingueculae. It is not known why some patients develop pterygia, whereas others have only pingueculae, but the prevalence of pterygia increases steadily with proximity to the equator.

SIGNS AND SYMPTOMS

- Redness
- Irritation
- Dryness
- Inflammation
- Tearing
- Foreign body sensation
- Occlusion of the visual axis
- Irregular astigmatism
- Painless area of elevated white tissue with blood vessels on the inner and/or outer edge of the cornea.

PTERYGIUM SURGERY

Microsurgical excision of a pterygium aims to achieve a normal, topographically smooth ocular surface

Multiple different procedures have been advocated in the treatment of pterygia **(Figure 2A).** These procedures range from simple excision to sliding flaps of conjunctiva with and without adjunctive external beta radiation therapy and/or use of topical chemotherapeutic agents, such as mitomycin C.

Surgery for excision of pterygia is usually performed in an outpatient setting under local or topical anesthesia with sedation, if necessary.

Bare Sclera

One of the most popular methods for the removal of primary pterygium is excision of all remnants of the pterygium, leaving the underlying bare sclera exposed. Sharp dissection from the corneal side and from the uninvolved perimeter of normal conjunctiva is necessary. The cornea is left as smooth as possible, and all of Tenon's capsule from beneath the pterygium is excised.

After excision, light thermal cautery is usually applied to the sclera for hemostasis. No sutures or fine, absorbable sutures are used to appose the conjunctiva to the superficial sclera in front of the rectus tendon insertion, leaving an area of exposed sclera. This procedure has a relatively high recurrence rate, with variable techniques, of 5 to 68% with primary pterygium and 35-82% with recurrent pterygium **(Figure 2B).**

Simple Closure

The free edges of the conjunctiva are secured together. This technique is effective only when the conjunctival defect is very small. It may also be used for pingueculae removal. There are few complications with this method. The most frequent complication is dellen (thinning of the cornea) that occurs from dehydration. Reported recurrence rates range from 45 to 69% **(Figure 2C)**.

Sliding Flap

An L-shaped incision is made adjacent to the wound to allow a conjunctival flap to slide into place. Reported recurrence rates range from 0.75 to 5.6%. The most frequent complications are flap retraction and cyst formation **(Figure 2D)**.

Rotational Flap

Rotation of a flap of superior conjunctiva is thought to prevent recurrence and provide a smooth surface at the limbus to encourage proper tear film distribution. A U-shaped incision is made adjacent to the wound to form a tongue of conjunctiva that is rotated into place. Reported recurrence rates range from 4 to 6% **(Figure 2E)**.

Conjunctival Graft

The most common indication for conjunctival graft is the management of advanced primary and recurrent pterygium **(Figure 3)**. This technique reduces the risk of pterygium recurrence to approximately 2 to 5% and ameliorates the restriction of extraocular muscle function frequently encountered after pterygium excision. Because the superior bulbar conjunctiva is usually normal and undamaged, conjunctival autograft tissue can be obtained from this area in the same eye. The free graft is excised to correspond to the size of the wound and is then moved and sutured into place **(Figure 2F)**.

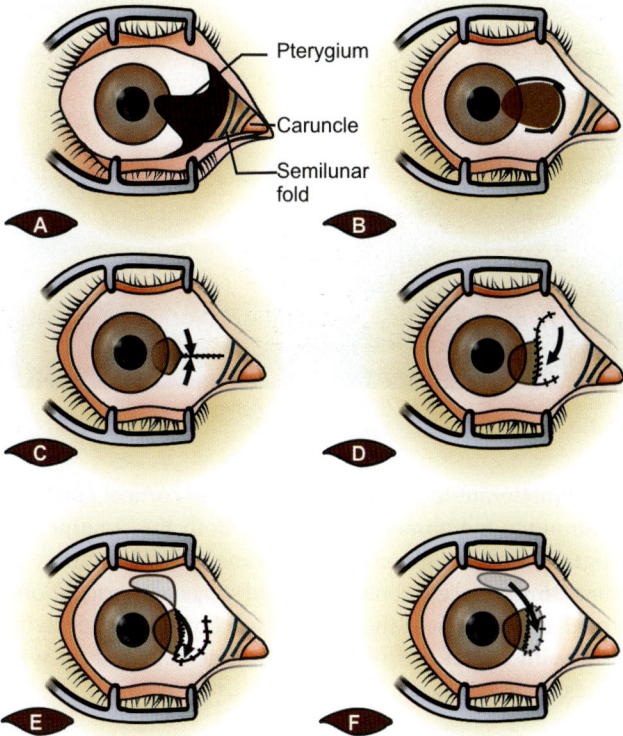

Figures 2A to F: Surgical wound closures following pterygium excision. (A) Pterygium; (B) Bare sclera; (C) Simple closure with fine, absorbable sutures; (D) Sliding flap that is closed with interrupted and/or running suture; (E) Rotational flap from the superior bulbar conjunctiva; (F) Conjunctival autograft that is secured with interrupted and/or running suture

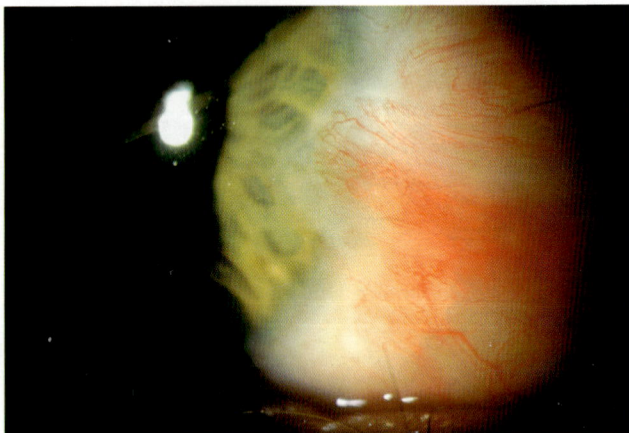

Figure 3: Recurrent pterygium

For moderate-to-severe pterygia, some corneal surgeons use amniotic membrane transplants. Both the conjunctival autografts and the amniotic membrane transplants may be sutured onto adjacent conjunctiva and subjacent cornea. Some corneal surgeons seal the graft tissue onto the underlying sclera with the aid of fibrin tissue glue rather than with sutures.

ADJUNCTIVE THERAPY

A number of adjunctive therapies have been described to decrease the risk of recurrence after the surgical removal of a pterygium. Each has its attractive features, but none is without drawbacks.

Corticosteroids

New vessels often herald the recurrence of a pterygium. Postoperative use of topical corticosteroids inhibits the inflammatory reaction and may reduce revascularization of the operative site. However, long-term corticosteroid treatment may cause relevant side effects: ocular hypertension, glaucoma, and cataract. Moreover, controlled clinical trials have not demonstrated any significant role of topical corticosteroids in pterygium recurrence prevention.

Thiotepa

Thiotepa (triethylene-thiophosphoramide) is a nitrogen mustard alkylating agent with antimitotic properties. It is a radiomimetic agent that presumably obliterates proliferating vascular endothelial cells. The most common dose is 1:2000 thiotepa given up to every 3 hours for approximately 6 weeks. It is usually used with the bare sclera method. The most frequent complication is scleral thinning (Recurrence rate: 10-16%).

Interferon Alpha-2b

Interferons are glycoproteins that have been shown to have antiproliferative and antiviral effects. Although the exact mechanism of action of interferons is unknown, the recombinant form of interferon alpha-2b (IFN-α-2b) has been used with good results in conjunctival intraepithelial neoplasia, conjunctival papilloma and as a lone therapy for early pterygium recurrence.

However, further studies are needed to delineate the ideal dosing and tapering schedule for topical Interferon alpha-2b administration in the treatment of early recurrent pterygium.

Mitomycin C

Mitomycin C (MMC), isolated from Streptomyces caespitosus, is an antibiotic with antineoplastic properties that blocks DNA synthesis. Although the recurrence rate was reduced by use of MMC, reports of side effects associated with its use (e.g. pyogenic granuloma, dellen of the sclera, perforation of the eye, glaucoma, cataract, corneal edema) have remained obstacles to its usefulness. MMC is used with bare sclera or single conjunctival closure, especially for recurrent cases. Most common concentration is 0.02%. Reported recurrence rates range from: 3-25% for intra-operative application (depending on the time of exposure) and 5-54% for postoperative application.

5-fluorouracil

The antiproliferative effect of 5-FU arises from its metabolites acting as metabolic blockers that inhibit thymidylate synthetase, which converts ribonucleotides to deoxyribonucleotides, thus inhibiting DNA synthesis. It acts selectively on the growth phases corresponding to DNA and RNA synthesis, respectively, in the cell cycle. Therefore, only those cells in the synthesis phase are affected, thus allowing the remaining cells to continue to proliferate after exposure to 5-FU. The topical use of 5-FU can cause epitheliopathy, ocular surface inflammation, pain and dry eye symptoms. Few studies, with limited number of patients, poor follow-up, and variable recurrence rates limit its application.

Beta Radiation

Inhibition of proliferating cells in the wound bed can also be accomplished by beta radiation, which presumably reduces mitosis in rapidly dividing vascular endothelial cell. However, the use of Beta radiation has been associated with late scleral melting in 13% of cases, cataract formation and conjunctival telangiectasia. Most common dosage is 15 Gy in single or divided doses. Reported recurrence rates range from: 4.3% to 35%, with bare sclera or single conjunctival closure. The most serious complications are scleral necrosis and endophthalmitis.

Amniotic Membrane

The use of amniotic membrane is useful for very large, conjunctival defects as in primary double-headed pterygium or to preserve superior conjunctiva for future glaucoma surgeries. It is associated with a recurrence rate of 3.0 to 40.9%, as well as the increased cost, stress and trauma of an additional surgical procedure.

SURGERY COMPLICATIONS

- Limitation of duction of the globe by subconjunctival scarring with resultant diplopia after primary resection of the pterygium.
- Inadvertent disinsertion of the medial rectus muscle or scleral perforation during pterygium excision.
- Corneal irregularity in the visual axis secondary to deep stromal excision of the pterygium.

CLINICAL PEARLS

- Pterygia are common ocular lesions, usually cured by primary excision.
- The surgeon should remain aware that relatively simple pterygium cases, if allowed to progress, can impair vision. This means that the pterygium need not cover the visual axis to inflict significant visual compromise. Surgery must be performed before vision is affected.
- Follow up on medium- to large-sized pterygia at least once or twice yearly, and include a manifest refraction, corneal

topography, slit-lamp evaluation with measurement of the pterygium, and photodocumentation if possible.

- When a pterygium recurs, more sophisticated surgery is necessary. Excellent microsurgical technique for the initial and secondary treatment of pterygium should keep these deleterious consequences to a minimum.
- Use of beta radiation and antimetabolites can be used with appropriate caution.

BIBLIOGRAPHY

1. Anduze AL. Pterygium surgery with mitomycin-C: ten-year results. Ophthalmic Surg Lasers 2001;32(4):341-5.
2. Bahar I, Weinberger D, Gaton DD, Avisar R. Fibrin glue versus vicryl sutures for primary conjunctival closure in pterygium surgery: long-term results. Curr Eye Res 2007;32(5):399-405.
3. Cogan DG, Kuwabara T, Howard J. The nonelastic nature of pingueculas. Arch Ophthalmol 1959;61:388.
4. Cohen RA, McDonald MB. Fixation of conjunctival autografts with an organic tissue adhesive. Arch Ophthalmol 1993;111(9):1167-68.
5. Coroneo MT, Di Girolamo N, Wakefield D. The pathogenesis of pterygia. Curr Opin Ophthalmol 1999;10(4):282-8.
6. Dougherty PJ, Hardten DR, Lindstrom RL. Corneoscleral melt after pterygium surgery using a single intraoperative application of mitomycin-C. Cornea 1996;15:537-40.
7. Elliot R. The aetiology of pterygium. Trans Ophthalmol Soc NZ 1961;13:22.
8. Esquenazi S. Treatment of early pterygium recurrence with topical administration of interferon alpha-2b. Can J Ophthalmol 2005;40:185-7.
9. Fernandes M, Sangwan VS, Bansal AK, Gangopadhyay N, Sridhar MS, Garg P, et al. Outcome of pterygium surgery: analysis over 14 years. Eye 2005;19(11):1182-90.
10. Jain AK, Bansal R, Sukhija J. Human amniotic membrane transplantation with fibrin glue in management of primary pterygia: a new tuck-in technique. Cornea 2008;27(1):94-9.
11. Kamel S. The Pterygium: its etiology and treatment. Am J Ophthalmol 1954;38:682.

12. Kheirkhah A, Casas V, Sheha H, Raju VK, Tseng SC. Role of conjunctival inflammation in surgical outcome after amniotic membrane transplantation with or without fibrin glue for pterygium Cornea 2008;27(1):56-63.

13. Lee JS, Oum BS, Lee SH. Mitomycin c influence on inhibition of cellular proliferation and subsequent synthesis of type I collagen and laminin in primary and recurrent pterygia. Ophthalmic Res 2001;33(3):140-6.

14. McDonald JE, Wilson FM. Ocular therapy with beta particles. Trans Am Acad Ophthalmol Otolaryngol 1959;63:468.

15. Miyai T, Hara R, Nejima R, Miyata K, Yonemura T, Amano S. Limbal allograft, amniotic membrane transplantation, and intraoperative mitomycin C for recurrent pterygium. Ophthalmology 2005;112(7):1263-7.

16. Oguz H. Amniotic membrane grafting versus conjunctival autografting in pterygium surgery. Clin Experiment Ophthalmol 2005;33(4):447-8.

17. Raiskup F, Solomon A, Landau D, Ilsar M, Frucht-Pery J. Mitomycin C for pterygium: long term evaluation. Br J Ophthalmol 2004;88(11):1425-8.

18. Rubinfeld RS, Pfister RR, Stein RM, Foster CS, Martin NF, Stoleru S, et al. Serious complications of topical mitomycin-C after pterygium surgery. Ophthalmology 1992;99(11):1647-54.

19. Saw SM, Tan D. Pterygium: prevalence, demography and risk factors. Ophthalmic Epidemiol 1999;6(3):219-28.

20. Singh G, Wilson MR, Foster CS. Long-term follow-up study of mitomycin eye drops as adjunctive treatment of pterygia and its comparison with conjunctival autograft transplantation. Cornea 1990;9(4):331-4.

21. Srinivasan S, Slomovic AR. Eye rubbing causing conjunctival graft dehiscence following pterygium surgery with fibrin glue. Eye 2007;21(6):865-7.

22. Starck T, Kenyon KR, Serrano F. Conjunctival autograft for primary and recurrent pterygia: surgical technique and problem management. Córnea 1991;10(3):196-202.

23. Tan D. Conjunctival grafting for ocular surface disease. Curr Opin Ophthalmol 1999;10(4):277-81.

24. Threlfall TJ, English DR. Sun exposure and pterygium of the eye: a dose-response curve. Am J Ophthalmol 1999;128(3):280-7.

25. Ti SE, Chee SP, Dear KB, Tan DT. Analysis of variation in success rates in conjunctival autografting for primary and recurrent pterygium. Br J Ophthalmol 2000;84(4):385-9.

26. Tsai YY, Lin JM, Shy JD. Acute scleral thinning after pterygium excision with intraoperative mitomycin C. Cornea 2002;21:227-9.

27. Uy HS, Reyes JM, Flores JD, Lim-Bon-Siong R. Comparison of fibrin glue and sutures for attaching conjunctival autografts after pterygium excision. Ophthalmology 2005;112(4):667-71.

28. Yao YF, Qiu WY, Zhang YM, Tseng SC. Mitomycin C, amniotic membrane transplantation and limbal conjunctival autograft for treating multirecurrent pterygia with symblepharon and motility restriction. Graefes Arch Clin Exp Ophthalmol 2006;244(2):232-6.

Pediatric Epiphora

14

AK Grover, Shaloo Bageja, Malvika Bansal (India)

INTRODUCTION

Congenital nasolacrimal duct obstruction is the most common cause of epiphora in children, occuring in approximately 2-6% of infants. Ophthalmologists should however be aware of the other causes of epiphora in thisagegroup. Thus information of the developmental anatomy, abnormalities of the nasolacrimal system and other congenital disorders is essential for appropriate diagnosis and management of the conditions encountered.

EMBRYOLOGY OF THE LACRIMAL SYSTEM

Lacrimal system comprises the secretory and the excretory system.

Secretory System

It is ectodermal in nature. It begins as epithelial buds from basal cells of bulbar conjunctiva in the superotemporal fornix. These buds form cord of cells, which is later enclosed by the mesenchyme. At 60 mm stage lumen begins to form, though development continues 3-4 yrs postnatally.

Accessory glands of Krause and Wolfring develop as non-keratinized buds of epithelium from conjunctiva.

Excretory System

The excretory system begins in the first trimester when two facial prominence derived from first branchial arch fuse. Fusion of lateral nasal prominence with maxillary process entraps two layer of surface ectoderm. The surface ectoderm forms solid epithelial lacrimal cord in rudimentary naso-optic fissure. The cord grows during fetal life and is later surrounded by mesenchyme. The canalization of cord begins at about 4th-5th month of fetal life. It extends both caudally and cephalad. The cephalic end forms canaliculi and sac while the caudal end grows towards the nasal cavity. The puncta open when eyelids separate. The last portion to canalize is the lower end of the duct at the inferior meatus. The valve of Hasner may rupture any time between 6th month of gestation to soon after birth or may be delayed to several months after birth.

Interruption in canalization at any stage of development may result in congenital nasolacrimal obstruction.

DEVELOPMENTAL ABNORMALITIES

Punctal and Canalicular Abnormalities

Punctal and canalicular abnormalities include punctal agenesis, stenosis and membranous occlusion of punctum.

Lacrimal sac fistula or diverticula of sac may occur.

Nasolacrimal duct obstruction is the most common congenital abnormality, seen in 50% of infants at birth. The level of obstruction may vary in congenital nasolacrimal duct obstruction.

1. The most common obstruction occurring at the lower end of the duct where it fails to perforate the mucosa of the inferior meatus **(Figure 1).**

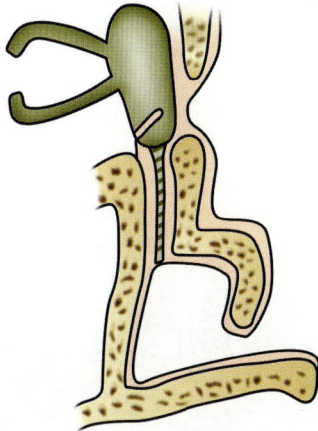

Figure 1: A diagram is showing nasolacrimal duct obstruction at or near the inferior meatus, due to nonperforation of the nasal mucosa

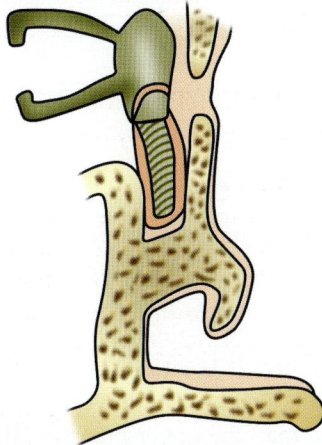

Figure 2: Diagram showing almost complete absence of the nasolacrimal duct

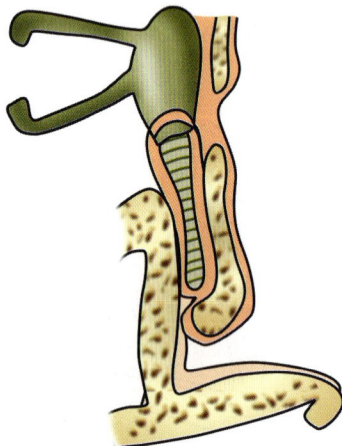

Figure 3: Diagram showing obstruction at the lower end of the duct due to impaction of inferior turbinate

2. Absence of duct due to failure to the osseous nasolacrimal canal to form, commonly seen with cleft palate anomalies **(Figure 2).**
3. Blockage of duct due to impaction of anterior end of inferior turbinate **(Figure 3).**

Anatomy of Excretory System

The drainage system comprises of puncta, upper and lower canaliculi, common canaliculus, lacrimal sac and nasolacrimal duct **(Figure 4).**

The excretory system begins with puncta which is about 0.3 mm in diameter. It is situated medially in line with meibomian glands orifice. The lower punctum is located lateral in postion than the upper punctum. Both puncta are ringed by avascular fibrous tissue. The punctum leads into canaliculus which comprises of 2 mm verical and 8 mm

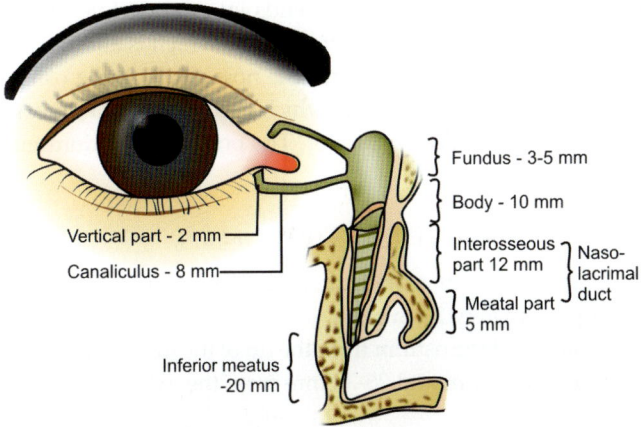

Figure 4: Diagram showing anatomy of
lacrimal excretory system

horizontal limb. The two canaliculi may converge into
common canaliculus in majority of cases. The two canaliculi
or common canaliculus enter the lacrimal sac 3-5 mm from
its apex. A fold of mucosa, i.e. valve of Rosenmuller, at the
junction of the canaliculi and sac prevents tear reflux from
the sac back into the canaliculi.

The lacrimal sac lies within the lacrimal sac fossa, formed
by the lacrimal bone and ascending frontal process of maxilla.
The lacrimal fossa is enclosed by anterior and posterior crus
of the medial canthal tendon. The lacrimal sac is about 15
mm in height.

The lacrimal sac drains into nasolacrimal duct. The
intraosseous part of nasolacrimal duct is approximately
12 mm. The duct traverses downward, laterally and
posteriorly. This is important to remember when surgeon is
probing the lacrimal system, otherwise may create a false

passage. The distal portion extends into the middle meatus forming the meatal portion of the duct, which is about 5 mm in length. The duct opens into the nose through the ostium under the inferior turbinate, which is covered by a mucosal fold called the valve of Hasner. The position of ostium may vary.

Important Points to Remember in Infants

1. Distance from punctum to the floor of the nose is approximately 20 mm.
2. Distance of the ostium from the tip of the inferior turbinate is about 15 mm and 25-30 mm from the external nares.

Physiology

Some amount of tear elimination occurs by evaporation along with physical factors like gravity and capillary action. However the blink mechanism play an important role in the tear flow. Jones' description of lacrimal pump mechanism was well accepted in the past. It reported that blink mechanism propels the tears into nasolacrimal duct by altering the intrasac pressure. However, Rosengren-Doane has described a better explanation based on cinematographic studies. On blinking, the apposition of eyelids and contraction of orbicularis creates a positive pressure in the tear sac, thus drawing fluid into the nose. On opening of eyelids, the puncta separate and negative pressure draws tears into the canaliculi and the sac.

The valve of Rosenmuller at common canaliculus and the valve of Hasner at the lower end of naso-lacrimal duct ensure unidirectional flow of tears. Paralysis of orbicularis result in epiphora due to lacrimal pump failure.

Evaluation

In evaluating a patient of paediatric epiphora, it is important to obtain a detailed history and to carry out a careful examination of the patient.

History

A thorough history from child's parents is essential as the child is not co-operative for proper examination. Parent's usually present with complaint of persistent watering with or without mucopurulent discharge **(Figure 5)**. Age of onset of symptoms is important as the tear production begins a couple of weeks after life. Thus the child may be asymptomatic for a month or so. History of trauma is necessary to rule out canalicular or bony injury. Symptoms of photophobia, watering, corneal haze or nystagmus should be enquired to rule out congenital glaucoma.

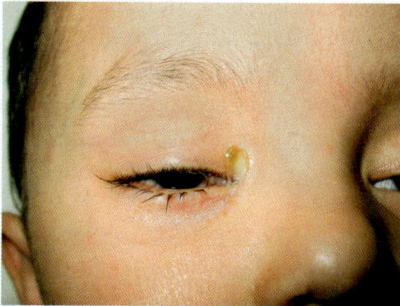

Figure 5: 13 months old child who presented with persistent watering and discharge

Examination

Eyelid margin—Eyelid margins are inspected for punctal position, its apposition to globe and its patency. It is important to exclude any lid abnormalities and any cause for reflex secretion like epiblepharon, conjunctivitis, trichiasis, blepharitis or meibomitis.

Medial canthal area—An ophthalmologist should look for any swelling over the medial canthal area like mucocele or congenital dacryocele. Pressure over the medial canthus may cause regurgitation of discharge from the punctum if blockage is distal to the sac. It is important to distinguish swellings above the medial canthal tendon which indicate conditions like anterior ethmoidal mucocele or encephalocele and one needs to perform a CT scan to identify the condition.

Investigations

In cases of congenital lacrimal system obstruction, the diagnosis is usually clear cut on history and examination as child present with watering, discharge, matting of eyelashes, inferior palpebral congestion. In doubtful cases, the dye disappearence test can be conducted. A drop of 2% fluorescein is placed in the inferior fornix. Tear film is observed with cobalt blue light. Delay in clearence of the dye after 5 minutes indicates outflow obstruction. This test is useful in children as diagnostic syringing cannot be performed in outpatient department.

Imaging has limited role in pediatric age though lacrimal scintigraphy or intraoperative dacryocystography can be performed in doubtful cases.

Management

Punctal and Canalicular Abnormalities

Punctal agenesis—Agenesis of punctum results due to failure of conjunctival dehisence overlying a canaliculus during eyelid separation. Thus leaving a persistent membrane across the punctum.

If papilla is visible, then the membrane can be punctured with a dilator. Syringing and probing following membrane rupture can restore the patency, if the remaining system is normal structurally.

If papilla is not seen, one may cut at the expected area of punctum and attempt probing. In case the passage is patent, intubation should of the lacrimal system is indicated. Canalicular agenesis is usually associated with punctal agenesis.

Single patent punctum, child may be asymptomatic especially in case of upper punctum involvement. If patient is symptomatic, surgeon should evaluate normal punctum and its passage.

Both punctum absent—Requires conjunctivodacryocystorhinostomy when patient is old enough to take care of the tube.

Lacrimal Sac Abnormalities

Dacryocystocele—A dilated sac without any signs of inflammation indicate congenital dacryocele or amniotocele. It is due to entrapment of mucus or amniotic fluid within the lacrimal sac due to nasolacrimal duct obstruction. It presents within first few weeks of life. An infant presents with tense swelling at the medial canthus inferior to the medial canthal tendon. Gentle massage over the sac along with topical antibiotics may relieve the obstruction. Syringing and probing is required if infant is symptomatic even after massage. Probing is done as early as 6 weeks of age.

Congenital Nasolacrimal Obstruction (CNLDO)

CNLDO is commonly due to membranous block of the opening into the inferior meatus at the valve of Hasner. Of the 50% of newborn infants who have obstruction at the inferior end of nasolacrimal duct, only 2-6% clinically presents with epiphora at 3-4 weeks of age. Spontaneous resolution occurs in approximately 90% of all patients in first year of life. Conservative management is therefore recommended in all cases.

Conservative Management

Parents are educated regarding maintenance of lid hygiene and lacrimal sac massage (Criggler massage).

Criggler Massage

Surgeon should demonstrate the proper technique of massage to the mother. It should be emphasized to use the little finger for this maneuver. One should first palpate the medial canthal tendon and move the finger downwards, feeling the anterior lacrimal crest. Massage is done with firm strokes over the lacrimal sac at least twice a day. Approximately 90% of the infants respond to massage in first year of life and 60% respond in their second year of life.

Topical antibiotics are advised at least thrice a day to reduce mucoid discharge. Infants who do not respond to conservative management are taken up for probing.

Acute dacryocystitis—Some cases of CNLDO may present with an acute episode of inflammation of lacrimal sac. It is often associated with cellulites and needs to be managed vigorously with systemic intravenous antibiotics. One should not attempt to drain the pus in acute stage as it may lead to lacrimal –

cutaneous fistula. Early syringing and probing is indicated once the acute stage subsides.

If lacrimal sac abscess is developed, surgical drainage is required.

Syringing and Probing

Timing of probing is controversial, most of the surgeons now prefer to wait till one year of age, while some surgeons advocate early probing.

Anesthesia—It is performed under general anesthesia with protected airway. Laryngeal mask may be used instead of Endotracheal intubation depending on the choice of the anesthesiologist.

Technique—Before starting the procedure it, the lacrimal sac needs to be evacuated either by performing massage over the sac area or syringing with saline **(Figure 6).**

Upper punctum is generally preferred for probing to prevent any damage to the lower punctum during the manipulation. Punctum is dilated with Nettleship dilator **(Figure 7A)** and then Bowman probe (size 0 or 00) is introduced into the punctum perpendicular to the eyelid

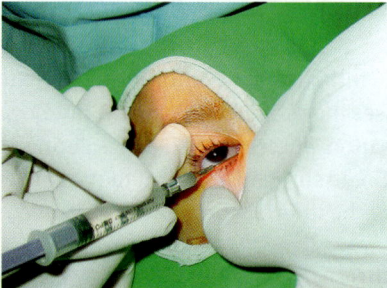

Figure 6: Syringing is performed prior to probing of the nasolacrimal duct to evacuate the lacrimal sac

margin **(Figure 7B)**. It first traverses the vertical 2 mm of the canaliculus and then the horizontal part while maintaining a lateral traction of eyelid ismaintained **(Figure 7C)**. The lateral traction of skin stretches the canaliculus and avoids any chance of damage to the canalicular mucosa and decreases the probability of creation of a false passage. If one feels the resistance while passing the probe medially, it may be due to kink of the canaliculus. Surgeon should withdraw the probe slightly and then proceed medially maintaining the lateral traction. As the tip reaches the medial wall of lacrimal sac and lacrimal bone, surgeon will feel a hard stop.

The probe is then slightly withdrawn and rotated superiorly against the brow and should come to rest over the supraorbital notch at the superior orbital rim **(Figure 7D)**. The probe is then passed downwards, posteriorly and slight laterally down the nasolacrimal duct. The probe should slide down smoothly. In case of any feel of resistance, withdraw the probe slightly and proceed forward. If the surgeon feels the firm stop at a distance of about 12 mm (distance fom punctum to nasolacrimal duct) and cannot manipulate further, it indicates a bony obstruction and absence of nasolacrimal duct. Dacryocystorhinostomy is indicated in such a situation. If probe pass down the nasolacrimal duct to about 20 mm, it indicates that it has reached the inferior meatus. Some resistance is felt due to membranous obstruction. Firm pressure passes the probe into the nasal cavity with a slight " pop up" sensation. Successful probing is verified by syringing **(Figure 7E)**. Some surgeons confirm the patency by passing a spatula under the inferior turbinate to have a metal on metal feel.

Availability of nasal endoscopes, may also assist in verifying the correct passage of probe. It aids rupturing of the membrane under direct visualization and thus avoids

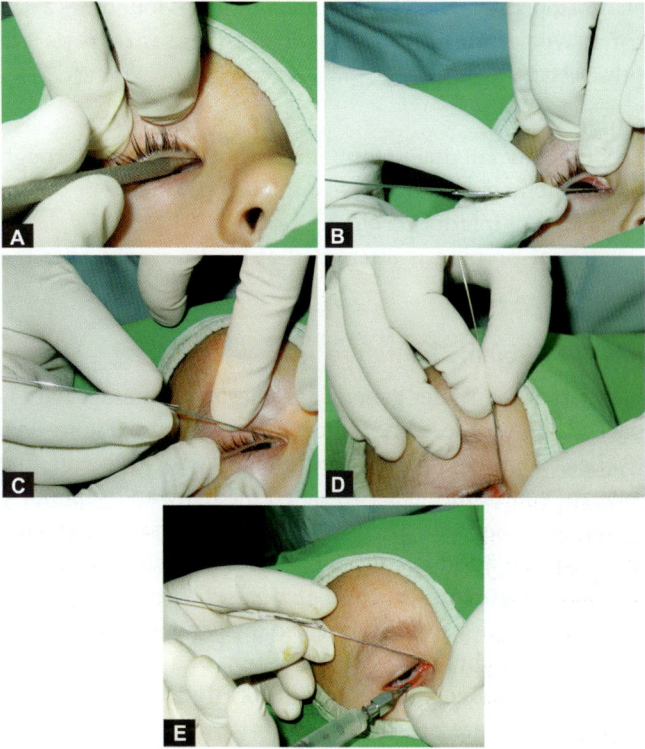

Figures 7A to E: (A) A Nettleship dilator is used to gently dilate the punctum. (B) Bowman Probe size 00 is introduced into upper punctum perpendicular to eyelid margin. (C) Bowman probe is advanced horizontally while maintaining lateral traction of eyelid. (D) Probe lies over the supraorbital notch at superior orbital rim and is advanced into the nasolacrimal duct. (E) Syringing of nasolacrimal system is done to check the patency

creation of false passage. Postion of inferior turbinate can be visualized and infracture of the turbinate can be done if inferior turbinate is impacted at the ostium.

Postoperatively, steroid—antibiotic drops four times a day for 2 weeks along with nasal decongesant drops are prescribed.

Failure

Probing may fail due to formation of small opening through the membrane, leading to closure postoperatively or due to impaction of inferior turbinate.

Repeat probing is attempted at least 6 weeks after the initial one.

Inferior Turbinate Infracture

It is performed under general anesthesia. The nasal cavity is packed before proceeding for turbinate infracture **(Figure 8A).**

Lens spatula is passed under the inferior turbinate, the anterior end of turbinate is rotated medially and superiorly towards the septum. Then the spatula is passed backwards and then the middle and the posterior part of turbinate are fractured **(Figures 8B and C).** Patency is checked by syringing **(Figure 8D).** Nasal cavity is packed for 24 hours as there may be a risk of slight bleed.

Postoperatively, steroid-antibiotic drops and nasal decongestants are prescribed.

Silicone Intubation

Indication—Silicone intubation is indicated in cases of recurrent failed probing with or without inferior turbinate infracture or in older children.

Various types of intubation sets like Crawford, Ritleng and others are available for the purpose.

It is performed under general anesthesia. Before intubation nasal packing is done to constrict the mucosa of the inferior turbinate. These silicone tubings have metal bodkins attached

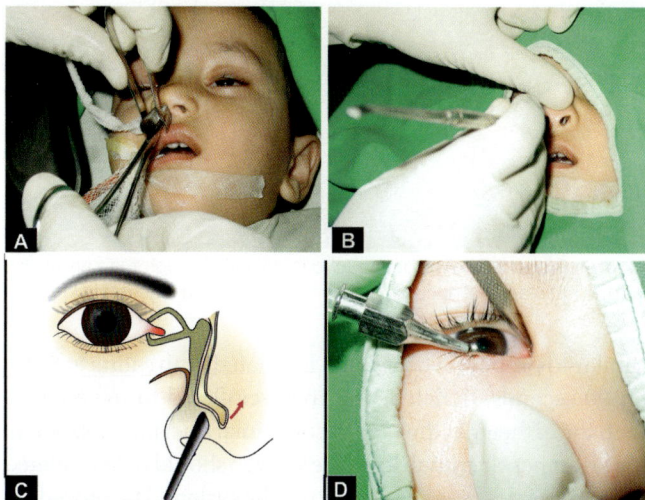

Figures 8A to D: (A) Nasal cavity is packed before proceeding for inferior turbinate infracture. (B and C) Inferior turbinate infracture with use of blunt spatula. (D) Syringing through inferior canaliculus to check patency

at each end. Punctum is dilated. If metal tube cannot be easily passed through the punctum, one or three snip procedure may be performed. The metal tubings are passed through each canaliculus into the nasolacrimal duct. They can be pulled into the nasal cavity with the help of an artery forceps. The silicone tubings are tied together in the nose near inferior meatus after removing the metal bodkins **(Figures 9A and B)**.

The procedure can be combined with inferior turbinate infracture. Stents are left in position for atleast six months.

Ballon Dacryoplasty

This is a new technique of management, where collapsed catheter is introduced into the nasolacrimal duct by a procedure

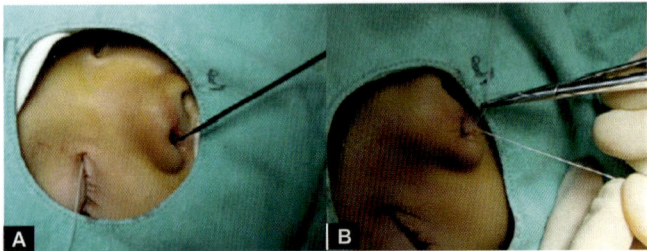

Figures 9A and B: (A) Silicone tube is passed through the canaliculus into the nasolacrimal duct. (B) Silicone tubing are tied together in the nose

similar to probing. The balloon is inflated with saline to 8 atm for 90 seconds, deflated, and then reinflated for 60 seconds with the catheter at the sac- Nasolacrimal duct junction and at the lower nasolacrimal duct. The balloon should not be inflated in the lacrimal sac as it may rupture the system. The procedure is not so popular due to dependence on the requirement of a catheter and its high cost.

Dacryocystorhinostomy (DCR)

Indication—DCR is indicated in cases of repeated failed probing with inferior turbinate infracture or silicone intubation or in cases where on the initial probing a bony obstruction is diagnosed. It is also indicated in traumatic cases leading to canalicular scarring or injury to intraosseous part of nasolacrimal duct and in craniofacial abnormalities, associated with nasolacrimal abnormalities.

Timing—Surgery is usually not performed before 3 years of age except in cases of persistent episodes of acyte dacryocystitis.

Anesthesia—The procedure is performed under general anesthesia. Mild hypotensive anesthesia may be preferred to minimize blood loss intraoperatively.

DCR in children is may be difficult owing to smaller size of the structures. The technique requires some modifications due to some anatomical differences from the adult lacrimal system. The anterior lacrimal crest and the lacrimal fossa are pooly developed and it is sometimes difficult to locate the site for osteotomy. Medial canthal tendon insertion provides an important landmark to identify the superior part of anterior lacrimal crest.

Due to thin bones, osteotomy is easily performed. One should prefer to have a larger osteotomy as there may be postoperative bony regrowth which may be a cause of failure.

Failures have been observed in the paediatric age group due to less well defined anatomy, postoperative bony growth and greater scarring.

Mitomycin C have also been tried intraoperatively by applying a soaked piece of cotton to the osteotomy site to reduce fibrosis and scarring postoperatively.

Endonasal DCR

Endonasal DCR, though technically difficult in young children offers a number of advantages over the external approach. It avoids the need for a skin incision and consequent scarring, enables creation of a large ostium even when the lacrimal sac is small and scarred. It has additional advantage of limited intraoperative bleeding.

SUMMARY

Abnormalities of lacrimal system are encountered frequently in the pediatric age group. Epiphora is a common condition in infancy and early childhood. Congenital nasolacrimal duct obstruction resolves spontaneously in 90-95% cases in first year of life. Inital management includes massage of lacrimal sac and application of topical antibiotics. Syringing and Probing alone or in combination with inferior turbinate infracture is performed in cases who does not respond to conservative therapy after one year of age. Silastic intubation is performed for repeated failed probing and finally DCR is indicated in cases of failed probing after 3 years of age.

BIBLIOGRAPHY

1. Chen PL, Hsiao CH. Balloon dacryocystoplasty as the primary treatment in older children with congenital nasolacrimal duct obstruction. J AAPOS 2005;9:546-9.
2. Chiesi C, Guerra R, Longanesi L, Fornaciari M, Morano RP. Congenital nasolacrimal duct obstruction: therapeutic management. J Paediatric Ophthalmol Strabismus 1999 Nov-Dec;36(6):326-30.
3. J E Marr, A Drake-Lee, HE Willshaw. Management of childhood epiphora. British Journal of Ophthalmology 2005;89:1123-26.
4. Jones LT, Wobig JL. Surgery of the eyelids and lacrimal system.Birmingham, Ala: Aesculapius Publishing Co; 1976
5. MacEwen CJ, Young JD, Barras CW, et al. Value of nasal endo-scopy and probing in the diagnosis and management of children with congenital epiphora. Br J Ophthalmol 2001;85:314-8.
6. Maheshwari R. Results of Probing for Congenital Nasolacrimal Duct Obstruction in Children Older than 13 Months of Age. Indian J Ophthalmol 2005;53:49-51
7. Nesi FA, Lisman RD, Levine MR, Brazzo BG, Gladstone GJ. Smith's Ophthalmic Plastic and Reconstructive Surgery. 2nd ed. St Louis, MO: Mosby Year Book, Inc; 1998.
8. Sekhar GC. Practical approach to a patient with epiphora. Indian J Ophthalmol 1994;42:157-61
9. Wesley RE. Inferior turbinate fracture in the treatment of congenital nasolacrimal duct obstruction and congenital nasolacrimal duct anomaly. Ophthalmic Surg 1985;16:368.

Congenital Tumors

15

AK Grover, Shaloo Bageja (India)

PIGMENTED LESIONS

Nevi (Figure 1)

These are benign congenital tumors. They may vary in size and may be sessile or pedunculated. The commonest location is along the lid border. Risk of malignancy is low. However in large tumors, there will be 4-6% risk of malignant transformation. Sudden increase in size and increase in pigmentation suggests concern regarding malignant transformation and requires excision.

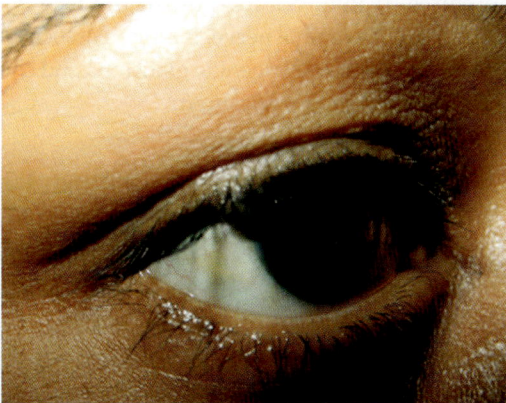

Figure 1: Showing nevus in upper eyelid

Management

Shave off flush with the lid margin if it involves the lid margin or if nevus does not involve the lid margin excision with direct repair with margin repair can be done.

Nevus of Ota (Oculodermal Melanocytosis)

It is characterized by patchy bluish or brownish pigmentation of periocular skin and sclera. The lesion is composed of dermal melanocytes and has malignant potential. Increased intraocular pigmentation contributes to risk of glaucoma. It is occasionally associated with Sturge-Weber syndrome.

Management

Ruby laser has been tried to lighten the cutaneous component.

ANGIOMATOUS TUMORS

Portwine Stain (Nevus Flammeus)

This condition is characterized by telangiectasia of the deeper skin capillaries. It involves the part of the face which is innervated by the trigeminal nerve. It is often associated with Sturge-Weber syndrome. Congenital glaucoma and choroidal hemangioma have strong association.

Strawberry (Capillary) Hemangioma (Figure 2)

These are benign tumors present at birth. 90% of these clinically manifest by age of 1 month.

Symptoms and Signs

The child may present with ptosis, refractive error, amblyopia and proptosis.

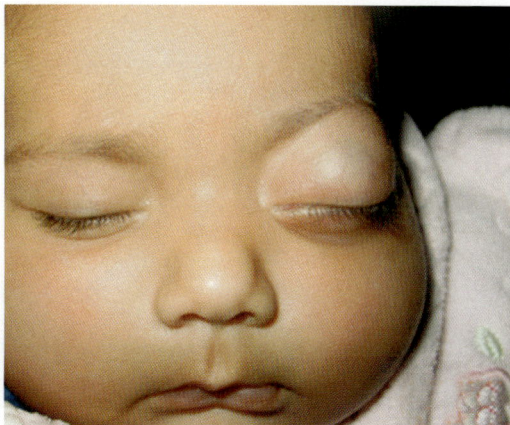

Figure 2: An infant with capillary hemangioma

Prognosis

These tumor grow for 3-6 months after birth and slowly regresses by second year of life. Spontaneous resolution occurs in 40% by 4 years of age and 80% by 8 years.

Management

Surgery is indicated in cases of total ptosis obscuring the visual axis and induced astigmatism and for better cosmesis.

Intralesional injection of 1-2 ml of corticosteroid. Betamethasone 6 mg/ml and triamcinolone 40 mg/cc combined in 1:1 concentration and is injected all around the lesion with 26 G needle deep into the lesion **(Figure 3)**. Rapid shrinkage occurs in first two weeks and then continues slowly for several months. Injection may be repeated after 6 weeks in case of residual mass. Depigmentation of overlying skin, eyelid necrosis and rarely central retinal artery occlusion are few complications seen with steroid injection.

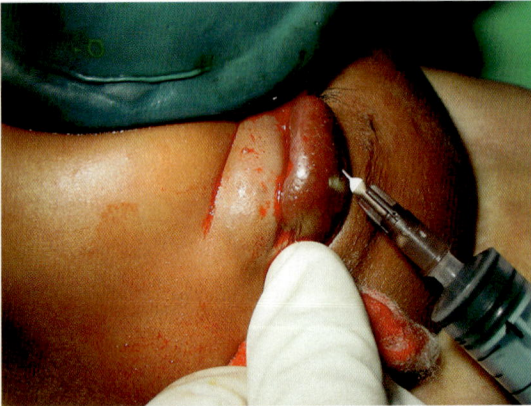

Figure 3: Injecting corticosteroid in the hemangioma

Dermoid and Epidermoid Cyst

Abnormal sequestration of surface ectoderm beneath the skin during embryonic development results in the cyst formation **(Figure 4)**. Lids are usually secondarily involved due to extension of the tumor from the orbits.

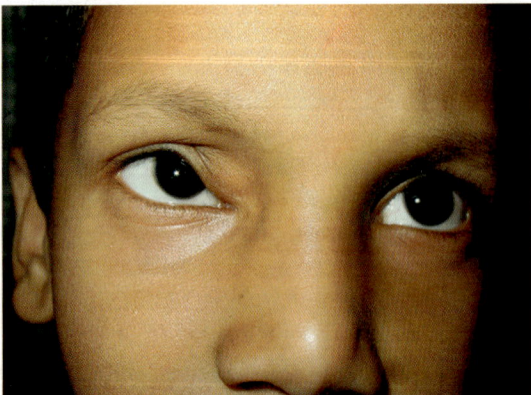

Figure 4: Showing swelling superonasally of dermoid

Signs

They are clinically evident by first year of life. Most common location is superonasal. On palpation, these are firm in consistency, nontender and are attached to underlying periosteum.

Investigation

Imaging is necessary to know the extension.

Management

Surgical excision is required in case of progressive enlargement of mass.

Plexiform Neurofibroma

Involvement of the lid with plexiform neuroma in cases of neurofibromatosis **(Figure 5)**. Café au lait spots are characteristic of neurofibromatosis.

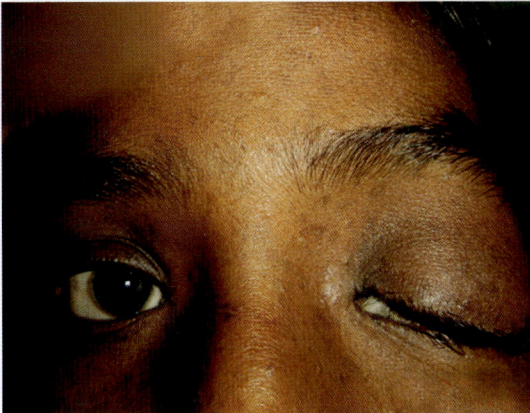

Figure 5: Showing plexiform neurofibroma of let upper lid

Management

Surgery is indicated in cases of significant mechanical ptosis and to improve cosmesis. Surgical debulking of the mass along with ptosis correction and lateral shortening may be performed.

Prognosis

These tumors cannot be fully excised and recurrence is common.

To conclude, pediatric abnormalities poses challenges for an ophthalmologist. Patient's cooperation is a limitation for adequate assessment in paedatric age group. Cosmetic consideration is also critical for child's psychological development. It is important to carefully assess and plan the technique of intervention for gratifying results.

Section *Two*

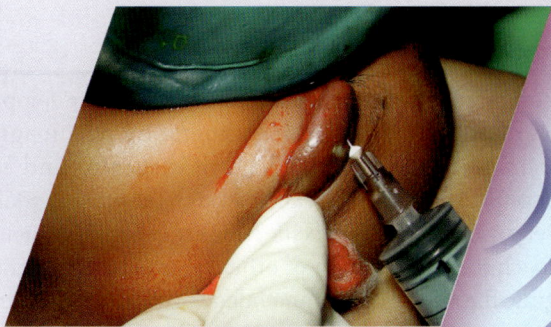

Orbital Diseases

Imaging of the Orbit

16

Roshmi Gupta, Savari Desai, Santosh G Honavar (India)

INTRODUCTION

The commonly used orbital imaging modalities are computed tomography (CT scan), ultrasonography and magnetic resonance imaging (MRI). The most useful and most commonly used is the CT scan, although the other modalities are very useful in some specific situations. For the systematic approach to interpretation of orbital computed tomography imaging, the reader is recommended to consult the references quoted. In this chapter, we shall discuss orbital imaging of selected orbital pathology with respect to computed tomography, and specific features best identified with MRI scanning or orbital ultrasound. All imaging has to be interpreted in context of the clinical presentation.

COMPARISON OF THE THREE MODALITIES

Computed Tomography

A thin collimated fan-shaped beam of X-rays emanate from the machine, pass through the tissue and are detected and converted into signals. Areas of greater density are depicted as brighter on the image, while lower density areas are depicted to be darker. CT scan of the orbit, at 2 mm slices shows orbital processes with high anatomical accuracy. Bones of the orbit are imaged well. A lesion which becomes brighter after intravenous injection of contrast material is said to be enhancing. Contrast-enhancement is seen in vascular and cystic lesions.

Magnetic Resonance Imaging

The part of interest is placed in a strong magnetic field, and the protons in the tissue rotate to align their magnetic fields to that of the superimposed field. When the field is switched of, the protons regain their previous orientation, emitting energy in the process. The emitted energy is detected and converted to signals. Any tissue that contains a higher number of free protons will emit a stronger signal, whereas cortical bone, which is nearly devoid of protons, shows up black in an MRI. Depending on the relaxation times and weightage given, the T1 weighted images show fat to be brighter, or hyper-intense, and water to be darker, or hypo-intense. The T2 image shows orbital fat as dark, and water, including vitreous humor and cerebrospinal fluid to be brighter, or hyper-intense. Lesions may enhance with the contrast agent Gd-DTPA, best seen on fat-suppressed T1-weighted images.

The MRI scan is able to image orbital soft tissues and their relationship in detail, but has poor histologic specificity. Most tumors are hypo-intense on T1-weighted images and hyper-intense on T2 weighted images. Vascular lesions enhance well on contrast injection. Lack of enhancement may be seen in cystic lesions or less vascular areas such as scar tissue. MRI scans can help in the differential diagnosis of hemorrhagic lesions, and can detail the optic nerve and orbital apex lesions.

Orbital Ultrasound

Sound waves with frequency in the ultrasonic range are transmitted through the tissues. The reflected waves are detected and converted into images, two-dimensional in case of the B-scan and linear in case of the A-scan. Highly reflective tissues are represented as being brighter.

Echography may be used as an adjunctive imaging modality, in lesions that involve the globe and adjacent orbit. It can detect cystic lesions of the orbit well.

EVALUATION OF CT SCAN ORBIT

The maximum information is elicited from an orbital imaging by evaluating it systematically:

The bony orbit: The orbital roof, floor, medial and lateral walls, orbital apex, optic foramen, inferior orbital fissure.

- Eyeball
- Extaocular muscles: size, shape, laterality and distribution of muscle enlargement, muscle margins, contrast enhancement.
- Extraconal tissues.

Intraconal tissues: Optic nerve, superior ophthalmic vein
- Sella and parasellar regions.

Any orbital space-occupying lesion is to be assessed in terms of its size, location, shape, circumscription, effect on surrounding soft tissue, effect on surrounding bone, internal consistency, contrast enhancement and extraorbital invasion.

THE ORBITAL BONES

The orbital bones are best imaged by a CT scan; MRI and Ultrasonography have little role to play. In this section we shall be discussing the bony lesions of the orbit. Changes in the bones secondary to disease processes will be mentioned with the relevant disease process.

Osteoma

Introduction: An osteoma is a tumor-like mass of bony tissue; in the vicinity of the orbit, they arise most commonly form the frontal sinus, followed by ethmoid, maxillary and sphenoid sinuses. The mass extends into the orbit and causes proptosis and globe displacement.

Computed tomography: The CT scan shows a well-defined, well-circumscribed mass, arising from the sinus and invading the orbit. They may have a bosselated surface, and may be sessile or pedunculated. The bone window shows a very dense periphery, and lower density inside, due to the cancellous internal structure **(Figures 1A and B).**

Differential diagnosis: An osteoma is to be differentiated from other bony tumors like ossifying fibroma and fibrous dysplasia.

Investigations: A patient should be evaluated for multiple osteomas, retinal pigment epithelial hypertrophy and soft tissue tumors. These are associated with Gardner's syndrome, which needs colonoscopy to rule out premalignant intestinal polyps.

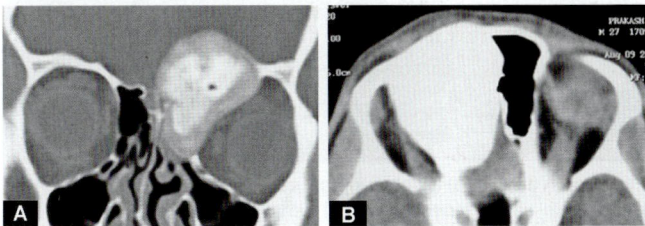

Figures 1A and B: (A) Coronal view of right frontal osteoma, bone window setting. (B) Axial view of same, in soft tissue window setting. The bony lesion appears uniformly dense

Treatment: If asymptomatic, osteomas may be treated conservatively. The tumor can be excised via orbitotomy.

Ossifying Fibroma

Signs and symptoms: Ossifying fibroma or fibro-osseous dysplasia involves a single bone; near the orbit, it affects the frontal, ethmoid or maxillary bones, and extends into the orbit. The lesion may cause asymptomatic proptosis.

Orbital imaging: There is a well-circumscribed mass, with a thin rim of high density sclerotic bone. The internal structure shows multi-loculated heterogeneous density due to the osteoblastic and osteolytic areas **(Figures 2A and B).**

Differential diagnosis: Histopathologically it is to be differentiated from fibrous dysplasia.

Investigation and management: The tumor tends to recur if removed incompletely. Total excision needs to be done; for a large tumor, combined orbital, neurosurgical and rhinological approaches are needed.

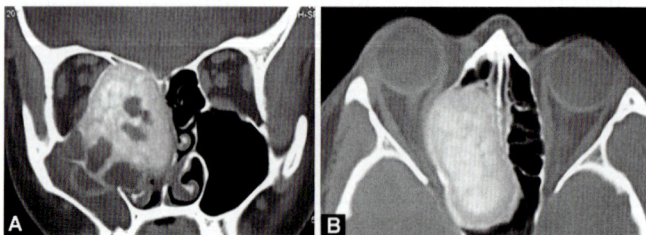

Figures 2A and B: (A) CT scan image, coronal section of the well-defined lesion, with heterogeneous internal density, involving the ethmoid and maxillary sinuses, the nasal cavity and the orbit. (B) Axial view of the lesion showing the lesion displacing the extraocular muscles and the optic nerve

Histopathological examination of the biopsied tissue confirms the diagnosis.

Orbital Fracture

Signs and symptoms: The patient has a history of trauma, and subsequent pain and diplopia. The eye is enophthalmic, with restriction of ocular movement in the vertical and occasionally the horizontal gaze.

Computed tomography: The blow-out fractures of the floor and medial wall of the orbit are best visualized with bone window settings. The medial wall fracture is best seen in the coronal and axial views, while the floor fracture is best seen in the coronal or re-formatted sagittal views. A discontinuity is seen in the orbital wall. The fractured fragment may be dislocated completely into the paranasal sinus, or may be rotated like a trap-door, hinged at one edge. The orbital soft tissues—fat, septa, or muscle may be entrapped in the fracture **(Figures 3A and B).**

Differential diagnosis: The orbital fracture should be clinically differentiated from mechanical limitation of movement due to tissue edema, and from traumation extraocular muscle paresis.

Investigation: Preoperative forced duction testing can confirm entrapment of extraocular muscle and soft tissues in the fracture.

Treatment: A small, asymptomatic orbital fracture may be treated conservatively. Surgical repair is required for a large fracture, or one causing diplopia by restriction of ocular motility **(Figure 3C).**

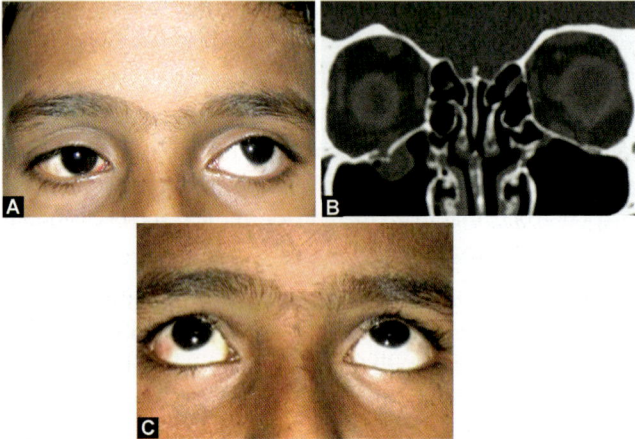

Figures 3A to C: (A) Clinical photograph of right orbital floor fracture, with right enophthalmos and restricted elevation of the right eye. (B) Coronal view of the CT scan orbit, showing trap-door deformity in the orbital floor, with soft tissue prolapsing into the maxillary sinus. The lateral edge of the inferior rectus muscle is trapped in the fracture. (C) Clinical photograph after surgical repair of the floor fracture, showing improved ocular elevation

EXTRAOCULAR MUSCLES

Thyroid Eye Disease

Signs and symptoms: Patients of thyroid orbitopathy present with unilateral or bilateral proptosis. There may limitation of ocular movement, eyelid changes such as lid retraction and lagophthalmos, corneal exposure and signs of optic nerve compression.

Computed tomography: On CT scan, thyroid eye disease is commonly bilateral, the eyes are proptosed. The optic nerves appear straightened. Pre-septal soft tissue edema may be seen. There is bilateral fusiform enlargement of the extra-ocular muscles, with smooth borders and sparing of the tendons. Multiple sections should be studied to detect posterior enlargement which may be compressing the optic nerve. Occasionally the orbital involvement may be asymmetrical, but some evidence of thyroid-related changes can be seen in the eye with milder disease also **(Figures 4A to C)**.

Differential diagnosis: Thyroid eye disease is to be differentiated from orbital inflammatory myositis, where there is a diffuse enlargement of one or more muscles; the enlargement conforms to the shape of the globe, and the tendinous insertion is involved. An inflammatory process may show contrast enhancement of the muscle.

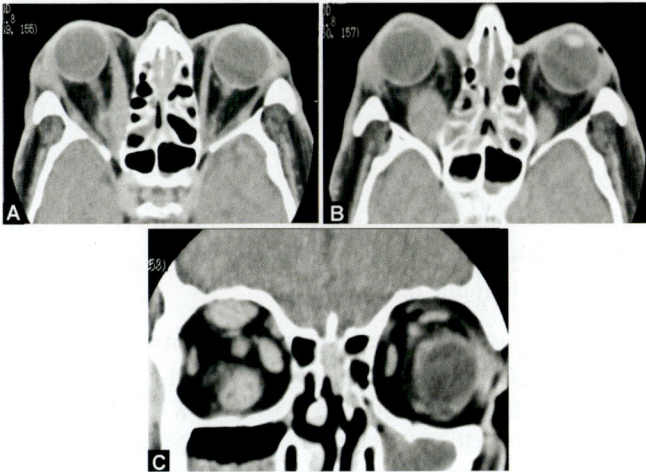

Figures 4A to C: Axial view of CT scan in thyroid orbitopathy, showing bilateral proptosis, straightening of the optic nerve, and enlargement of the extraocular muscles without tendon involvement. (B) Axial view of the same in a more inferior section. The enlarged inferior rectus may be mistaken for a space-occupying lesion. (C) Coronal view of the same, depicting enlargement of all extraocular muscles

Arteriovenous fistulas may also show enlargement of multiple extraocular muscles, proptosis, and some contrast enhancement. The dilated superior ophthalmic vein is a differentiating feature.

Cavernous sinus thrombosis would cause bilateral enlargement of multiple extraocular muscles. The superior ophthalmic vein would be enlarged. The cavernous sinus would enhance with contrast, and demonstrate enlargement, and loss of the concavity of the lateral border as seen on an axial section.

Investigations: Ultrasound B scan of the orbit may confirm enlarged size of the extra-ocular muscles.

Systemic evaluation for thyroid abnormalities should be performed. Thyroid function tests for T3, T4, TSH, and anti-thyroid antibodies may confirm the diagnosis in a previously undetected patient. However, in about 10% of the cases, Graves' orbitopathy may present in a euthyroid patient.

Myositis

Orbital myositis is a non-specific inflammatory condition of the extraocular muscles, though it may be associated with underlying immune disease.

Signs and symptoms: The patient presents with periorbital pain, which increases on ocular movement, and orbital inflammatory signs such as periocular and lid edema, and conjunctival chemosis. The episodes may be recurrent, and involve different muscles in the recurring episodes.

Investigation

Computed tomography: The CT scan shows enlargement of one or more extraocular muscles, commonly unilateral. The muscle borders are irregular, and the diffuse inflammatory shadow extends to the tendon and the orbital fat **(Figures 5A to C)**.

Differential count of leucocytes may help to rule out eosinophilia, which is associated with trichinellosis causing myositis.

Differential diagnosis: In thyroid orbitopathy, the involvement of the muscles is bilateral, and in multiple extraocular muscles. There is a fusiform dilatation of the muscle, but the tendon is usually spared. The commonly affected muscles are the inferior, superior and medial recti.

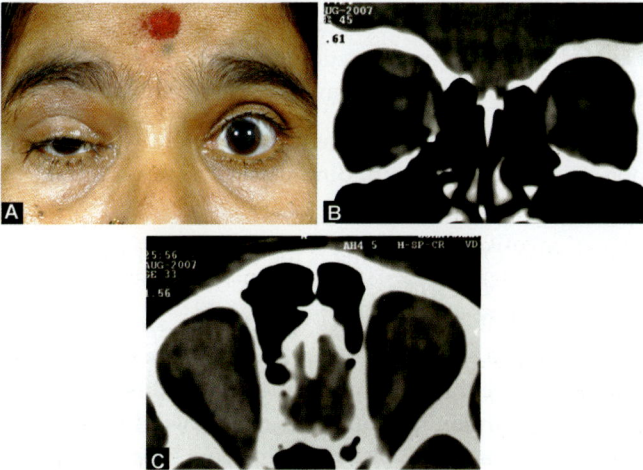

Figures 5A to C: (A) Clinical photograph of patient with right orbital myositis involving the superior rectus and levator palpebrae superioris. The patient presented with right ptosis and limitation of elevation. (B) The coronal section of the CT scan shows isolated enlargement of the right superior rectus. (C) Axial section showing the the thickened superior rectus, with irregular outline depicting an inflammatory process. The thickening extends anteriorly to the tendon

In an intracranial arteriovenous fistula, all muscles will be enlarged. The superior ophthalmic vein will also be dilated, seen on axial as well as coronal views.

Other infiltrative disease, including lymphoma may cause enlargement of extraocular muscles.

Treatment: Depending on the severity and extent of the disease, myositis may be treated with systemic nonsteroidal anti-inflammatory drugs, low dose steroids, or high dose steroids. Recurrent disease may need intravenous pulses of steroids.

Orbital Cysticercosis

Introduction: Orbital cysticercosis occurs in the extraocular muscles and may migrate anteriorly and subconjunctivally. Depending on the exact location, the clinical presentation is varied. The inflammatory signs may be moderate or severe.

Signs and symptoms: The patient may present with axial or non-axial proptosis; pain, diminished vision, limitation of ocular motility and ptosis.

Investigation: Orbital imaging is the mainstay of diagnosis in orbital myocysticercosis.

Computed tomography orbit will show a well-circumscribed lesion within an extraocular muscle. The muscle may be thickened and have surrounding soft tissue shadows of inflammation. The cyst shows low internal density, with a high density internal spot representing the scolex **(Figures 6A and B).**

Magnetic resonance imaging will depict a well circumscribed cystic lesion within an extraocular muscle, which is hypo-intense on T1 sequences, and hyper-intense on T2-weighted sequences, with an internal hypo-intense spot representing the scolex **(Figure 7A).**

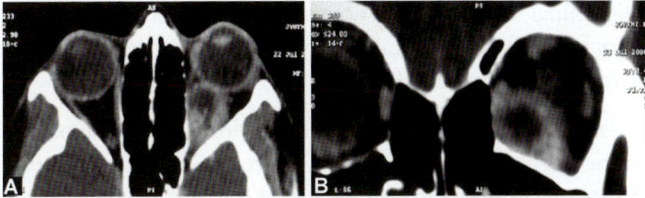

Figures 6A and B: (A) Axial CT scan of orbital myocysticercosis showing cystic lesion with low internal density, with a high density internal spot representing the scolex, surrounded by inflammatory soft tissue shadow. (B) The coronal section confirms the location in the inferior rectus muscle

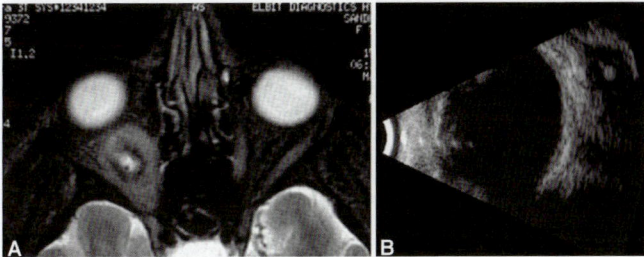

Figures 7A and B: (A) T1 –weighted MRI of orbital myocysticercosis, showing hyper-intense lesion with surrounding inflammatory changes and internal hypo-intense spot of the calcified scolex. (B) USG B-scan of orbital myocysticercosis shows an echo-lucent cystic structure in an extraocular muscle, with the internal scolex showing high echo-reflectivity

Ultrasound B scan of the orbit will show a low-echo reflective cystic structure in relation to an extraocular muscle. The cyst will show internal high-echo reflective area of the scolex. Te adjacent muscle will also demonstrate thickening. Sometimes only the cyst is visualized, without the scolex. **(Figure 7B).**

For a patient on medical management, requesting serial ultrasound B scans is a good way of monitoring improvement. The scolex disappears, and the cyst gradually grows smaller in size and finally collapses.

Differential diagnosis: The appearance of myocysticercosis is very characteristic. If only the cyst is seen, the differentiation is from other cystic lesions.

Treatment: Medical management comprises the use of oral anthelminthic, albendazole, and steroid. Surgical excision of the cyst is rarely required.

EXTRACONAL LESIONS OF THE ORBIT

Dermoid Cyst

A dermoid cyst is the commonest cystic space-occupying lesion of the orbit. The dermoid cyst may be superficial, as external and internal angular dermoids, or deep dermoid cysts.

Signs and symptoms: Superficial dermoid cysts present early in life with gradually enlarging periorbital cystic lesion. Deep dermoid cysts present later in life, with progressive proptosis. If the dermoid cyst is bilobular, and is dumbbell shaped, and has a component in the temporal fossa, the patient may present with intermittent proptosis.

Ultrasound B scan: The dermoid cyst has a smooth well-circumscribed shape. There may be erosion of the adjacent bone. The internal reflectivity of the dermoid cyst is variable.

Computed tomography orbit will show a smooth rounded lesion, with or without fossa formation of the adjacent bone. The internal consistency of the cyst is heterogeneous, due to the variable nature of the contents. Occasional deep dermoid cysts are dumb-bell shaped, with components in both the orbit and the temporal fossa, and erosion of the lateral wall of the orbit **(Figures 8 and 9).**

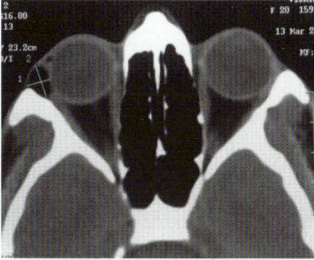

Figure 8: Axial CT scan of superficial dermoid cyst, showing well-defined lesion with low internal density, with a shallow fossa formation in the adjacent bone

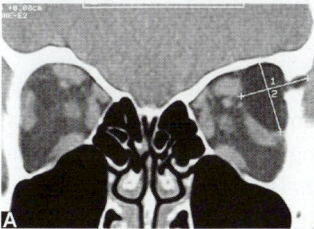

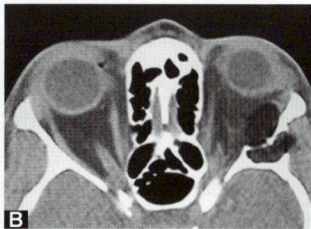

Figures 9A and B: (A) Coronal CT scan of deep dermoid cyst, showing well circumscribed extraconal lesion, with low internal density, with extension to the temporal fossa through a defect in the lateral orbital wall. (B) Axial CT scan of the same, showing the deep dermoid with a dumb-bell shaped extension into the temporal fossa

Differential diagnosis: The clinical and imaging features are characteristic of dermoid cysts. A cyst with inflammation needs to be distinguished from other orbital inflammatory disorders.

Treatment: The progressively enlarging dermoid cyst is excised surgically.

Sphenoid Wing Meningioma

Sphenoid ridge meningiomas are intracranial tumors, but affect the orbit secondarily to have significant orbital and visual effects. They comprise 18-20% of all intracranial meningiomas, and are commoner in women.

Signs and symptoms: The more medially arising tumors compress the optic nerve and structures in the superior orbital fissure, and present more often with visual loss and limitation of ocular motility. The visual loss is slowly progressive, and may be bilateral. Defects in color perception are early indicators.

The tumors arising from the lateral part of the greater wing of sphenoid bone tend to enlarge before they are symptomatic. They cause progressive proptosis and fullness of the temporalis fossa **(Figure 10A).**

Computed tomography: The tumor is well defined, and shows intracranial, intraorbital and temporalis fossa components, the orbital component extending at the apex and along the posterolateral wall of the orbit. The bones may show lysis **(Figure 10B)** or hyperostosis **(Figure 11).** The tumor enhances on contrast.

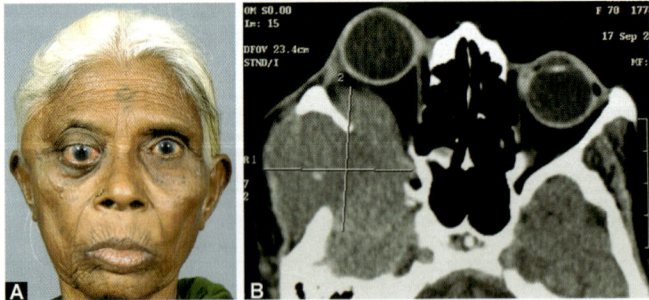

Figures 10A and B: (A) Clinical photograph of patient with sphenoid ridge meningioma, with proptosis and fullness of the right temporal region. (B) Axial CT scan of the same patient, showing large tri-radiate soft tissue lesion extending intracranially, into the temporal fossa and the orbit. The lesion is centered on the area of the sphenoid ridge, which shows bone destruction

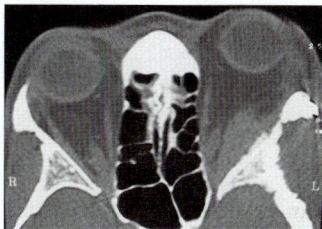

Figure 11: Axial CT scan of sphenoid ridge meningioma, showing hyperostosis of the sphenoid bone and soft tissue lesion adjoining the lateral wall of the orbit

Differential diagnosis: Rarely, other tumors with both orbital and intra-cranial components, and showing lysis of the sphenoid bone, may mimic sphenoid ridge meningiomas.

Investigations: Neuroimaging may pick up other intracranial meningiomata. The definite diagnosis is by histopathological examination if a biopsy specimen.

Treatment: if the tumor is well-defined, it may be excised completely. Otherwise debulking of the tumor can provide relief from the symptoms. Residual or recurrent tumor after surgery can be treated by external beam radiotherapy.

Lymphoproliferative Disease of the Orbit

Signs: Lymphoproliferative disease of the orbit presents as a gradual onset of mass effect in the orbit. The eye may or may not show significant proptosis.

Computed tomography: There will be presence of orbital lesion bilaterally in 30% of the patients. The lesion is often extra-conal, and superotemporal orbit is a common location. The lymphoproliferative lesions have smooth, regular outlines. The lesion extends into tissue spaces, conforming to the existing orbital structures. This 'molding' around structures is a very characteristic feature of lymphoproliferative disease, whether reactive lymphoid hyperplasia, atypical lymphoid hyperplasia or lymphoma **(Figures 12A and B)**.

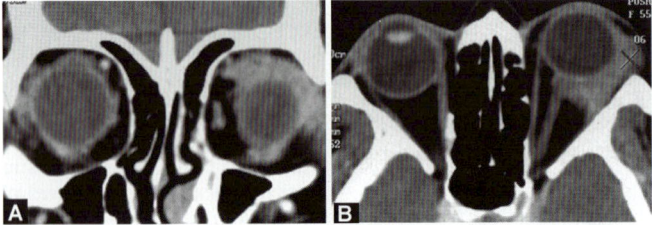

Figures 12A and B: Axial and coronal CT scans of non-Hodgkin lymphoma in superolateral orbit, moulding around the globe without indentation

Differential diagnosis: Specific or non-specific orbital inflammatory disease must be differentiated from lymphoproliferative disorders.

Investigations: Biopsy of the suspicious lesion is the investigation of choice. Further systemic evaluation and choice of tests depends on the histopathological features of the biopsied specimen.

Treatment: Isolated orbital disease is treated by locoregional radiotherapy. Systemic involvement with lymphoma requires chemotherapy.

Lacrimal Fossa Tumors: Pleomorphic Adenoma

Signs and symptoms: The patient presents with eccentric proptosis and inferomedial displacement of the globe. Often there is a palpable mass in the superotemporal orbit.

Computed tomography: On a CT scan, a benign lacrimal tumor like pleomorphic adenoma will appear as a globular enlargement of the lacrimal gland, with smooth borders and homogeneous internal consistency. The large lacrimal gland may displace the globe inferomedially. A long-standing tumor would cause fossa formation in the adjacent bone **(Figure 13).**

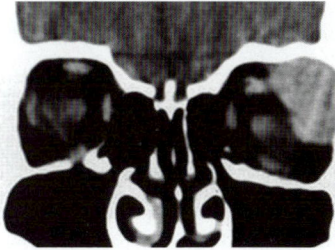

Figure 13: Coronal CT scan of pleomorphic adenoma shows well-defined lesion in the superolateral orbit, with smooth outline, heterogeneous internal density, separat from extraocular muscles, with fossa formation in the frontal bone

Differential diagnosis: Inflammations and lymphoproliferative disease of the lacrimal gland would have a more diffuse outline, and tend to conform to the contours of surrounding structures.

Malignant lacrimal gland tumors may have irregular borders. They may extend posteriorly in the orbit, as well as extend beyond the midline in the coronal plane. There can be erosion of the adjacent bone. Any malignant tumor may infiltrate the orbital structures such as the extraocular muscles; hence the muscle may not be distinguishable from the mass on a CT scan **(Figure 14A and B)**.

Investigation: Any suspicion of malignancy should be followed up with biopsy and histopathological examination of the lesion.

Management: A pleomorphic adenoma of a lacrimal gland may be removed in toto through a suitable orbitototmy incision.

Orbital Invasion of Paranasal Sinus Disease

Signs and symptoms: A secondary tumor or fungal granuloma commonly extends to the orbit from an adjoining paranasal sinus. The patient presents with pain, progressive non-axial proptosis, dystopia of the globe, and limitation of ocular motility.

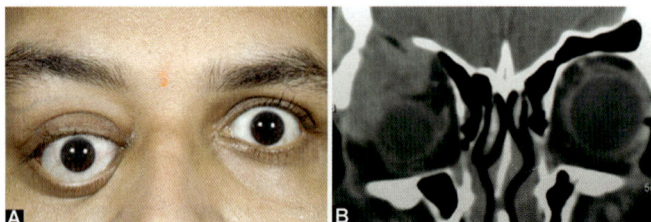

Figures 14A and B: (A) Clinical photograph of patient with adenoid cystic carcinoma of the right lacrimal gland, showing proptosis with inferior and medial displacement of the globe, superior sulcus fullness, and visible enlargement of the right lacrimal gland. (B) Coronal CT scan of the same patient, showing soft tissue lesion in right superolateral orbit, with irregular outline, infiltrating right superior and lateral recti, with erosion of the orbital roof

Computed tomography: A homogeneous irregular mass would be seen extending from the paranasal sinus, most commonly the maxillary sinus. The mass enhances only slightly with contrast. The bony orbital wall between the sinus and the orbit is seen eroded. The mass lesion is seen displacing the globe in the opposite direction. The mass may be infiltrating the corresponding rectus muscle, which can no longer be identified separately on the image **(Figures 15A and B).**

Differential diagnosis: A lesion eroding the bony wall of the orbit and entering from the sinus may also be a mucocele. A sinus mucocele is however, smooth in outline.

Investigation: A biopsy specimen obtained by endoscopic sinus surgery or through an orbitotomy is essential for the histopathological diagnosis.

Management: The treatment of the condition varies according to the diagnosis obtained on histopathologic examination, and the extent of the disease.

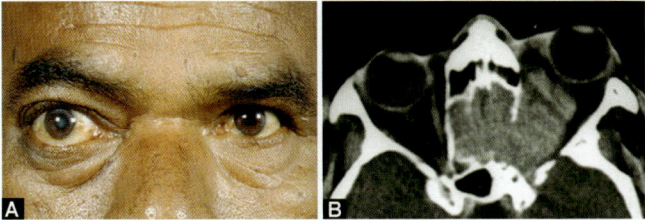

Figures 15A and B: (A) Clinical photograph of patient with fungal granuloma of the right paranasal sinus and orbit, showing right proptosis with lateral displacement of the globe. (B) Axial CT scan of the same patient showing the soft tissue shadow of the fungal granuloma in the ethmoid sinuses, eroding the medial wall of the orbit and extending into the orbit

COMBINED INTRACONAL AND EXTRACONAL PATHOLOGY

Orbital Hemorrhage

Signs and symptoms: The patient usually presents with a history of trauma. There is rapid and progressive proptosis, pain, periorbital edema, ecchymoses, and limitation of ocular motility. The mass effect on the optic nerve may cause diminished vision.

Computed tomography: An orbital hemorrhage is seen as a diffuse or well-defined shadow of soft-tissue density on computed tomography. There may be associated fracture of orbital bones **(Figure 16).**

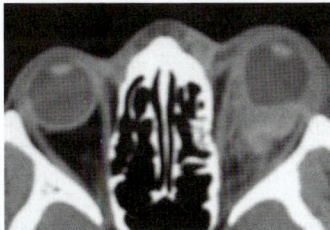

Figure 16: Axial CT scan showing soft tissue density shadows in orbital hematoma. The extreme proptosis of the globe has stretched the optic nerve and caused tenting of the globe at the posterior pole

Magnetic resonance imaging: A diffuse or well-defined soft tissue shadow may be present in the orbit. The hematoma may be intraconal, extraconal, or combined. A sub-periosteal hematoma is seen as a well-demarcated lesion adjacent to the bony orbital wall, and delimited by the extent of the bony sutures. The intensity of the hematoma depends on the age of the hemorrhage: an acute hemorrhage is iso-intense on T1-weighted sequences, and hypo-intense on T2-weighted sequences. A sub-acute presentation, within 2 days of the hemorrhage, shows hyper-intensity in both T1- and T2-weighted images. A chronic hemorrhage is hyper-intense in T1 sequences, and hypo-intense in T2 images **(Figures 17A and B).**

Differential diagnosis: An orbital hemorrhage is to be differentiated from tissue edema due to trauma. The trauma may also be accompanied by an orbital fracture.

Treatment: An orbital hematoma causing significant mass effect and compromising the visual function should be drained surgically.

Lymphangioma

Signs and symptoms: The deep lymphangiomas present with spontaneous, rapidly progressing proptosis; this is due to

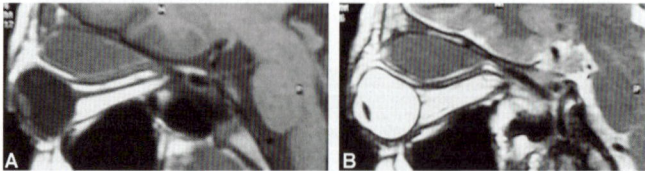

Figures 17A and B: (A) Sagittal view of T1-weighted sequence or sub-periosteal hematoma orbit. The hematoma is delimited, adjacent to the orbital roof, is hyper-intense to vitreous but hypo-intense to the orbital fat, and stretching the optic nerve. (B) Sagittal view of the same in T2-weighted sequence, where the hematoma is hypo-intense to the vitreous

hemorrhage into a previously undetected lesion. There may be restriction of ocular motility and strabismus. There may be features of optic nerve compression such as disc edema or relative afferent pupillary defect. The combined lymphangiomas are extensive, with both superficial and deep components. There may be prolonged history of proptosis, and episodes of hemorrhage. The superficial lesions in the periocular skin or conjunctiva may show clear fluid or blood.

Computed tomography: A long-standing lesion will cause enlargement of the bony orbit. The lymphangioma is a diffuse non-encapsulated soft tissue shadow, which may extend in both the intraconal and extraconal compartments, as well as in the preseptal area. The internal consistency is non-homogeneous, with some areas of low-density cyst-like appearance. Blood levels may be seen in some views. Circumscribed lymphangiomas resemble cavernous hemangiomas, and may even show phleboliths. On contrast injections, there may be irregular areas of enhancement, or rim enhancement **(Figure 18).**

MRI scan: MRI scan will depict a diffuse lesion, with multiple cystic spaces. The spaces may show fluid-fluid levels, which have different intensities due to difference in paramagnetic properties of blood of various ages. After contrast injection, there may be enhancement of some of the solid parts of the tumor **(Figures 19A and B).**

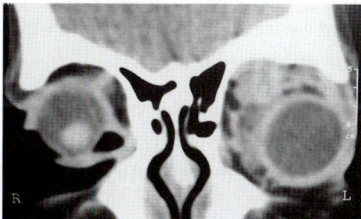

Figure 18: Coronal CT scan of orbital lymphangioma, showing diffuse lesion with heterogeneous density in the superior orbit, and fossa formation in the adjacent bone

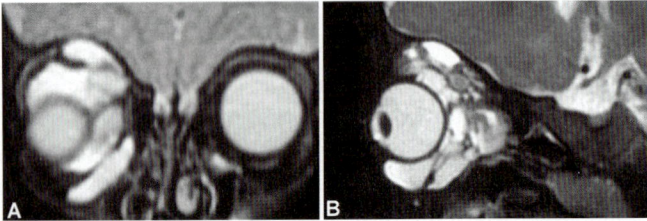

Figures 19A and B: Coronal and sagittal views of T2-weighted MR imaging in orbital lymphangioma, shows diffuse multi-loculated lesion, with variable intensity in different areas

Differential diagnosis: The lymphangioma should be distinguished from other vascular lesions of the orbit. A circumscribed lymphangioma may closely mimic a cavernous hemangioma.

Treatment: A lymphangioma with bleeding, or one causing a mass effect, is surgically debulked. Due to diffuse involvement of orbital tissues, complete excision may not be possible.

Orbital Varix

Orbital varices are distensible venous malformations of the orbit.

Signs and symptoms: A deep orbital varix causes intermittent proptosis enophthalmos due to fat atrophy, occasional bruising, and expansion on bending or Valsalva maneuver. There may be an accompanying superficial component with dark, tortuous Epibulbar or lid vessels. There may extensive involvement of peri-orbital or intracranial regions.

Imaging: An orbital varix has a smooth fusiform or globular appearance, and enhances strongly with contrast, increases in size during Valsalva maneuver during dynamic CT scanning.

Other investigation: Increased size of the lesion is seen on A- and B-scan ultrasonography. Venography can demonstrate abnormal saccular vessels flowing out through venous channels in the face, pterygopalatine fossa and cavernous sinus.

Differential diagnosis: The orbital varix is to be distinguished from other vascular lesions of the orbit.

Treatment: Most orbital varices can be safely observed. Surgical excision is technically difficult. Intraoperative venography and glue embolisation may be helpful, followed by excision.

INTRACONAL LESIONS OF THE ORBIT

Vascular Lesions of the Orbit

Orbital Hemangioma

Signs and symptoms: cavernous hemangiomas present in adults with gradually progressing proptosis. There may be associated globe indentation, choroidal folds and optic nerve displacement.

Computed tomography: Cavernous hemangiomas are well-circumscribed smooth ovoid intraconal masses that enhance with contrast. Long-standing extraconal masses may cause bony fossa formation **(Figure 20A)**. The globe is proptosed, and may show indentation **(Figure 20B)**. The optic nerve is displaced in a large intraconal lesion. Small areas of high density representing calcification are seen in the presence of phleboliths.

Magnetic resonance imaging: The MRI scan shows a well-circumscribed intraconal mass, which is round or ovoid. In T1 weighted sequences, it is hypointense relative to orbital fat, and isointense to muscle. In T2 weighted sequences, it is hyper-intense to fat and muscle. The tumor shows marked

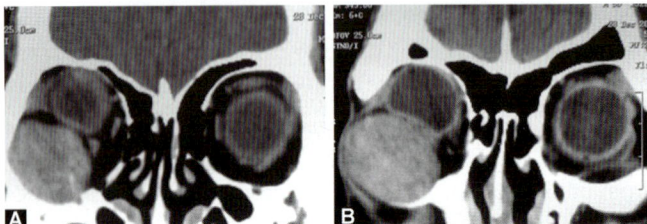

Figures 20A and B: (A) Coronal CT scan of orbital cavernous hemangioma showing ovoid lesion with smooth outline, with fossa formation in adjacent bone. (B) Coronal CT scan of the same patient, showing indentation of the globe by the tumor

enhancement after contrast injection in T1 weighted images **(Figures 21A and B).**

Differential diagnosis: Cavernous hemangioma should be differentiated from hemangiopericytoma and circumscribed lymphangioma. The latter may have phleboliths, but will have heterogeneous internal density. Diffuse lymphangiomas are heterogeneous with irregular margins.

Treatment: Cavernous hemangiomas can easily be excised in toto by a suitable orbitotomy approach.

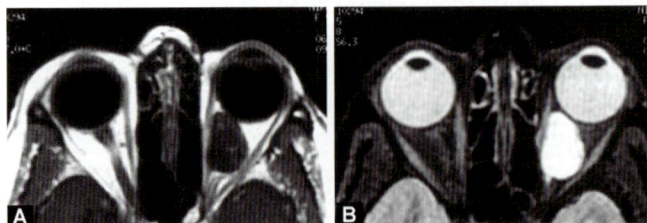

Figures 21A and B: (A) T1-weighted MRI of intraconal cavernous hemangioma, hypo-intense tumor with smooth outline. (B) T2-weighted MR image of the same tumor: the tumor appears hyper-intense in T2 sequences

NEUROGENIC LESIONS OF THE ORBIT

Optic Nerve Sheath Meningioma

Introduction: Optic nerve meningiomas are slow growing tumors. They may be extradural, subdural, or combined.

Signs and symptoms: The primary symptom is the diminished visual function. In early stages, it may be subtle such as defective color vision, enlargement of the blind spot, and transient obscuration of vision. The advanced disease, the visual acuity is diminished, and there is constriction of the visual fields.

The patient may have mild proptosis. The fundus examination may show choroidal folds, optic nerve head edema and opticociliary shunt vessels.

Computed tomography: The optic nerve on CT scan is enlarged, in a tubular or globular fashion. There may be a central low-density linear 'tram-track' appearance, which denotes the optic nerve. There may be a nodular appearance where the tumor breaks through the dura into the orbital tissues. It may sometimes grow eccentrically and produce amass on one side of the optic nerve. Some tumors may show flecks of high-density calcification, or adjacent hyperostosis. About 6% may be bilateral **(Figure 22A).**

MRI Imaging: On T1 weighted images, the meningioma is a tubular or fusiform lesion, iso-intense or hypointense to the optic nerve. Fat suppressed T1 images better demonstrate the tumor and its extension into the orbital soft tissue, distinct from the optic nerve. On T2 weighted images, the tumor is isointense or hyper-intense to the orbital fat **(Figure 22B)**.

T1 weighted sequences after contrast injection show the enhancement of the tumor, and are the best for detecting intracanalicular or intracranial extension of the tumor.

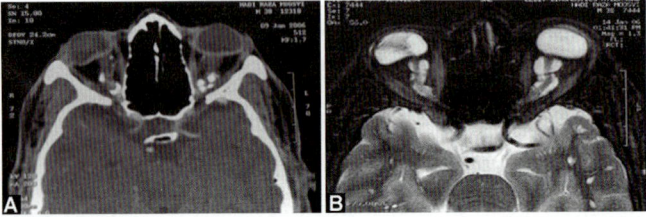

Figures 22A and B: (A) Axial CT scan of bilateral optic nerve sheath meningioma, showing thickening of optic nerve, with few flecks of calcification. (B) Axial view of the same in a T2-weighted MRI sequence, showing hyper-intense thickening of the optic nerve sheath bilaterally, with central hypo-intense shadow of the optic nerve

Investigation: Imaging of the brain is required to rule out other intracranial meningiomata, which are found in 5% of bilateral meningiomas.

Differential diagnosis: Optic nerve meningioma should be differentiated from optic nerve glioma on imaging, because both may cause fusiform enlargement of the optic nerve. However, the optic nerve glioma has a smooth outline, while the meningioma has a nodular appearance due to the extradural extension. Further, optic nerve glioma may show a buckling or kinking, which a meningioma will not.

Treatment: An isolated anterior meningioma may be resected. A meningioma causing progressive visual loss may be treated with external beam radiotherapy. An eye with no visual prognosis, with severe proptosis is occasionally exenterated along with resection of the intracranial tumor.

Optic Nerve Glioma

Optic nerve gliomas are low-grade astrocytomas that present early in life. They may be confined to the orbit, or have chiasmal and extrachiasmal involvement.

Signs and symptoms: The patient may present with visual loss, progressive proptosis and strabismus. On examination, the child may have optic disc edema, optic atrophy, or constricted visual fields.

Approximately 30% of patients with optic nerve glioma may have features of neurofibromatosis type 1.

CT scan imaging: CT scan appearance of an optic nerve glioma is generally characteristic, with fusiform swelling, which has smooth outlines. The optic nerve may be kinked. The lesion may have a few low density areas of cystic degeneration **(Figure 23A)**.

MRI scan: On MRI, the enlargement of the optic nerve shows a fusiform appearance, with iso-intense to nervous tissue. The lesion may have a hypo-intense surrounding arachnoid hyperplasia. The T2 weighted image is hyper-intense, occasionally heterogeneous, and has peripheral hypo-intense arachnoid hyperplasia. The tumor shows enhancement on contrast injection. Contrast enhancement also helps to identify the extension of the glioma intra-cranially **(Figure 23B)**.

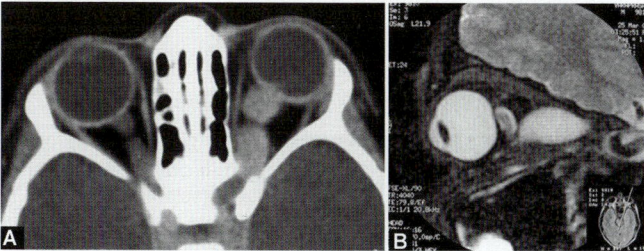

Figures 23A and B: (A) Axial CT scan of bilateral optic nerve glioma shows fusiform swellings of the optic nerve, and proptosis. (B) Sagittal view, T2-weighted MR imaging of optic nerve glioma. The Optic nerve shows fusiform enlargements, which are hyperintense, with a small hypo-intense area, and kinking of the optic nerve

Investigation: A biopsy may be required to distinguish an optic nerve glioma from a meningioma, in which case it should be remembered that the surrounding arachnoid hyperplasia may give a confounding histopathologic diagnosis.

Treatment: If there is a visual deterioration, the condition may be treated with chemotherapy or radiotherapy. A rapidly growing tumor may need tumor resection, with a tumor-free proximal end of the optic nerve.

Extraocular Extension of Intraocular Tumor

Signs and symptoms: The patient presents with proptosis and diminished vision. Retinoblastoma is a common cause of orbital extension of intraocular tumor. The child in an advanced stage of retinoblastoma would present with leucocoria, as well as proptosis and limitation of extraocular movement. The condition may be painful, and inflammatory signs such as lid edema may be present.

Computed tomography: The intraocular tumor is visible within the globe. In a retinoblastoma, the CT scan will show an intraocular tumor with high density areas of calcification. There may be a discontinuity in the sclera, and the tumor is seen to extend into the orbital tissues as a homogenous irregular mass lesion. A thickened optic nerve denotes optic nerve extension of the tumor **(Figure 24).**

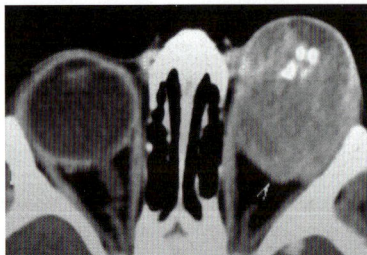

Figure 24: Axial view of CT scan in orbital extension of retinoblastoma. The globe is filled with a soft tissue density shadow of the tumor, with a few high density spots of calcification. The posterior contour of the globe is disrupted, and the tumor extends into the orbit

Investigations: the clinical features and imaging are characteristic. In doubtful cases incision biopsy may be performed.

Bone marrow biopsy, CSF cytology and CT scan brain are performed to rule out remote spread of tumor.

Treatment: The prognosis is poor. High dose chemotherapy along with enucleation and external beam radiotherapy can reduce the mortality.

Optic Neuritis

Signs and symptoms: Optic neuritis presents with diminution of vision; the color vision and contrast sensitivity are affected earlier than the visual acuity. There may be recurrent episodes, other cranial nerve palsies associated.

Magnetic resonance imaging: The MRI shows an abnormality in 54 to 85% of the patients with optic neuritis. The optic nerve may show Demyelination in the intraorbital, intracanalicular or intracranial segment. Lesions may be missed if they are smaller than the section thickness. On the T1 sequence, the affected segment of the nerve is iso-intense to normal nerve tissue; it becomes hyper-intense in the fat suppressed Gd-DTPA enhanced sequences, or on T2- weighted images **(Figure 25).**

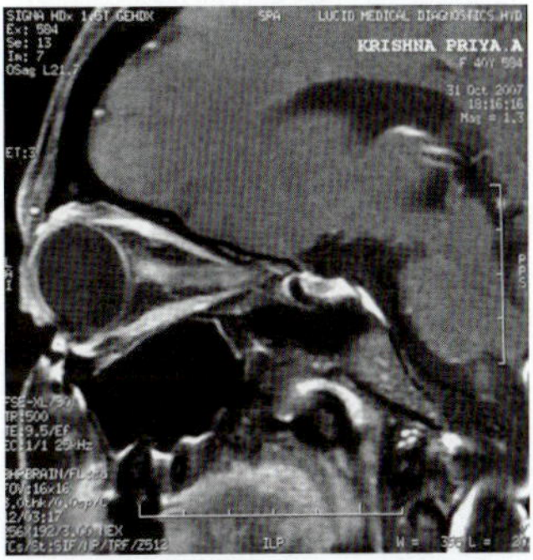

Figure 25: T1-weighted, fat-suppressed sagittal view after Gd-DTPA injection showing enhancement of a segment of intraorbital optic nerve in optic neuritis

Investigation: MRI of the brain may demonstrate other demyelinating plaques.

Management: The management may be conservative, intra-venous steroids or administration of interferon. The reader is advised to consult specific texts for guidelines.

BIBLIOGRAPHY

1. Byrne SF, Green RL. Ultrasound of the Eye and Orbit. Mosby-Year Book, St Louis, 1992.
2. Cockerham KP, Kennerdell JS. In Smith's Ophthalmic Plastic and Reconstructive Surgery, 2nd edition. Mosby-Year Book, St Louis, 1998.
3. De Potter P. Advances in imaging in oculoplastics. Curr Opin Ophthalmol 2001;12:342-6.
4. De Potter P, Flanders AE, Shields CL, Shields JA. Magnetic resonance imaging of orbital tumors. Int Ophthalmol Clin 1993;33(3):163-73.
5. Lemke AJ, Kazi I, Felix R. Magnetic resonance imaging of orbital tumors. Eur Radiol 2006;16:2207-19.
6. Naik MN, Tourani LT, Chandra Sekhar G, Honavar SG. Interpretation of computed tomography imaging of the eye and orbit. A systematic approach. Ind J Ophthalmol 2002;50:339-53.
7. Rootman J. Diseases of the Orbit. A Multidisciplinary Approach. 2nd edition. Lippincott Williams and Wilkins, Philadelphia, 2003.

Orbital Neoplasms

17

Jes Mortenson (Sweden)

INTRODUCTION

Until the computed tomography (CT) was introduced the orbit was considered the "black box" in ophthalmology. The magnetic resonance imaging (MRI) has even put the spotlight on the orbit, which has made it possible to early diagnosing neoplasms of the orbit promising theoretically a better prognosis. That has not been fulfilled as the neoplasms are often seen in an elderly population that will seek help late. The neoplasms have also often a slow growth bringing the patient late to his ophthalmologist, due to symptoms from the visual organs as proptosis, diplopia, ophthalmoplegia, ptosis, anisocoria and pain. Changes in vision due to neuropathy or astigmatism from pressure on the bulb or compression of the bulb inducing choroidal folds are often symptoms coming later.

A completely history especially covering earlier cancers as breast cancer in women and prostate cancer in men, thyroid disorders, autoimmune disease, infectious diseases and medical treatment with immune suppressive treatments.

A complete neuro-ophthalmologic evaluation of the patient with problems from the orbit is mandatory. Exophthalmos is easily measured by a Hertel exophthalmometer; protrusion more than 21 mm and a difference of more than 2 mm between the two eyes is pathologic. The displacement of the eye can give a suspicion where to look for the tumor in the orbit.

A palpation of the orbit will tell if the resistance is soft or hard if any pain is felt which might differ infection/inflammation from a solid neoplasm.

The ophthalmologist is often the first physician but the evaluation and treatment is multidisciplinary involving otorhinolaryngologist, radiologist, oncologist, plastic surgeon and oromaxillofacial surgeon. If metastases to the orbit is suspected further specialists are involved in the search for diagnosis and treatment.

It is not the purpose of this chapter to give a fully description of all neoplasms seen in the orbit, but rather to give a short presentation of the most common types seen by the author and even a very rare type will be presented, the Merkel cell carcinoma.

The adult orbital neoplasms differ from the neoplasms seen in childhood. Most neoplasms are seen late in life and many invade from the paranasal sinus. The neoplasms can primarily arise from the tissue in the orbit itself or secondary from the paranasal sinus and by invasion from neoplasms of the paraorbital skin (eyelids) and metastatic.

Lymphoid tumors are the most common neoplasm of the orbit seen in 10 to 13%. In a population over the age of 60 the incidence accounts for 24% of orbital neoplasms. Many patients have or will developed systemic lymphoma of non-Hodgkin type. The most common seen malignancy in the paranasal sinus is squamous cell carcinoma. Squamous cell carcinoma is seen in 9% of tumors of the eyelids and 10% of carcinomas involving the orbit, but represent one of the most seen skin cancers. In two-thirds of the patients orbital invasion is seen, pointing to a poor prognosis. Adenocarcinomas and adenoid carcinomas make up 5% all of tumors involving the orbit and are highly invasive.

Half of the lacrimal glad tumors are epithelial neoplasms, the other half are malignant lymphoma, benign lymphoid hyperplasia and leukaemia. Inflammatory lesions and lymphoid neoplasms of the lacrimal gland are assessing to be seen 2 to 3 times more common than the epithelial neoplasms.

Orbital meningiomas and schwannomas are most often seen in the fourth to seventh decade of life. 70% of the meningiomas invade the orbit from the cranium. This type of tumor has often a very slow growth, so in the old patient an excision of the tumor might never be needed. The prognosis for good visual acuity after an operation is very poor as the tumor often growth along the optic nerve.

A schwannomas is a benign neoplasm arising from a nerve in the orbit. Seen between 20 to 70 years of age. The therapy is surgical removal of the tumor.

A relatively common vascular lesion of the orbit is the cavernous hemangioma. Most often seen in adults with peak incidence around 40 years of age. It shows a slowly, painless growth over several years with a progressing proptosis. The treatment is surgical excision.

The metastatic tumors represent approximately 8% of all orbital tumors **(Figures 1 and 2)**. Breast carcinoma followed by lung metastasis in women. In the men the most common metastatic tumors are lung and prostate. The mean age is seventy years of age.

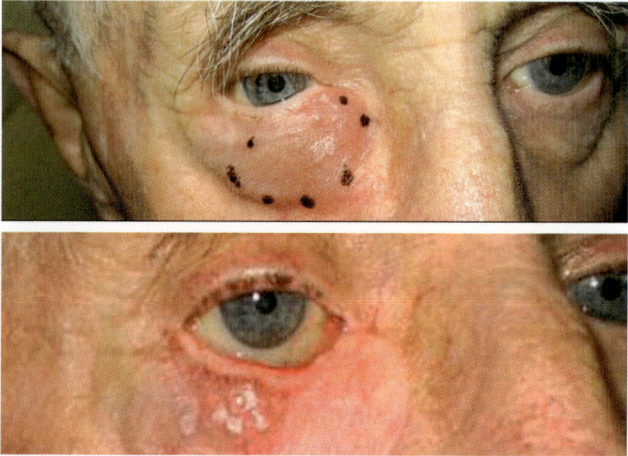

Figures 1 and 2: Recurrence adenocarcinoma

PRIMARY TUMORS OF THE ORBIT

Orbital Lymphoma of the Orbit

Introduction

The most common primary tumor of the orbit is the orbital lymphoma, 10% of the tumors of the orbit, and 40-60% of the lymphoproliferative diseases of the orbit. The lymphomas are often unilateral most often starting in the lacrimal gland.

The new diagnostic positron emission tomography (PET) and gastrointestinal endoscopy will often unveil a systemic non-Hodgkin's lymphoma (NHL) with a secondary spread to the orbit. The majority is NHL and is mainly seen after 50 to 70 years of age **(Figures 3A and B).**

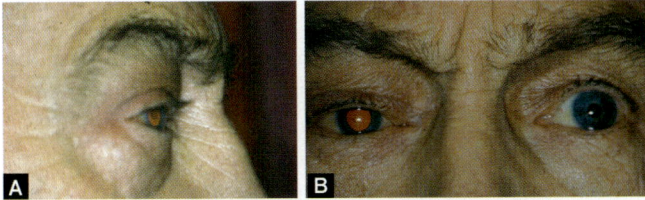

Figures 3A and B: Old man with exophthamos right eye due to slowly growing lymphoma

Clinical Signs and Symptoms

The patient develops a painless proptosis, eyelid edema and the bulb is suppressed downward. The first sign could be diminished vision due to optic neuropathy by compression of the lymphoma at the orbital apex. The growth of the tumor is often very slowly so the patient adapt to the tumor for a long time.

Investigation

MRI (magnetic resonance image) shows a homogeny mass in the superior part of the orbit caste to the bulb and orbital bones. CT (computed tomography) shows a homogeneous texture.

Fine-needle cytology will often give the diagnosis. PET and MRI of the body to look after systemic involvement by the lymphoma.

Differential Diagnosis

The REAL (Revised European-American Classification of Lymphoid Neoplasms) classify the lymphomas in categories based on morphology, immunophenotype, and genotype as indolent, aggressive and highly aggressive.

Treatment

Radiotherapy is advocated in local low-grade orbital lymphoma only, but if any suspicion on systemic involvement systemic chemotherapy is advocated to control the lymphomas. For the more aggressive type systemic chemotherapy and local radiation therapy is advocated. A new treatment is monoclonal immunotherapy in low-grade lymphomas especially in very old and weak patients.

In the most aggressive lymphomas aggressive chemotherapy followed by stem cells transplantation has been used.

Inference

Orbital lymphomas are the most common tumor of the orbit, often unilateral. The tumor is insidious bringing the patient to the ophthalmologist first after long time. The visual acuity might be reduced, and a painless proptosis is seen. MRI and fine-needle cytology will give the diagnosis in most cases. Systemic involvement should always be looked for.

Squamous Cell Carcinoma

Introduction

Squamous cell carcinoma (SCC) **(Figure 4)** is seen in 9% of tumors of the eyelids and 10% of carcinomas involving the orbit, but represent one of the most seen skin cancers. SCC inflicts mostly elderly individuals. Seen most often in fair-skinned individuals who have been exposed to sunlight as the skin of the face, hands and the scalp. Australian has again as in basal cells cancer the highest incidence in the world: 166 per 100,000 persons. It can metastasize and can locally spread aggressively.

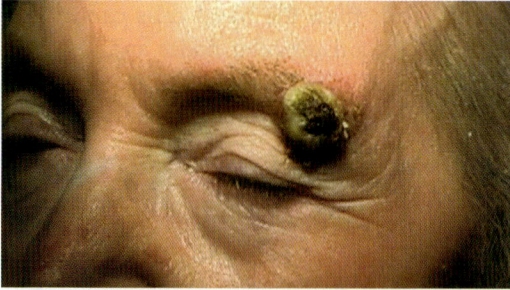

Figure 4: Squamous cell cancer

Predisposing factors of SCC is ultraviolet lightment treatments, chronic skin inflammation and in immunosuppressed individuals.

Clinical Signs and Symptoms

Often seen as an ulcerated lesion with induration and erythema of the inflicted skin **(Figure 5)**. The spread is locally invasive, deep into the connective tissue. It can spread via the lymphatic glands. The SCC tends to have a more

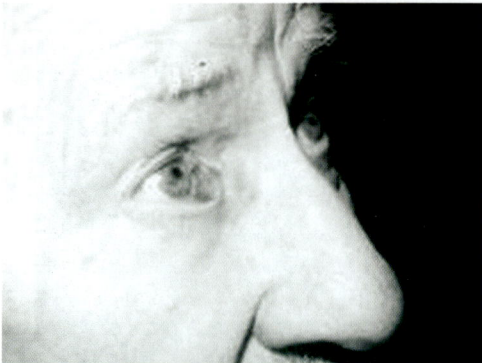

Figure 5: Recurrence of squamous cell canthus carcinoma

aggressive spread than the basal cells cancer. Look for involvement of the preauricular nodes and submandibular nodes.

Investigation

The same as with the basal cells cancer: Computed tomography (CT) and magnetic resonance imaging (MRI) **(Figure 6)**. The CT is the best tool for determining the bone destruction and MRI will show the invasion into soft tissue especially if perineural spread of the tumor is suspected. Perineural spread points at a solemn prognosis.

In the SCC the risk for spread via the lymph glands must be investigated.

Patients with the orbital apex syndrome or superior orbital fissure syndrome: pain, complete ptosis, and ophthalmoplegia indicate that the spread of the SCC is far reached.

Differential Diagnosis

Other cancers involving the eyelids, canthus and epicanthus and even the conjunctiva, basal cells cancer, melanoma

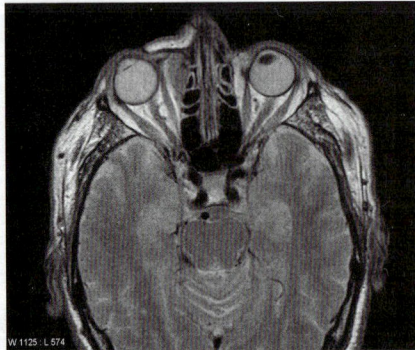

Figure 6: Recurrence of squamous cancer right orbita

especially the amelanotic type even lymphoma, sebaceous gland tumors and metastatic tumors with ulceration can be difficult clinically to different from squamous cell carcinoma.

Treatment

Radical surgery guided by the frozen section to be sure that the margins are free of tumor cells. Exenteration if the SCC is invasive into the orbit followed by radiotherapy. As said perineural spread is a very bad prognostic sign. The mortality rate is as high as 40% in squamous cell cancers involving the eyelids. Delayed diagnosis and inadequate, primary treatment are the factors that lead to invasive growth into the orbit.

Inference

The squamous cell cancer is a very common seen cancer of the skin. As the basal cells cancer seen in a fair-skinned individual exposed for sunlight.

The squamous cell cancers are 9% of the cancers involving the eyelids and 10% of the cancers involving the orbit.

The mortality rate is as high as 40% in squamous cell cancers involving the eyelids due to the risk of metastases and aggressive growth of the tumor. It is of the highest importance that the primary surgery shall be radical as inadequate treatment leaving cancer cells, often leads to recurrence of the tumor in spite of radiotherapy.

Basal Cell Carcinoma

Introduction

Basal cells carcinomas represent 90% of periocular tumors with orbital invasion. The exposure to sunlight is thought to be the major cause particularly in fair-skinned people. Especially seen in a fair-skinned population, which have migrated to a sunny climate as the white population in Australia, which have the highest incidence of skin cancers in the world, ranging from 650 to 1560 cases per 100,000 persons.

Clinical Signs and Symptoms

The BCC is classified into 4 types: Nodular ulcerative BCC, sclerosing BCC, superficial BCC and basosquamous BCC.

The nodular ulcerative BBC **(Figure 7)** is the most common type seen in 75% of the BBC tumors. The tumor start as a little papule, further growing form a central necrosis with a sclerosing round border, a rodent ulcer, which seldom invade the orbit.

The sclerosing BCC present as the name tells an indurated plaque without distinct borders often with a deep invasion into the dermis. This type is invasive into the orbit and accounts for near 15% of all BCC **(Figure 8)**.

The superficial BCC looks like dermatitis of chronic type **(Figure 9)**.

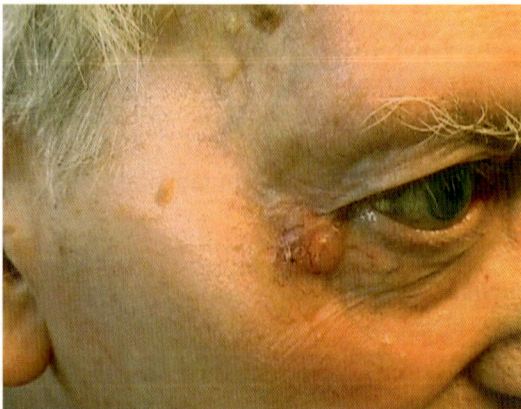

Figure 7: Nodular basal cells carcinoma

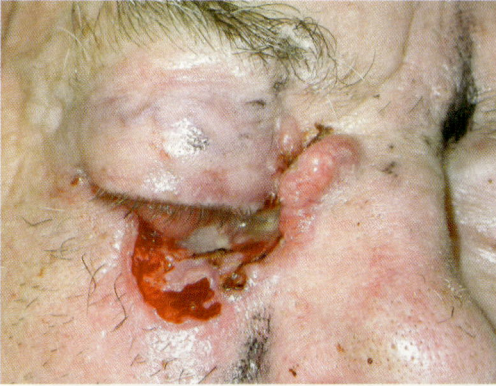

Figure 8: Basal cells cancer ingrowth orbit

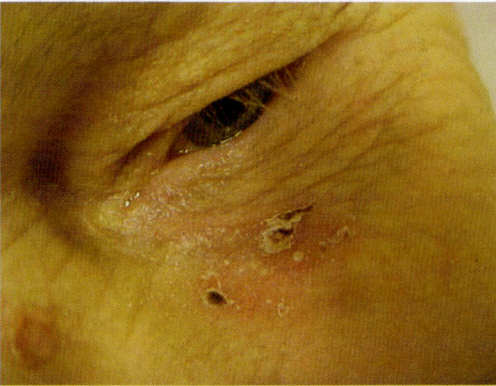

Figure 9: The superficial BCC

The basosquamous type of BCC may clinically look like the nodular type but is most more liable to grow invasive and even to metastasize **(Figure 10)**.

The typical patient is middle-aged person who has been working in the open air or has been exposed to actinic radiation for a long time.

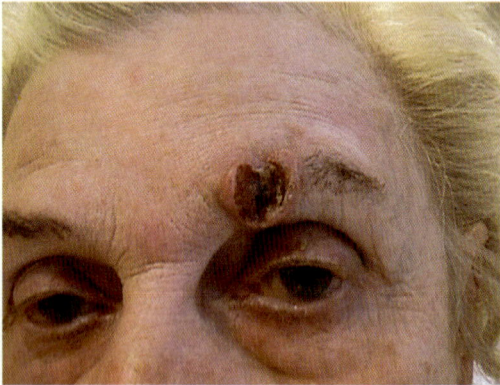

Figure 10: Highly aggressive BCC morphea basaliom

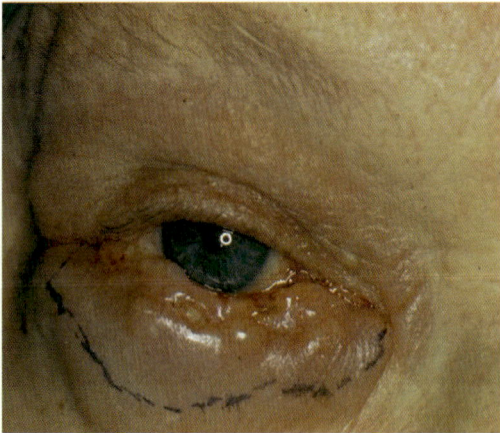

Figure 11: BCC inferior eyelid

The tumor is often seen in the lower eyelid **(Figure 11)**, medial canthus and more seldom the lateral canthus and upper eyelid.

If the complain is pain and restricted movement of the bulb or proptosis invasion into the orbit should be suspected.

Investigation

Computed tomography (CT) and magnetic resonance imaging (MRI). The CT is the best tool for determining the bone destruction and MRI will show the invasion into soft tissue especially if perineural spread of the tumor is suspected.

Differential Diagnosis

Melanoma especially amelanotic can be difficult to distinguish from BCC. Squamous cell carcinoma and sebaceous gland tumors can even be difficult to distinguish clinically. Metastatic tumors involving the skin, e.g. breast carcinoma.

Treatment

The best treatment is surgical excision of the tumor with clear margins verified by the pathologist. In orbital invasion exenteration is the preferred technique to be sure that the tumor is totally removed. Radiation is not recommended as a high risk of recurrence of the tumor is seen after radiotherapy. The recurrent tumor is often much more biologically aggressive **(Figure 12)**.

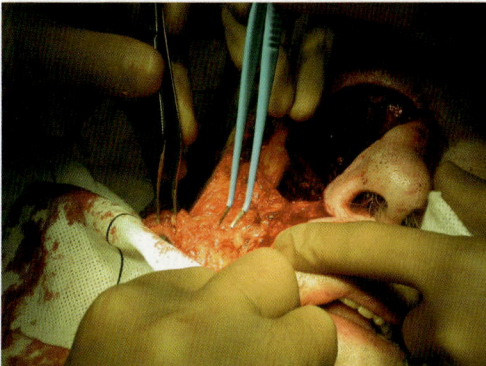

Figure 12: Exenteration of invasive BCC

Inference

The basal cell carcinoma account for 90% of the periocular skin tumors with orbital invasion. Four subtypes are described: Nodular ulcerative BCC, sclerosing BCC, superficial BCC and basosquamous BCC.

The BCC is seen in a fair-skinned individual who has been exposed for a long time to bright sunlight. The highest incidence of BCC in the world is seen in Australia in the white population. Treatment is surgically excision, excenteration if invasion to the orbit is seen. Radiotherapy is not advocated, as the risk for recurrence of a biologically aggressive BCC is very high.

Melanoma

Introduction

Melanoma affecting the eyelids accounts for 1% of the cancers afflicting the periocular skin and is 1% of melanomas seen elsewhere in the skin of the body.

Three types are described, melanoma arising from a Hutchinson's melanotic freckle or lentigo maligna **(Figure 13)**, nodular melanoma **(Figure 14)** and from premalignant melanosis or cutaneous melanoma in situ **(Figures 15 and 16)**.

The incidence of malignant melanoma is the fastest growing in Sweden. The cause to that is the popularity to have tanned skin. The risk for developing melanoma increases if the child has heavy sunburn early in life. The risk is higher in individuals with red or fair hair and freckled skin.

Clinical Signs and Symptoms

Lentigo maligna is seen in an elderly Caucasian that has been exposed to sunlight. Often seen in skin with degeneration

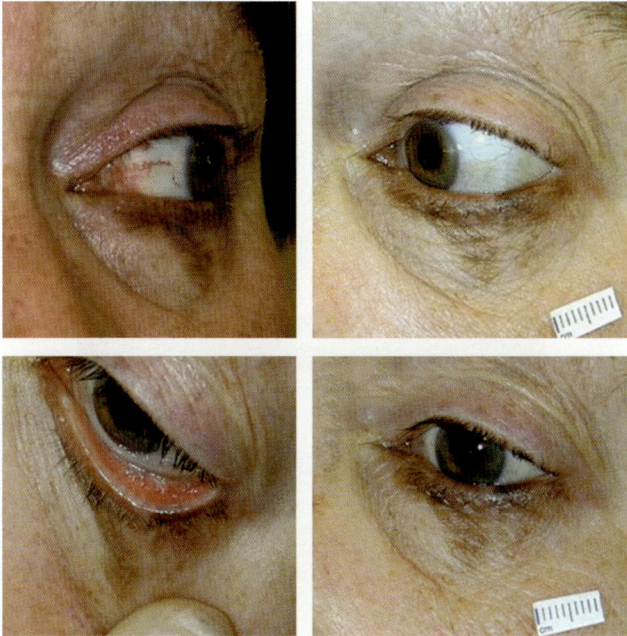

Figure 13: Lentigo maligna

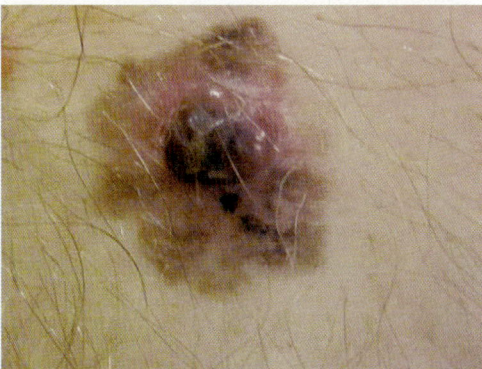

Figure 14: Nodular melanoma

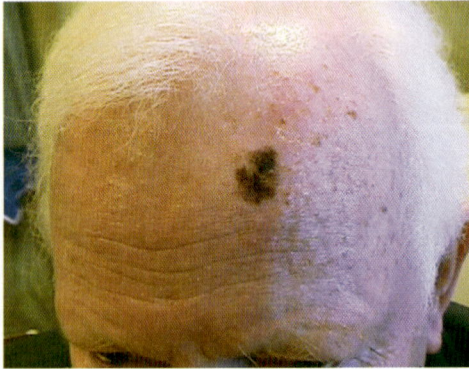

Figure 15: Melanoma *in situ*

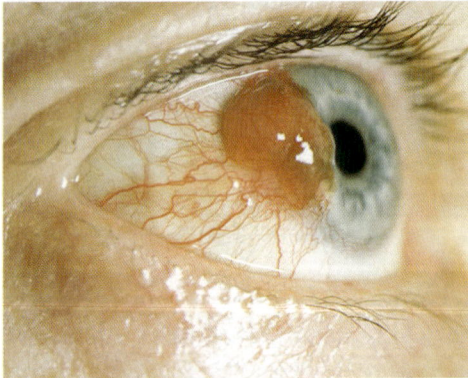

Figure 16: Nodular melanoma in conjunctiva

after solar exposure. Look as a nodular invasive area with pigmentation and an irregular outline. Is most likely to be inflicting the lower eyelid and canthus. Low grade of malignancy is seen, but the risk for developing into malignant melanoma is estimated to be 25 to 30%. Suspicion for malignant transformation should be when a change in color or shape is seen.

The premalignant melanosis is seen in the skin and the conjunctiva and is often more demarcated than the lentigo maligna indicating invasion of the dermis. The tumor is seen both in sun-exposed and unexposed skin.

Nodular melanoma can develop from a pre-existing junctional nevus. The melanoma can be no pigmented **(Figure 17),** but is usually pigmented. Seen in sun-exposed and unexposed skin, conjunctiva and mucosal membranes. Has a rapid growth and is highly invasive.

Investigation

CT scans and MRI is essential as shown in the other tumor types. As the melanoma has a high risk of sending metastases, a systemic screening especially investigation of the lungs, liver and lymph node mapping. The prognosis depends on the thickness of the melanoma the degree of invasion and metastases found.

Differential Diagnosis

Basal cells cancer can be pigmented **(Figure 18)** and difficult to distinguish from melanoma. Squamous cell carcinoma can

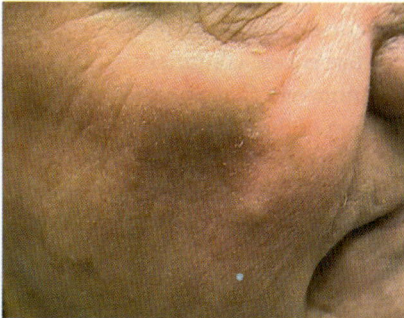

Figure 17: Amelanotic melanoma

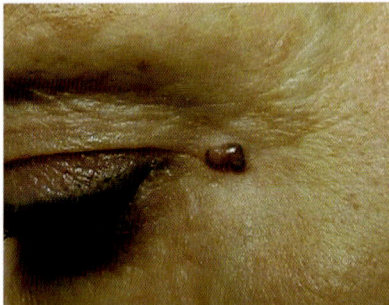

Figure 18: Pigmented BCC

be confused with an amelanotic melanoma as the tumor can be bleeding and the surrounding skin showing inflammation. A very rare type of melanoma can be confused with recurrent chalazion: desmoplastic malignant melanoma, which has an aggressive growth with potential to invade the orbit.

Treatment

Complete surgical excision with wide margins is recommended as soon as possible; do not wait for answer from a biopsy. If orbital invasion is found, the treatment is exenteration. If suspicion of spread to the regional lymph glands a neck dissection followed by chemotherapy or radiation. In superficial conjunctival melanomas topical therapy with mitomycin C can be tried.

Early detection of the melanoma is very important, if the melanomas has reached an invasive growth and send metastases, the prognosis for cure is very poor.

Inference

Melanoma of the periocular skin and conjunctiva is a rare tumor. Three subtypes are described, lentigo maligna, nodular melanoma and premalignant melanosis. Melanomas of the eyelids occur in Caucasian. The melanomas have a high risk of distant metastases. Early detection is very important for a good prognosis.

Surgical excision of the melanoma with a broad margin as soon as possible is mandatory.

Merkel Cell Carcinoma

Introduction

Merkel cell carcinoma is a very rare type of cancer of the skin. The Merkel cell carcinoma is a neuroendocrine carcinoma arising from uncontrolled growth of Merkel cells in the skin. Predominantly seen in fair-skinned individuals over the age of 60 years. Seen in sun-exposed areas. The patient is seeking the doctors due to a fast growing skin tumor with red to blue colour **(Figure 19)**.

Clinical Signs and Symptoms

A fast growing firm, painless, flesh-colored tumor on the neck, head, eyelid, arms.

Investigations

Biopsy of the tumor will give the diagnosis. A thorough investigation follows in the search for metastases as even small

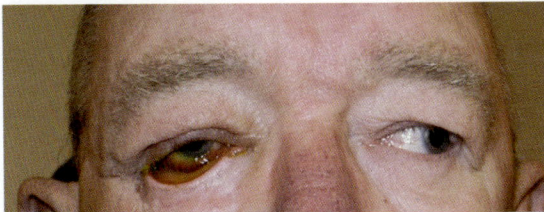

Figure 19: Recurrence of Merkel cell carcinoma restricted eye movement due to orbital invasion

Merkel cell carcinomas have the potential to metastasizing firstly to the regional lymph nodes later to liver, bone, lungs and brain.

Differential Diagnosis

Other neuroendocrine tumors and other infiltrative tumors as melanoma, basal cell cancer and squamous cell cancer are candidates.

Treatment

It is important to know the stage of the Merkel cell carcinoma.

Stage 1: The primary tumor has not spared to lymph nodes or other distance parts of the body.

Stage 2: The cancer has spread to nearby lymph nodes.

Stage 3: The cancer has spread to nearby lymph nodes and other distance parts of the body.

Recurrent stage: The cancer has recurred after treatment

Wide surgical excision, radiation and chemotherapy are recommended in stage 2. In stage 1, surgery followed by regional radiation to the lymph nodes. In stage 3, chemotherapy. In recurrent stage all three treatments might be tried.

The mortality is extremely high, increasing with age.

Inference

Merkel cell carcinoma is very uncommon, highly aggressive with an alarming mortality.

CONCLUSION

The evaluation and treatment of neoplasms of the orbit is a multidisciplinary task involving otorhinolaryngologist, radiologist, oncologist, plastic surgeon, oromaxillofacial surgeon and ophthalmologist. In bigger hospitals orbital teams are already organized to cope with the task so no time is loosed.

An increase in incidence has been reported of the most common seen tumor, lymphoma in most countries. In some parts of the world HIV (human immunodeficiency viruses) has been the cause to the increase. In Denmark a study over the period 1974 to 1996 has shown a steady increase in the incidence of both benign and malignant orbital neoplasms. The more widely use of immunosuppressants is thought to be the course.

(Courtesy to my colleagues at the otorhinolaryngeal department University Hospital Örebro for providing information and pictures: Hans Gertze'n,MD, Christer Nilsson,MD, Hans Gustafsson,MD, Svante Hugosson,MD.

Courtesy to Jan-Erik Axelsson,MD Dermatology Clinic Korsta. For providing pictures.

Literature: Orbital Tumors. Diagnosis and Treatment, Editor Zeynel A. Karcioglu).

Orbital Disorders — Vascular Abnormalities 18

AK Grover, Shaloo Bageja (India)

INTRODUCTION

Orbital lesions in pediatric age group are of extreme concern. Most orbital tumors in children are benign and familiarity with the more common orbital lesions is required to aid the clinician in making a timely and accurate diagnosis.

CAPILLARY HEMANGIOMA

It is most common orbital tumor of childhood. It is diagnosed at birth or in the first six months of life **(Figure 1A).**

Symptoms and Signs

They are most commonly situated in the upper lid or orbit. Cutaneous lesions are known as strawberry nevus **(Figure 1B).** Depending upon their location these tumors can cause proptosis, ptosis, strabismus, astigmatism and amblyopia.

Investigations

CT scan shows homogenous soft tissue density **(Figure 1C).** Enhancement is variable according to the vascularity of the lesion.

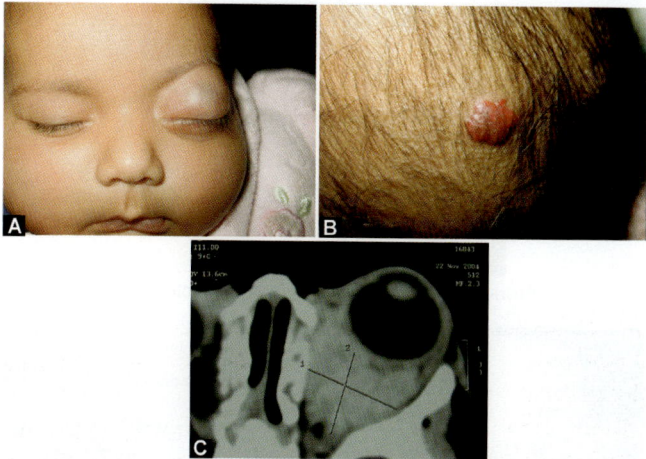

Figures 1A to C: (A) 8-month-old child presented with proptosis. (B) Showing telangiectatic vessels on the scalp (C) CT scan showing diffusely infiltrating non-encapsulated mass in intraconal and extraconal spaces

Management

Most of them does not require treatment. Amblyopia is the most common indication for treatment. Intralesional corticosteroid, i.e a combination of triamcinolone and dexamethasone is a preferred treatment **(Figure 2).**

Prognosis

These lesions increase in size in the first year of life and spontaneously regresses over the years. Complete surgical resection may not be possible.

LYMPHANGIOMA

It is a benign vascular tumor that become apparent in the first decade of life. It may involve eyelid, conjunctiva and orbit **(Figure 3A and B).**

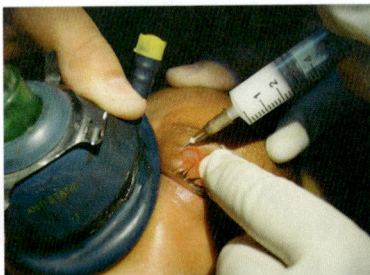

Figure 2: Inj. Triamcinolone being injected

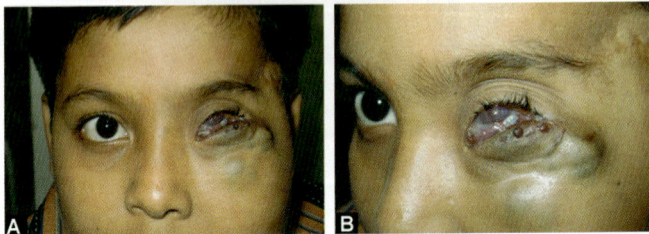

Figures 3A and B: An 8-year-old boy with multiloculated lymphangioma

Symptoms and Signs

They may present as a slowly progressive proptosis or sudden presentation due to hemorrhage following a trivial trauma. It may be associated with ptosis, strabismus, amblyopia, glaucoma and optic nerve compression.

Investigations

Imaging studies show the multicompartmental nature of the venous-lymphatic malformations. MR imaging is preferred over CT scan as it delineates the internal structure of the various cysts of the lesion.

Management

Surgical debulking is the treatment of choice.

Prognosis

It is difficult to remove tumor en toto, due to its nonencapsulated nature. Surgery may be complicated with bleeding and recurrence.

CAVERNOUS HEMANGIOMA

These are benign well encapsulated vascular tumor.

Symptoms and Signs

They may be present at birth but usually present later **(Figure 4A)**. They gradually increase in size manifesting as proptosis and visual impairment.

Investigations

Diagnosis is established by ultrasonography and CT scan, which demonstrates well encapsulated intraconal cystic lesion **(Figure 4B)**.

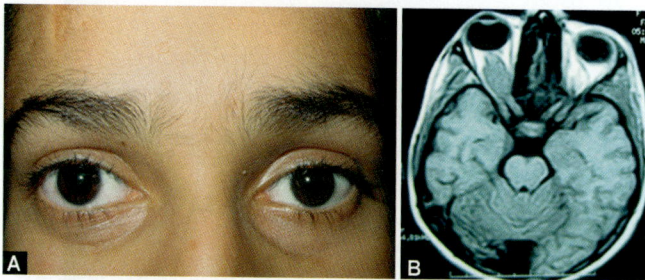

Figures 4A and B: (A) A 13-year-old girl presented with R/E axial proptosis. (B) CT scan showing well encapsulated intraconal mass

Management

Removal of mass en toto via orbitotomy.

Prognosis

Prognosis is excellent. Recurrence are rare even with incomplete resection.

ORBITAL VARICES

It is the most common congenital venous malformation.

Symptoms and Signs

It usually present as intermittent proptosis with dilated conjunctival or lid vessels **(Figure 5)**. They grow slowly during childhood and rarely cause visual problems, unless spontaneous hemorrhage occurs. The proptosis increases with Valsalva maneuver or while straining. It may present with bruit and pulsating exophthalmos mimicking caroticocavernous fistula **(Figures 6A and B)**.

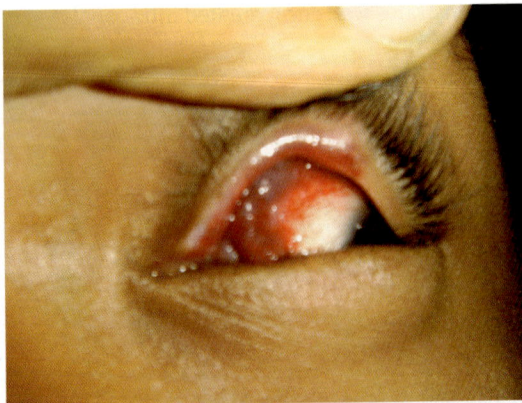

Figure 5: Showing dilated conjunctival vessels

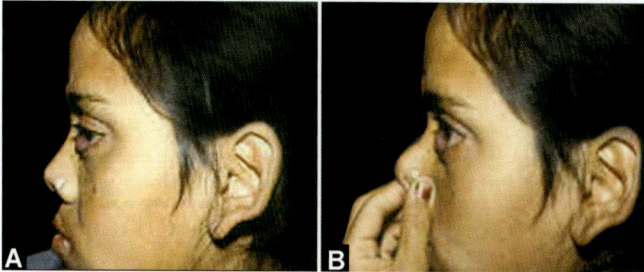

Figures 6A and B: Showing increase in proptosis following Valsalva maneuver

Investigations

Diagnosis can be established by orbital venography or CT scan.

Management

Observation is warranted for small lesions. Surgical intervention may be necessary in non-resolving episodes of thrombosis, severe proptosis and optic nerve compression. Surgery can be extremely difficult, as varices are very friable and intimately intermixed with normal orbital structures.

Prognosis

Complete removal is not possible. There is also a significant risk of visual loss as a result of hemorrhage or optic nerve damage.

SUGGESTED READING

1. Henderson JW. Orbital tumors. Philadelphia:WB Saunders 1973.
2. Rootman J, Graeb DA. Vascular lesions. In: Rootman J, ed. Diseases of the Orbit. Philadelphia: Lippincott, Williams and Wilkins 1988:553-7.
3. Shields JA, Shields CL. Vascular and hemorrhagic lesions. In: Shields JA, Shields C, eds. Atlas of Orbital Tumors. Philadelphia: Lippincott, Williams and Wilkins 1999.

Roshmi Gupta, Savari Desai, Santosh G Honavar (India)

ORBITAL CELLULITIS

Introduction

Bacterial orbital cellulitis is one of the common causes of inflammatory proptosis. It is commonly associated with sinusitis. Other sources of infection are spread of infection to the orbit from the eyelid, after penetrating injury, endogenous in an immunocompromised or debilitated patient, or from a tooth infection.

Signs and Symptoms

The patient presents with acute onset, progressive painful proptosis, axial or non-axial. The patient may be febrile. The eyelids will show edema and mechanical ptosis. Ocular mobility will be limited. The conjunctiva may show chemosis, congestion, and conjunctival prolapse. In severe cases, pupil may show relative afferent pupillary defect. Fundus may show venous congestion, disc hyperemia and disc edema **(Figure 1A).**

Investigation

Nasal swab and sinus drainage may yield material for identification of infective agent and antibiotic sensitivity.

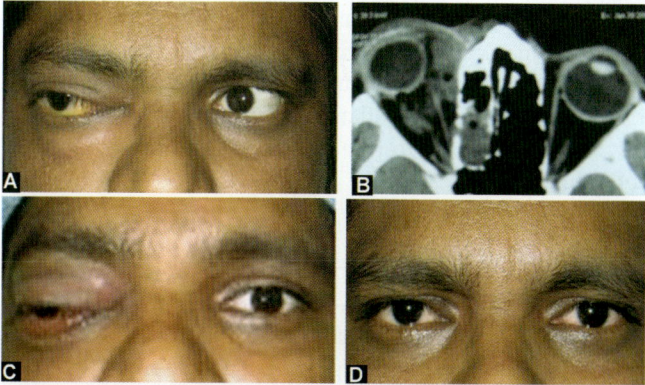

Figures 1A to D: (A) Clinical picture of patient with orbital cellulitis, showing proptosis, chemosis, restricted ocular movement, periocular edema and erythema. (B) Axial view of CT scan of orbital cellulitis, showing diffuse shadow with heterogeneous density and lucent pockets of gas formation, extraconal and intraconal. The ethmoid sinuses are opacified. (C) Clinical picture of same patient, deteriorating to orbital abscess. Proptosis, chemosis, limited ocular motility and periorbital edema are increasing. There is a localized, tense, fluctuant area of orbital abscess in the superonasal quadrant of the orbit. (D) Clinical picture of complete recovery of the patient after systemic antibiotics and drainage of orbital abscess

Orbital imaging helps to confirm the diagnosis and rule out orbital abscess formation. The optic nerve will appear straightened due to proptosis. The lids will be thickened and show soft tissue shadows. The orbit will show ill-defined soft tissue shadows, with increased density of intra-conal and extra-conal orbital fat. Anaerobic infection may show gas in orbit. The sinuses may show opacification or mucosal thickening **(Figure 1B).**

Differential Diagnosis

The condition should be differentiated from other causes of inflammatory orbital disease, and orbital abscess.

Other non-inflammatory rapidly progressive painful proptosis may caused by orbital hematoma after trauma, or by hemorrhage into an orbital lymphangioma.

In children, orbital inflammation with proptosis should be carefully assessed to rule out an atypical presentation of retinoblastoma.

Treatment

Orbital cellulitis is treated by parenteral antibiotics. If the causative organism can be isolated, specific therapy should be started. Otherwise, the choice of antibiotic is empirical depending on the patient profile. Further investigations should be done, or abscess formation suspected if there is no improvement after 48 hours of starting therapy. The paranasal sinuses may need drainage, which will also aid in identification of causative organism.

The correct choice of antibiotics assumes greater importance due to the change in patterns of causative organisms in recent years. First, after the introduction of hemophilus vaccine, *Hemophilus influenzae* is no longer the commonest organism in children. Secondly, there is a growing prevalence of methicillin-resistant *Staphylococcus aureus* as a causative organism.

In childhood, sinusitis and orbital cellulitis tend to be due to a single aerobic organism such as *Streptococcus, Moraxella or Hemophilus*. In adults, the infection is often polymicrobial with mixed gram-positive and gram-negative bacteria, and aerobic and anaerobic organisms. *Streptococcus* and *Staphylococcus* are common. Frequently used antibiotics are the third generation cephalosporins, and vancomycin combined with gram-negative coverage. In methicillin-resistant *Staphylococcus aureus*, the treatment is with trimethoprim-sulfamethoxazole, rifampin, clindamycin or vancomycin.

ORBITAL ABSCESS

Introduction

Orbital abscess is usually a complication of orbital cellulitis. An orbital sub-periosteal abscess may develop rapidly from the adjacent paranasal sinus with minimal previous orbital cellulitis.

Signs and Symptoms

Progressive non-axial proptosis, worsening lid edema and chemosis of conjunctiva, severe limitation of ocular motility will be seen. Visual acuity may be diminished, with relative afferent pupillary defect. There may be a palpable fluctuant mass. The fundus examination may show disc edema and perivasculitis **(Figure 1C).**

Systemically, the patient may have increased fever spikes and malaise.

Investigation

On a CT scan a subperiosteal abscess is commonly adjacent to the paranasal sinuses, against the bony walls of the orbit, with homogeneous low density internal appearance, and smooth convex surface with contrast-enhancing capsule. An orbital abscess will have an intra-orbital mass with lower density areas internally, with or without a contrast-enhancing capsule; gas may be present in the orbit. Sinus opacification may be present **(Figure 2).**

Attempt should be made to isolate the organism as in orbital cellulitis. The organism can be better isolated from the purulent material obtained by draining the abscess.

Treatment

An orbital abscess in an adult or older child needs surgical drainage. After draining the pus completely, the abscess cavity

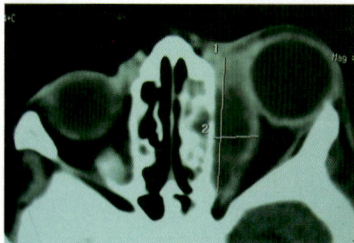

Figure 2: Axial view of CT scan of subperiosteal orbital abscess. The abscess is located at the medial wall adjacent to the ethmoid sinus, has a low internal density, convex shape and enhancement of its rim after contrast injection

should be irrigated with antibiotic solution, and a tube drain placed. Children responding to antibiotics do not need sinus or abscess drainage.

Intensive systemic antibiotics as discussed under orbital cellulitis are administered.

Complications

Orbital cellulitis and orbital abscess may lead to visual loss, cranial nerve paresis, brain abscess and subdural empyema, superior ophthalmic vein thrombosis and cavernous sinus thrombosis.

CAVERNOUS SINUS THROMBOSIS

Introduction

Cavernous sinus thrombosis is a dreaded complication of orbital cellulitis, with high morbidity.

Signs and Symptoms

The patient is febrile, and may complain of headache. The sensorium may be affected in the late stages of the disease.

The patient has increasing proptosis, periorbital edema, chemosis and limitation of ocular movement. All extraocular muscles as well as the sphincter pupillae are affected. On fundus examination, papilledema, hyperemia and retinal hemorrhages are seen. Limitation of motility of the contralateral eye in a previously unilateral orbital cellulitis is indicative of cavernous sinus thrombosis. There may be loss of sensation in the distribution of the maxillary division of the trigeminal nerve, unlike in orbital cellulitis.

Investigations

Imaging of the orbit and parasellar region by CT scan or MRI will show bilateral enlargement of multiple extraocular muscles. The superior ophthalmic vein would be enlarged. The cavernous sinus would be enlarged and enhance with contrast; loss of the concavity of the lateral border of the sinus would be seen on an axial section. An MRI would show the loss of blood flow within the sinus **(Figure 3).**

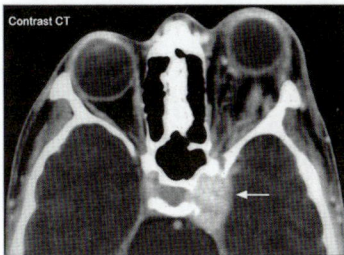

Figure 3: Axial view of CT scan showing dilated cavernous sinus, enhancing with contrast; the lateral concavity is replaced by a convexity in cavernous sinus thrombosis

Treatment

Treatment of cavernous sinus thrombosis entails a team effort in conjunction with internal medicine, neuromedicine and infectious disease specialists. The therapy requires intravenous antibiotics and supportive care. In selected cases of sinus thrombosis from an infective cause, anticoagulants have a role in reducing the morbidity.

ORBITAL TUBERCULOSIS

Introduction

Worldwide, tuberculosis causes significant morbidity and mortality; the incidence of tuberculosis, particularly multi-drug resistant varieties has been on the rise. Orbital involvement with tuberculosis is rare. Orbital involvement is either secondary to hematogenous spread or by direct spread from neighboring structures such as the sinuses.

Signs and Symptoms

Orbital tuberculosis progresses slowly. It may present as a space-occupying lesion, causing proptosis, limitation of ocular motility, and a hard palpable mass. The mass effect may be caused by a tuberculoma or a cold abscess **(Figures 4A and B)**.

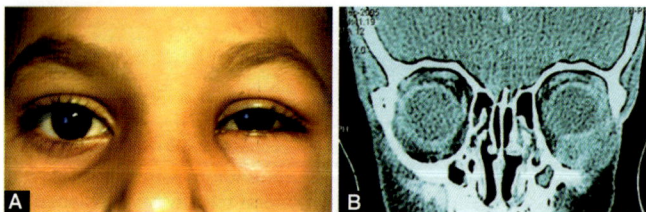

Figures 4A and B: (A) Clinical picture of patient with tubercular granuloma left orbit, showing inferior orbital mass which is tense and erythematous. (B) Coronal CT scan of same patient, showing soft tissue density irregular mass in inferior orbit, with hypodense area corresponding to area of necrosis

Tuberculosis may also affect the orbital bones, causing osteomyelitis, with inflammation and discharging sinuses. Necrotizing infiltrating lesions may develop cutaneous fistulas **(Figures 5A to D)**.

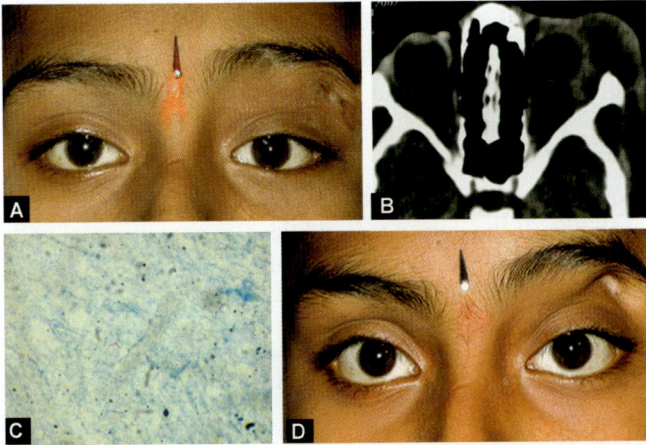

Figures 5A to D: (A) Clinical photograph of patient with tubercular osteomyelitis left orbit, showing left proptosis, fullness of superior sulcus, and discharging sinus. (B) Axial CT scan of the same patient, showing well-circumscribed soft-tissue density mass in left superolateral orbit. (C) Acid fast bacillus detected with Ziehl Nielson staining. (D) Healed orbital tuberculosis after treatment. The site of the sinus is scarred

Investigation

Orbital biopsy: the biopsy shows caseating or non-caseating granulomatous inflammatory changes. Histopathological examination of biopsied material may rarely reveal acid fast bacilli. The biopsied material inoculated on culture media may rarely grow AFB. It may be useful to subject biopsied material to Polymerase chain reaction (PCR) for *Mycobacterium tuberculosis* DNA.

Concomitant active tuberculosis elsewhere in the body may or may not be present. A chest X-ray may be helpful. Strongly positive tuberculin test in presence of an orbital lesion may be corroborative evidence.

Management

Management of orbital tuberculosis is systemic therapy with antitubercular drugs.

Inference

Diagnosis of orbital tuberculosis requires a high index of suspicion. If the evidence is subtle, a therapeutic trial with anti-tubercular drugs may be beneficial.

ORBITAL FUNGAL INFECTION

Orbital fungal infection is by predominantly two classes of fungi—*Mucor* and *Aspergillus*.

ORBITAL MUCORMYCOSIS

Introduction

Orbital mucormycosis, by species of rhizopus, is commonly seen in debilitated, immunocompromised patients. Uncontrolled diabetics are a susceptible group of patients, as are patients on chemotherapy for hematological malignancies. Orbital disease is frequently associated with sinus or cerebral disease

Sign and Symptoms

The condition is painful in about 40% of patients, with ocular as well as facial pain. The patient may be febrile. There is facial and periocular edema. Vision is diminished; there may be proptosis and ptosis. Orbital apex involvement will cause total ophthalmoparesis. Other cranial nerves involved are the fifth and seventh nerves. Inflammatory signs such as conjunctival congestion and chemosis are present. The pupil

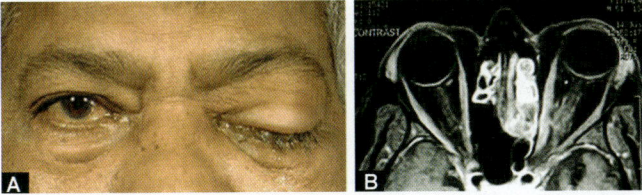

Figures 6A and B: (A) Clinical photograph of patient with uncontrolled diabetes, with pain, proptosis, ptosis, complete ophthalmoparesis and diminished vision. (B) Axial contrast-enhanced T1-weighted MRI scan of same patient, showing soft tissue density shadows in the ethmoid sinus and orbital apex

may have relative afferent pupillary defect. Blackened areas of necrosis and eschar are visible in the external nares or palate. The periocular and facial skin shows necrosis with advanced disease **(Figures 6A and B).**

Investigations

Suspected mucormycosis warrants orbital imaging, preferably with CT scan. CT scan shows homogenous, well circumscribed or diffuse irregular soft tissue density mass in the orbit, extending to paranasal sinus or intracranially. The imaging will also show any bone erosion. MRI scan better visualizes intracranial extension into the frontal lobe or into the carotid artery siphon.

Diagnosis is by biopsy from the affected tissue, the biopsy specimen showing fungal filaments on staining, or growing mucor species on inoculation into culture media. Biopsy material may be obtained by endoscopic sinus surgery or from the orbit, and stained by both hematoxylin-eosin and specific fungal stains.

Investigations also demonstrate the underlying systemic condition: historically, mucormycosis has been associated with diabetic ketoacidosis. Appropriate investigations should be undertaken for diabetes, hematological malignancies, chronic renal failure and other immunosuppressed states.

Treatment

Mucormycosis is best treated by a multi-specialty team of infectious disease specialist, orbital surgeon, neurosurgeon and ENT surgeon. Patients with rhino-orbito-cerebral mucormycosis require extensive and repeated debridation of the sinuses, orbit and other infected areas. The aim is to remove all unhealthy tissue. Orbital extension may be required in nearly half the patients with severe orbital disease.

The mainstay of treatment is intravenous amphotericin B, at the dose of 1 to 1.5 mg/kg body weight per day. Prolonged treatment may be required. Liposomal amphotericin B has been shown to be more effective. Newer systemic antifungals such as posaconazole and voriconazole have been used in addition. Hyperbaric oxygen may aid in the treatment. Supportive therapy is required for the concurrent systemic conditions.

ORBITAL ASPERGILLOSIS

Introduction

The saprophyte Aspergillus can infect the orbit insidiously, and affects both immunocompetent and immunocompromised individuals. It may also be related to drug addiction, renal transplants, alcoholism and diabetes mellitus.

Signs and Symptoms

Orbital aspergillosis presents with a slowly progressive mass extending into the orbit from the adjacent paranasal sinus. The patient may have progressive proptosis and globe

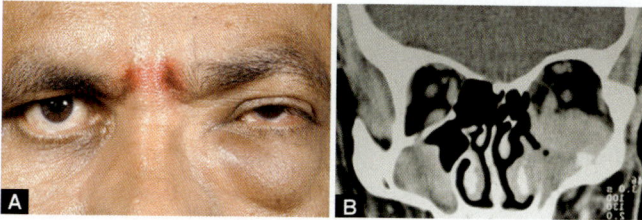

Figures 7A and B: (A) Clinical photograph of patient with maxillary sinus fungal granuloma extending into the orbit. There is left eye proptosis, hyperglobus, chemosis and inferior orbital palpable mass. (B) Coronal CT scan shows bilateral maxillary sinus opacity, with diffuse soft tissue mass extending from left maxillary sinus into the orbit, eroding orbital floor, and involving the inferior rectus

displacement. There may be an orbital apex syndrome, with visual loss, ptosis and ophthalmoparesis. The patient has orbital pain and headache. The orbital inflammatory signs are less marked. The vision is relatively better preserved unless there is orbital apex involvement. Occasionally there may be abscess formation. Rarely, the condition may be rapidly progressive.

In the disseminated form, endophthalmitis may occur. **(Figures 7A and B).**

Investigation

CT scan imaging of the orbit and paranasal sinuses will detect localized mass from a sinus with bony erosion and infiltrating into the orbit. Rarely there may be an isolated orbital mass. An MRI scan will help early detection of cranio-cerebral spread of the disease.

Biopsy of the sinus or orbital mass will show septate fungal filaments by hematoxylin-eosin and special fungal stains. The confirmation of the diagnosis is by culture of aspergillus from the biopsy material.

The patient should undergo an evaluation for any underlying predisposing factor-systemic conditions mentioned earlier, or pre-existing sinus disease such as polyps.

Differential Diagnosis

Aspergillosis should be differentiated from other mass lesions arising from the sinus and extending into the orbit. A fulminant presentation of aspergillosis may mimic mucormycosis. Secondary orbital invasion by paranasal sinus malignancies can also have a similar presentation.

Treatment

Disseminated aspergillosis responds poorly to treatment. Local disease can be managed by surgical debridement and irrigation with amphotericin B. The patient needs adjuvant systemic therapy with amphotericin B, ketoconazole or itraconazole. The patients may be followed up with endoscopy and CT scan to detect recurrences early.

ORBITAL CYSTICERCOSIS

Introduction

Orbital infection with cysticercosis is not uncommon in endemic areas of the world. The cysts occur in the extra-ocular muscles and may migrate anteriorly and sub-conjunctivally. Depending on the exact location, the clinical presentation is varied. The inflammatory signs may be moderate or severe.

Signs and Symptoms

The patient may present with axial or non-axial proptosis; the pain may be only mild or more severe. Visual acuity may be diminished due to rare involvement of the optic nerve by a cyst, or due to compression. There may be limitation of ocular motility; the restriction of ocular motility is often worst in the direction opposite the muscle involved. Presentation may be that of an isolated rectus weakness; acquired Brown syndrome has been reported in cysticercosis involving the superior oblique. A cyst in the levator palpebrae- superior rectus complex would present with ptosis and restricted elevation of the globe. Cysticercosis in the area of the lacrimal gland presents with a picture like dacryoadenitis. A cyst which has migrated subconjunctivally may present at the insertion of the muscle. Occasionally a cyst may migrate anteriorly and be palpable in the periorbital region as a cystic mass. A cyst may extrude spontaneously. If the cyst ruptures within the orbit, it sets up an intense inflammatory reaction, with pronounced signs and symptoms **(Figures 8A and B).**

Investigation

Orbital imaging is the mainstay of diagnosis in orbital myocysticercosis.

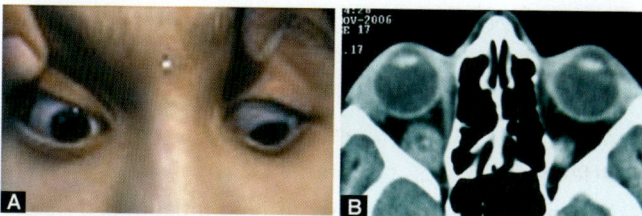

Figures 8A and B: (A) Clinical photograph of patient with right inferior rectus myocysticercosis. The patient had pain, limitation of depression and diplopia. (B) Axial CT scan of same patient, showing cystic lesion with low internal density, with single high density area representing the scolex. The soft tissue density shadow surrounding the cyst is inflammatory in nature

An ultrasound B scan of the orbit is a sensitive tool. It will show a low-echo reflective cystic structure with an internal high-echo reflective area of the scolex. A CT scan or MRI scan of the orbit will also detect a cyst with a scolex.

If only the cyst is visualized, but no scolex, a good clinical response to the appropriate therapeutic trial will confirm the diagnosis.

Serum ELISA test for cysticercus antigens has a low sensitivity, but may be corroborative if a cyst without a scolex is detected on imaging.

Management

Medical management comprises the use of oral anthelminthic, albendazole, 15 mg/kg body weight/day, for two weeks. Systemic corticosteroids, 1-2 mg/kg body weight/ day is started concurrently to reduce the inflammatory effects. The steroid is tapered over 6 weeks. Serial USG B scan imaging can document the collapse and ultimately the disappearance of the cyst.

Surgical excision of the cyst is rarely required. The cyst should be removed in toto; rupturing the wall would cause an intense inflammatory response.

Inference

Any patient with proptosis, with mild inflammatory signs and an unusual pattern of ocular motility restriction should be suspected of having orbital myocysticercosis, particularly if the patient has been residing or travelling in the endemic geographical distributions.

ORBITAL HYDATID CYST

Introduction

Involvement of the orbit by *Echinococcus* cysts is found in the endemic areas of the world. Orbital hydatid cyst comprises about 1% of all hydatid cysts.

Signs and Symptoms

The patient presents with progressive proptosis, axial or non-axial. There may be associated pain, diminished vision, limitation of ocular movements and chemosis in addition. There may be edema of the optic disc, and even loss of vision in long-standing cases **(Figures 9A and B).**

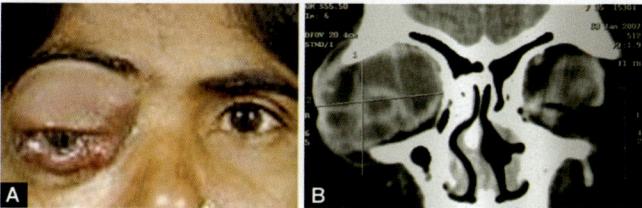

Figures 9A and B: (A) Clinical picture of patient with orbital hydatid cyst, presenting with proptosis, chemosis and periocular edema. (B) Coronal CT scan of same patient, showing multiple cystic lesions in orbit, with low internal density and rim enhancing with contrast

Investigation

An ultrasound B scan will identify a single cyst or multi-lobulated cysts with echo-lucent centers. MRI scan CT scan will identify clear cystic structures, which may have some calcification on the cyst wall. Additional supportive evidence is from a positive indirect hemagglutinin test (IHA) and eosinophilia.

Hydatid cysts may involve multiple locations in the body, particularly in children. The common sites are liver, lung and brain, and USG abdomen and CT scan brain may be helpful.

Treatment

The cyst is to be removed surgically by orbitotomy. Care is to be taken not to rupture the cyst during removal. Accidental spillage of the cyst contents into the orbit may cause seeding.

Sytemic albendazole at the dose of 15 mg/kg body weight has been used of recurrent hydatid cysts.

BIBLIOGRAPHY

1. Ambati BK, Ambati J, Azar N, Stratton L, Schmidt EV. Periorbital and orbital cellulitis before and after the advent of *Haemophilus influenzae* type B vaccination. Ophthalmology 2000 Aug; 107(8):1450-3.

2. Andronikou S, Welman CJ, Kader E. Classic and unusual appearances of hydatid disease in children. Pediatr Radiol 2002 Nov; 32(11):817-28 Epub 2002 Aug 16.

3. Bennett JE, Mucormycosis. In Harrison's Principles of Internal Medicine, 14th Edition, Mcgraw-Hill 1998.

4. Biswas J, Roy Chowdhury B, Krishna Kumar S, Lily Therese K, Madhavan HN. Detection of *Mycobacterium tuberculosis* by polymerase chain reaction in a case of orbital tuberculosis. Orbit 2001 Mar;20(1):69-74.

5. Blomquist PH. Methicillin-resistant *Staphylococcus aureus* infections of the eye and orbit (an American Ophthalmological Society thesis). Trans Am Ophthalmol Soc 2006; 104:322-45.

6. DiNubile MJ. Septic thrombosis of the cavernous sinuses. Arch Neurol 1988 May;45(5):567-72.

7. Diseases of the orbit, a multidisciplinary approach. Rootman J, 2nd Edition, Lippincott Williams and Wilkins, Philadelphia,2003

8. Hargrove RN, Wesley RE, Klippenstein KA, Fleming JC, Haik BG. Indications for orbital exenteration in mucormycosis. Ophthal Plast Reconstr Surg 2006 Jul-Aug; 22(4):286-91.

9. Kaur A, Agrawal A. Orbital tuberculosis—an interesting case report. Int Ophthalmol 2005 Jun; 26(3):107-9.

10. Levin LA, Avery R, Shore JW, Woog JJ, Baker AS. The spectrum of orbital aspergillosis: a clinicopathological review. Surv Ophthalmol 1996 Sep-Oct;41(2):142-54.

11. Levine SR, Twyman RE, Gilman S. The role of anticoagulation in cavernous sinus thrombosis. Neurology 1988 Apr;38(4):517-22.

12. Mahesh L, Biswas J, Subramanian N. Role of ultrasound and CT-scan in diagnosis of hydatid cyst of the orbit. Orbit 2000 Sep;19(3):179-88.

13. Mauriello JA Jr, Yepez N, Mostafavi R, Barofsky J, Kapila R, Baredes S, Norris J. Invasive rhinosino-orbital aspergillosis with precipitous visual loss. Can J Ophthalmol 1995 Apr;30(3):124-30

14. McKinley SH, Yen MT, Miller AM, Yen KG. Microbiology of pediatric orbital cellulitis. Am J Ophthalmol 2007 Oct; 144(4):497-501.

15. Mohindra S, Mohindra S, Gupta R, Bakshi J, Gupta SK. Rhinocerebral mucormycosis: the disease spectrum in 27 patients. Mycoses 2007 Jul;50(4):290-6.

16. Panda NK, Balaji P, Chakrabarti A, Sharma SC, Reddy CE. Paranasal sinus aspergillosis: its categorization to develop a treatment protocol. Mycoses. 2004 Aug;47(7):277-83.

17. Pushker N, Bajaj MS, Betharia SM. Orbital and adnexal cysticercosis. Clin Exp Ophthalmology Oct 2002;30(5):322-33.

18. Shome D, Honavar SG, Vemuganti GK, Joseph J. Orbital tuberculosis manifesting with enophthalmos and causing a diagnostic dilemma. Ophthal Plast Reconstr Surg 2006 May-Jun;22(3):219-21.

19. Siddiqui AA, Bashir SH, Ali Shah A, Sajjad Z, Ahmed N, Jooma R, Enam SA. Diagnostic MR imaging features of craniocerebral aspergillosis of sino-nasal origin in immunocompetent patients. Neurochir (Wien) 2006 Feb;148(2):155-66.

20. Sihota R, Honavar SG. Oral albendazole in the management of extra-ocular cysticercosis. Br J Ophthalmology 1994;78:621-3.

21. Sihota R, Sharma T. Albendazole therapy for a recurrent orbital hydatid cyst. Indian J Ophthalmol 2000;48:142.

22. Turgut AT, Turgut M, Ko°ar U. Hydatidosis of the orbit in Turkey: results from review of the literature 1963-2001. Int Ophthalmol 2004 Jul;25(4):193-200.

23. Uy HS, Tuano PM. Preseptal and orbital cellulitis in a developing country. Orbit 2007 Mar;26(1):33-7.

24. Youssef OH, Stefanyszyn MA, Bilyk JR. Odontogenic orbital cellulitis. Ophthal Plast Reconstr Surg. 2008 Jan-Feb;24(1):29-35.

Orbital Implants

20

INTRODUCTION

Orbital implants are devices, natural or synthetic, used to replace the orbital volume lost after enucleation or evisceration procedures.

An ideal implant should have the following features:

1. Mimics the normal globe as much as possible.
2. Must replace sufficient orbital volume.
3. Non-antigenic and biologically inert.
4. Light weight and simple in construction.
5. Allow for prosthesis of adequate anterior chamber depth.
6. Porous structure to allow fibrovascular ingrowth and better stability.
7. Provide socket motility transmitted to the prosthesis to simulate normal globe and socket as much as possible.
8. Buried and placed in intraconal space with good surgical technique to produce good cosmetic and functional results.
9. Minimal rates of exposure, extrusion, infection and inflammation.

Types of Implants

- Integrated/non-integrated
- Buried/exposed.

Non-integrated → no direct attachment to extraocular muscles or prostheses.

→ single spheres of inert material buried beneath the conjunctiva and Tenon's capsule in the muscle cone

→ the recti may or may not be imbricated or incorporated into the soft tissue closure

Examples → spherical implants made of PMMA, glass, silicon, acrylic etc

Status of non-integrated *implants*—have low complication rates (infection, extrusion) but poor motility. To improve motility they can be wrapped with sclera/fascia lata/vicryl mesh which provides an anchor for extraocular muscles attachment and an extralayer between the implant and prosthesis resulting in low extrusion rates. It does not allow fibrovascular ingrowth thereby increasing the chances of implant migration.

Integrated → is designed in a manner to allow attachment of extraocular muscles and has anterior surface projections to push the prostheses in synchrony to the implant.

Examples → Allen, Iowa and Universal implants (non-porous)

→ hydroxyapatite, polyethylene, alumina, etc. (porous)

Status of integrated implants—porous implants allow ingrowth of fibrovascular tissue providing greater stability and increased resistance to extrusion (Is supplied with host immune defences thereby reducing infection, migration, extrusion). Allows placement of motility/support peg providing excellent motility, decrease of weight of prostheses on lower lid and minimizes sagging.

Proper sizing of the implant at the time of insertion is important; if too small—will cause enophthalmos and superior sulcus deformity; if too large – will produce exophthalmos/staring appearance and increase the incidence of dehiscence, entropion of lids and lack of proper lacrimal lubrication of the anterior prosthetic surface. Implant sizer kit is available to find the optimal size preoperatively. Insertors are available to ease the procedure of inserting the implant without infolding the surrounding soft tissue.

NEWER GENERATION ORBITAL IMPLANTS (Figures 1 to 19)

Hydroxyapatite

Hydroxyapatite implant is close to being an ideal buried integrated implant. Hydroxyapatite is a calcium phosphate hydroxide compound made up of multiple interconnecting pores of diameter 500 microns. The implant material (corralline hydroxyapatite) is biocompatible, non-toxic and non-allergenic. The body's tissue recognizes the material as similar to human cancellous bone and because of the porous nature, tissue will grow into it. The implant becomes more fixed and therefore resists migration. The implant allows attachment of the extraocular muscles which in turn leads to improved orbital implant motility. The orbital implant can also be directly attached to the prosthesis through a peg, protruding from the implant allowing a wide range of prosthetic movement as well as the darting eye movements commonly seen when people are engaged in conversation. Once vascularized, the chances of infection/extrusion/migration are minimized. To offset the high costs of preparing the natural coral, an artificial variant has been made for a cheaper price.

Polyethylene (Medpor)

Polyethylene (Medpor) implant is a porous high density alloplastic material with pore sizes 100-400 microns. Its unique, highly porous texture allows vessels to incorporate into the enhancement shape, integrating the implant into a patient's tissues. The shape and size can be customized by the surgeon to fit individual needs. The material is inexpensive allowing wider use. A new variant with Titanium mesh embedded is also available for better attachment of extraocular muscles. Ingrowth can be seen as early as 1.5 months providing rapid stability.

Alumina (Bioceramic) Implant

Alumina (Bioceramic) implant is made of porous, strong, non-brittle biomaterial Alumina Al203. It has highly uniform interconnected pores approximately 500 microns size enhancing fibrovascular ingrowth thereby allowing secure attachment of extraocular muscles preventing migration and improving motility.

Dermis Fat Graft

Dermis fat graft is composed of subcutaneous fat and overlying dermis generally harvested from the lower abdomen/outer gluteal quadrant. Being an autologous graft, is highly biocompatible with negligible cost. It is specially useful in children where fat may proliferate with time and provide a stimulus for commensurate growth of the bony socket. It can be used as a primary graft or as a replacement for an extruded implant. Complications include fat atrophy, central graft ulceration, granuloma formation, keratinization with hair growth and donor site morbidity.

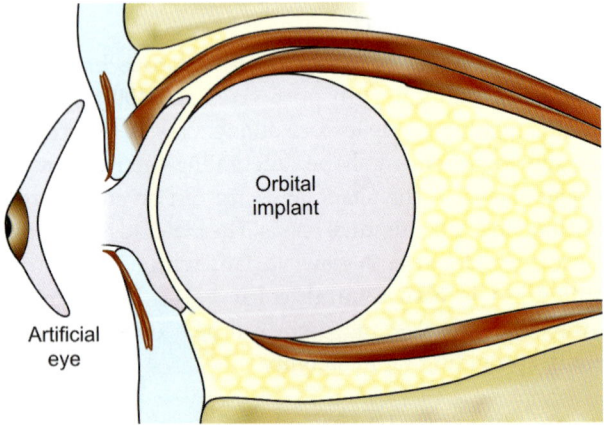

Figure 1: Orbital implant

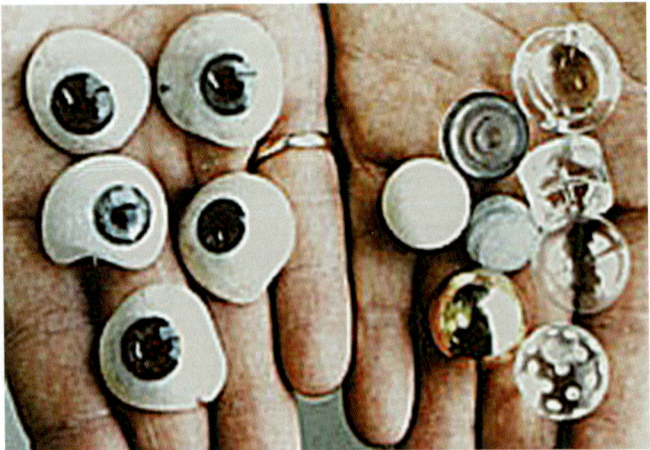

Figure 2: Older generation of implants

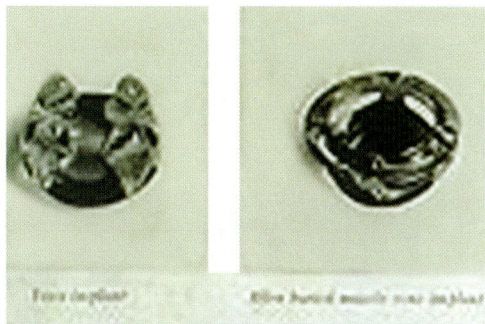

Figure 3: Iowa and Allen implant

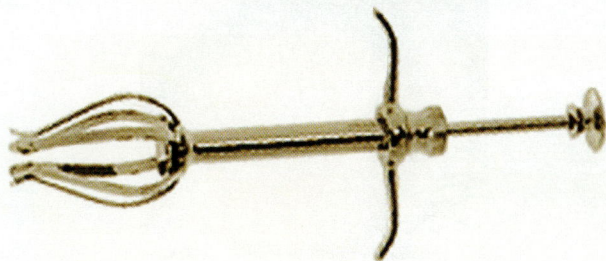

Figure 4: Sphere-introducer

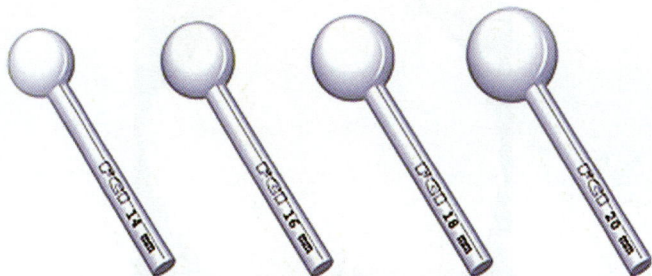

Figure 5: Orbital-sizers

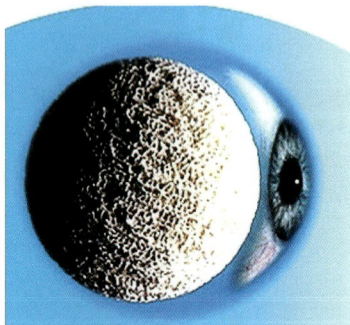

Figure 6: Hydroxyapatite

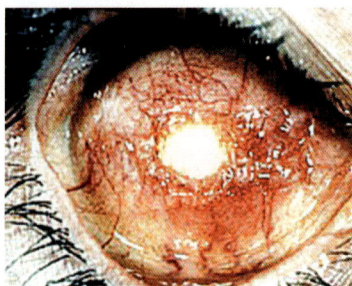

Figure 7: Exposure of hydroxyapatite implant

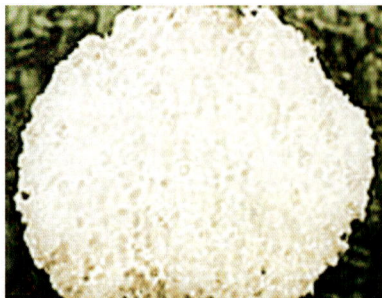

Figure 8: Synthetic hydroxyapatite

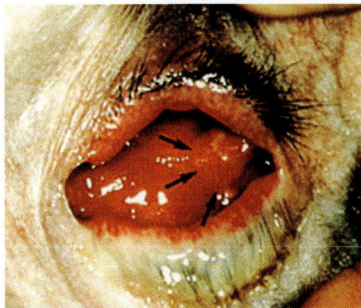

Figure 9: Pyogenic granuloma

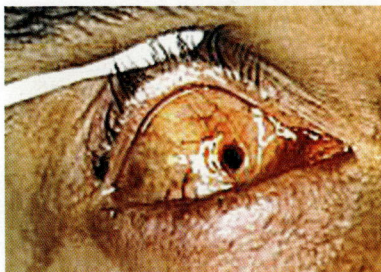

Figure 10: Coral implant with peg hole

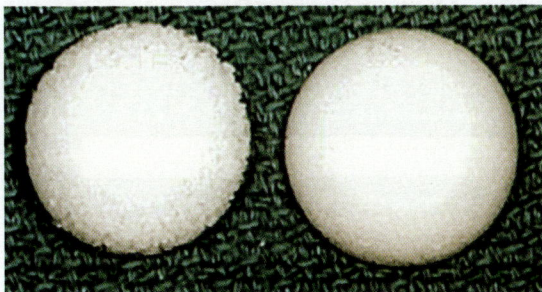

Figure 11: Medpor

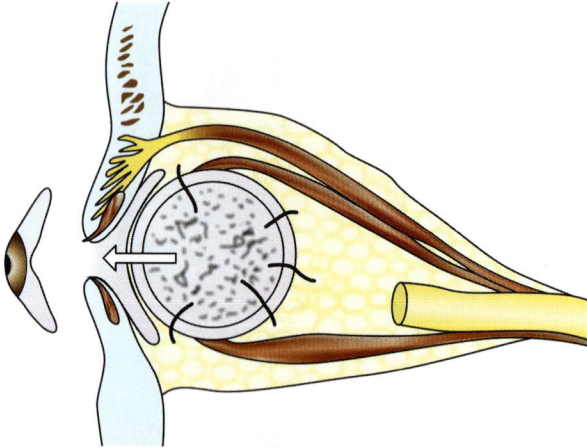

Figure 12: Pegged porous implant

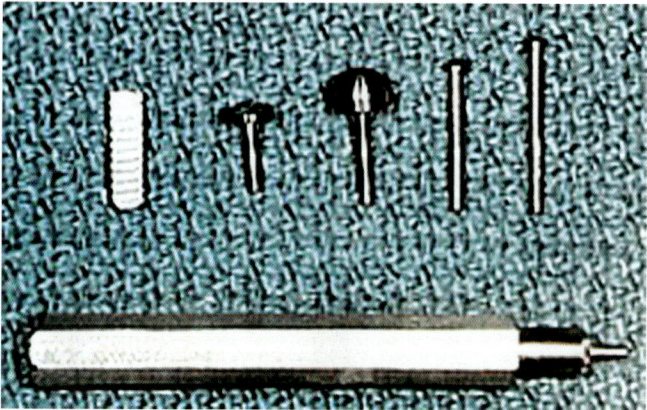

Figure 13: Titanium pegs

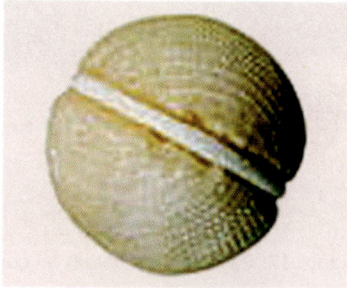

Figure 14: Alumina with vicryl mesh wrapping

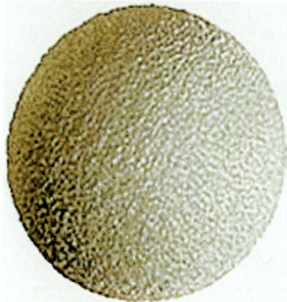

Figure 15: Bioceramic-orbital

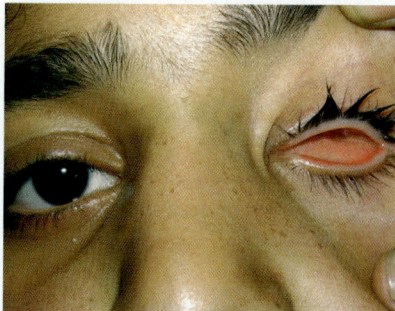

Figure 16: Preoperative dermis fat graft

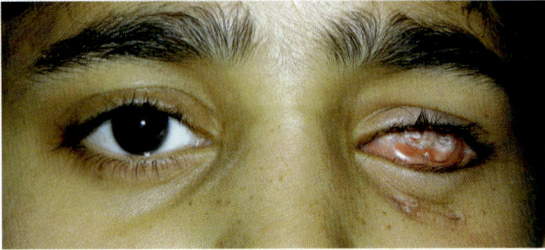

Figure 17: Postoperative dermis fat graft

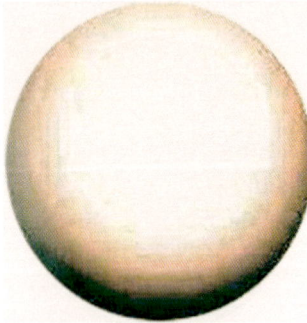

Figure 18: Silicone-orbital

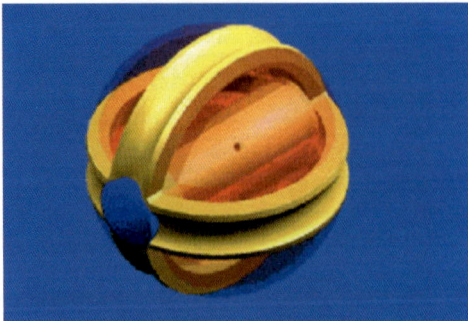

Figure 19: Expandable implant

Expandable Orbital Implant

Expandable orbital implant has an anterior injection portal, rectus muscle placement grooves, and 4 independently expandable/deflatable quadrants. An expandable orbital implant will have the capacity to be enlarged as the surrounding orbital tissues atrophy. An enlarging prosthesis should help correct ptosis (drooping eyelid), enophthalmos (sunken eye) and motility (movement). It is still in the pipeline for commercial production but seems to be a promising choice.

Management of Orbital Trauma and Fractures

21

Rania Abdel Salam, Essam El Toukhy (Egypt)

INTRODUCTION

Orbital injuries may be part of panfacial trauma that range from mild even non significant to severe and debilitating, however, such injuries are of secondary importance to securing airway, stabilizing the circulation and protecting the cervical spine. Trauma to the orbit can involve the globe, eyelid, sinuses and the brain. The nature and severity of the injury depend on the mechanism of trauma.

After securing the lifesaving measures, a team approach incorporating a plastic surgeon, otolaryngologist, a neurosurgeon in addition to the ophthalmologist is needed for the facial trauma patient's evaluation. A systematic ocular and orbital examination is necessary to delineate any subtle injuries as delay in the diagnosis of orbital and ocular problems may worsen the prognosis.

ANATOMIC CONSIDERATIONS

The orbit is a four-sided conical structure with its base directed forwards and apex projecting medially towards the optic foramen. The base or the orbital rim is outlined by thick strong bone: the supraorbital arch of the frontal bone above, the zygoma and maxilla inferiorly, the zygoma laterally and the frontal process of the maxilla medially. The walls of the orbit consist of relatively thin bone. The orbital volume is about 30 ml and the orbital depth is approximately 4.5 cm. Consequently, slight change in the bony anatomy will be reflected on soft tissue and globe position.

The medial wall is formed of the frontal process of the maxilla and the lacrimal bone forming the lacrimal fossa behind which is the extremely thin, less than 0.5 mm, lamina paparycea of the ethmoids and finally the lesser wing of the sphenoid and the optic foramen **(Figure 1)**. Being exceptionally thin and fragile, medial wall fractures are usually subtle and accompany many orbital injuries. The medial wall transmits the anterior and posterior ethmoidal arteries and nerves at the junction between the ethmoidal bone and the orbital plate of the frontal bone. Trauma to this wall

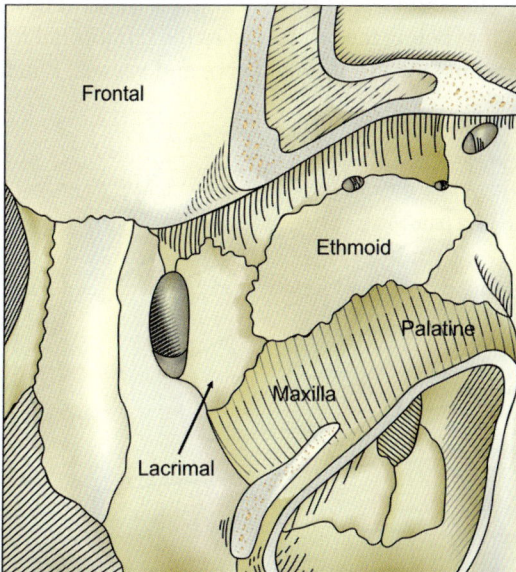

Figure 1: Bones forming the medial wall

is frequently associated with orbital hemorrhage, epistaxis and surgical emphysema.

The roof is composed mainly of the orbital plate of the frontal bone and posteriorly the lesser wing of sphenoid separating the orbit from the frontal lobes of the brain. It is thinnest anteriorly where it is related to the frontal sinus.

The orbital floor is composed of the orbital plates of the maxilla and zygomatic bones with a small contribution from the palatine bone posteriorly. The posterior limit of the floor is defined by the inferior orbital fissure and a small vertical component of the palatine bone posteromedially. Near the apex the inferior orbital fissure transmits venous channels as well as the infraorbital and zygomatic nerves. Contained entirely in the maxilla, the infraorbital groove posteriorly becomes the infraorbital canal as it gains a roof **(Figure 2)**. It opens 4 mm below the orbital rim as the infraorbital foramen that transmits the infraorbital nerve and vessels. The floor is

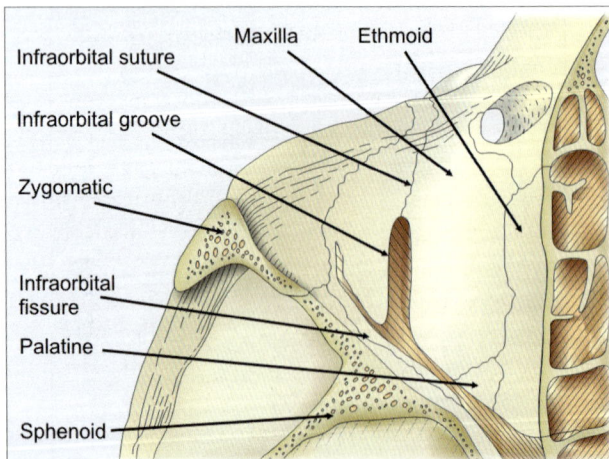

Figure 2: Diagram of the orbital floor

also thin, 0.5 to 1.0 mm thus it easily fractures especially medial to the infraorbital canal.

The lateral wall is thick formed of the frontal process of the zygomatic bone and the frontal bone anteriorly and the greater wing of sphenoid posteriorly. It transmits the zygomatic nerve and artery which often splits into the zygomaticotemporal and zygomaticofacial branches before entering the bone.

EVALUATION OF ACUTE ORBITAL AND PERIORBITAL INJURIES

Initial evaluation starts with *complete history* to determine the circumstances of the present injuries. Low velocity impact such as a human punch usually produces injury limited to the region of impact. High velocity injury such as motor vehicle accidents is often associated with soft tissues and skeletal injuries that are more extensive and may be remote from the impact. With projectile injuries such as with shattered glass or missiles, intraocular, subcutaneous and orbital foreign bodies should be ruled out.

It is better to remove blood and debris as well as any superficial foreign bodies to do *a careful and precise examination of the injured area as well as the surrounding areas.* Blunt low velocity trauma usually cause edema and contusions and the extent of the facial fractures is often more than in cases associated with extensive lacerations as the energy of the impacting force in the former is dissipated by the skeleton rather than soft tissue. Palpation of the orbital rims, malar eminences, zygomatic arches and nose may show fractures and surgical emphysema.

A complete ophthalmic examination is a must to rule out globe injuries and present medicolegal problems. If the patient is conscious, the visual acuity and field by confrontation should be documented. Pupil diameter and responses to light as well as swinging flash light test should be also documented. Presence of afferent papillary defect denotes optic nerve injury, however if both optic nerves are equally damaged, this sign may be absent. The lid, adnexa, conjunctiva, cornea, anterior chamber, iris and lens should be examined with magnification either by slit lamp or a magnifying loupe for lacerations, tissue loss, hemorrhage, opened globe injuries, presence of foreign bodies or lens displacement. When ocular rupture is suspected, globe exploration should take place before any fracture repair.

The retina and optic nerve should be examined on both sides using the ophthalmoscope looking for retinal edema or hemorrhages as well as optic nerve pallor or edema. The caliber of the retinal vessels comparing arteries to veins is also evaluated. Engorged non-pulsatile veins may signify increased orbital pressure, similarly central retinal artery pulsations denotes increased ocular or orbital pressure. B scan ultrasound can be performed if media opacity precludes the visualization of the retina.

The *position of the globe* on the affected side in comparison to contralateral one should be noted and measured, if possible, by the exophthalmometer. The eye positions should be evaluated from the vertex prospective; however, significant lid edema may cause bias. Vertical globe displacement can be estimated by putting a ruler across the medial canthi and noting the point at which it crosses the globe at each side. A depressed orbital floor fracture leads to globe ptosis. Enophthalmos occurs with increased orbital volume such as in wall fractures. While proptosis occurs due to increased soft tissue contents such as hemorrhage and /or reduction of orbital volume associated with inward displacement of one or more of its walls. If the condition is associated with reduced vision or afferent papillary defect, computed tomography (CT) examination is immediately done and intervention should not be delayed. Presence of pulsatile proptosis suggests abnormal vascular communications or transmission of dural pulsations through a fractured displaced orbital roof.

In a conscious cooperative patient with minimal lid edema *eye movements* all directions of gaze should be examined. The patient is asked to report any diplopia at any direction of gaze. Gaze restriction can be caused by nerve injury, soft tissue swelling, direct muscle injury or entrapped muscle within a skeletal fracture. Forced duction and diplopia fields are performed when indicated.

Hyposthesia in areas around the orbit should be looked for especially in the cheek which is supplied by the commonly injured infraorbital nerve. *Upper lid position* should be noted and documented as ptosis may occur as a result of nerve injury, levator aponeurosis laceration or dehiscence or later from fibrosis.

Soft tissue landmarks of the orbit such as canthal angles may be displaced by fractures of the underlying bone. For example, increased intercanthal distance suggests nasoethmoidal fractures involving the reflected part of the medial canthal tendon while inferiorly placed lateral canthus suggests inferior dislocation of the zygoma. If the medial wall is involved, the lacrimal drainage system should be evaluated

RADIOLOGICAL EVALUATION

Radiological studies especially computed tomography (CT) play an indispensable role in evaluating the orbital trauma and detecting radio-opaque foreign bodies. Both axial and coronal CT sequences are required.

Coronal images in 2 mm sections delineate the orbital floor, roof, medial and lateral walls, the nasoethmoid region, the orbital rim and the face surrounding the orbit. It helps delineate the size, shape and location of fractures and associated soft tissue injuries.

Axial scans permit evaluation of the lacrimal drainage pathways, nasal and paranasal sinuses, medial and lateral walls of the orbit, superior and inferior orbital rims, zygomatic arch, pterygoid plates, temporomandibular joint, base of the skull, superior orbital fissures and optic canal. It allows to show globe placement in comparison to the unaffected side.

The combination of axial and coronal scans can give most of the needed information in trauma cases. Three-dimensional scans are helpful in obtaining a more accurate evaluation and understanding of the situation, hence help in deciding the best line for treatment. They are generated from the reformatting 1.5 mm slices on conventional CT scan using a special software computer program. They are very helpful in old trauma cases as they show the deformity, the site, size and appearance of bony defects as well as bone fractures

Problems Associated with Orbital Trauma

- Orbital hemorrhages and emphysema
- Traumatic optic neuropathy
- Orbital fractures
- Septic cavernous sinus thrombosis
- Carotid cavernous fistula
- Orbital foreign bodies

PROBLEMS ASSOCIATED WITH ORBITAL TRAUMA

Orbital Hemorrhages

Bleeding is frequently associated with periorbital trauma and fractures. Blood may be found in the eyelid anterior to the orbital septum due to direct tissue injury. These tissues afford extensive hemorrhage that may extend to the lid margin and even cross the nasal bridge to the uninvolved eyelid.

Mild to moderate orbital hemorrhage commonly accompany orbital trauma. Both conditions can cause variable degrees of proptosis, globe displacement and motility disturbance. If severe, they may cause increased intraocular pressure, central retinal artery occlusion, marked proptosis with corneal exposure as well as compressive optic neuropathy leading to vision loss.

Blood may also accumulate in the subperiosteal space. The extent of the blood is limited by bone suture lines where periorbita becomes firmly adherent. If the periotrbita is intact, the patient may present with mild proptosis and globe displacement. If the periorbita is disrupted the hemorrhage becomes extensive and moves towards the orbital septum and bulbar conjunctiva.

If there is mild proptosis with normal or minimally elevated intraocular pressure with no visual compromise, follow up can be safe and the hemorrhage will gradually resolve over 1 to 3 weeks usually without sequelae.

In sudden and extreme orbital hemorrhage threatening vision, lateral canthotomy and cantholysis of the superior or inferior crura should be performed. If this is not effective, the hematoma should be drained either through lid crease incision if placed superiorly or though lower lid blepharoplasty incision if inferiorly placed. In either condition, the orbital septum must be opened to allow the egress of the blood from the socket. The stab incisions and canthal tissue could be repaired when swelling decreases.

Surgical Emphysema

This means accumulation of air in the subcutaneous tissue. This is a common finding in medial wall and floor fractures as they involve walls of the paranasal sinuses. The condition usually increases when the patient blows his nose and there is a crepitus felt on palpation. Reassurance of the patient and instruction not to forcibly blow his nose are usually enough till the symptoms are relieved provided there are no associated orbital or ocular problems detected **(Figure 3)**.

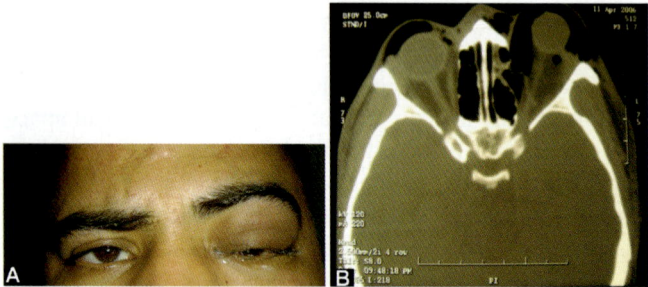

Figure 3: Fracture in the medial wall associated with surgical emphysema and air could be seen within the orbital cavity

TRAUMATIC OPTIC NEUROPATHY

Optic neuropathy may accompany orbital and head injuries.This is diagnosed by presence of decreased vision, afferent papillary defect with otherwise normal eye in a patient with trauma history. The cause of this problem is multifactorial including direct or indirect mechanisms.

Direct optic neuropathy results from compression along the course of the optic nerve by bone fragments **(Figure 4)**, retrobulbar or subperiosteal hematoma, and foreign body or by fractures that narrow the optic canal. Rarely, the optic nerve may be avulsed. When clinically suspected, CT evaluation of the orbit, optic canal and sinuses can identify the cause.

Indirect optic neuropathy is diagnosed when there are no radiologic findings of abnormalities damaging the nerve. It

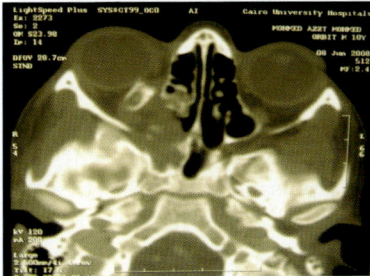

Figure 4: A case of a 7-year-old child with trauma to the sinuses and fracture of the ethmoid and sphenoidal bones. There is a bony fragment that is pressing the optic nerve

may be caused by abrupt brain deceleration with forwards movement causing compression of the intracranial optic nerve. It can also be due to contusion and edema resulting from deformation of the optic canal. The small arterioles in the intracanalicular optic nerve my rupture leading to infarction or hematoma of the optic nerve or sheath. Edema and vasospasm are thought to cause nerve ischemia.

Patients may suffer from sudden complete loss of vision after trauma which is usually caused by actual tear or primary complete optic nerve necrosis. These patients have poor prognosis in spite of treatment. Other patients experience delayed visual loss (hours to days) or partial visual loss usually due to partial ischemic infarction or compression by edema or hemorrhage, however, these patients have better prognosis.

Treatment remains controversial. High-dose corticosteroids are used in treating indirect optic neuropathy. Extracranial transethmoidal optic canal decompression is an alternative treatment especially if the vision drops while on steroid treatment. Direct optic neuropathies attributable to mechanical nerve compression usually require surgical treatment and removal of the offending factor such as repair of floor fracture, intracranial optic canal decompression, hematoma drainage and optic nerve sheath fenestration.

Carotid Cavernous Fistula

It results from shearing of intracavernous carotid artery during deceleration injuries, or direct artery injury by foreign body or bone shrapnel. They develop shortly after trauma but the onset of symptoms may be delayed. They present with progressive proptosis usually pulsatile with subjective and objective bruit. IOP is usually elevated with engorged retinal veins. Brain CT scans with contrast confirm the diagnosis. The fistula can be closed using endovascular occlusion with coils which is the preferred technique.

Septic Cavernous Sinus Thrombosis

Fracture of the posterior ethmoidal or sphenoidal sinuses may allow concomitants with the paranasal sinuses to reach the cavernous sinuses. They usually have a rapid presentation and associated with low grade fever, headache, orbital pain or diplopia. This is followed by progressive proptosis, mydriasis, ophthalmolplegia due to nerve palsy and eventually visual loss due to compressive optic neuropathy. If not treated, septic thrombosis may spread to the cerebral veins leading to increased intracranial tension.

MRI may show a mass caused by thrombus in the sinus compressing the intracavernous part of the internal carotid. Cerebral arteriography and venography may be used however MRA presents a good alternative. Early diagnosis is of extreme importance as it improves the prognosis. Systemic antibiotics are the main line of treatment. Anticoagulant treatment is used to prevent progressive thrombosis if not controlled by antibiotics within 48-72 hours; however, they should not be used if a fungal etiology is suspected due to increased risk of mycotic aneurysm formation.

Orbital Foreign Bodies

A high index of suspicion may lead to discovery of intraorbital foreign bodies. The patient usually reports a history of trauma to the face with a foreign body entering the eye or the orbit. In case of loss of consciousness, or psychiatric illness, the patient may fail to give a helpful history. Foreign bodies may be found without any antecedent history of trauma where the initial injury is thought to be insignificant and usually forgotten. Such patients may remain asymptomatic for long periods of time until the foreign body provokes a reaction, forms an abscess or begins to extrude.

Some foreign bodies may inflict immediate, sometimes irreversible, damage to the globe, extraocular muscles, orbital bone, optic nerve as well as cranial nerves. Infection and inflammation can result secondary to contaminated foreign body entering the globe or penetrating an adjacent sinus. The latter can present with associated surgical subcutaneous emphysema. The long-term effects of the foreign body can be due to chronic inflammation, migration and scar tissue formation. Chronic inflammation causes foreign body granuloma that can be of significant size causing mechanical effects with globe displacement and limitation of its motility. The latter can also result form extraocular muscle fibrosis or soft tissue scarring. A fistula to the skin or conjunctiva may be formed with pus drainage or extrusion of the foreign body

The anatomic structure of the orbit allows large pieces of metal or organic material to be imbedded without significant signs or symptoms unless one of the orbital contents is involved. The location of the foreign body within the orbit influences the presenting picture as well as the management decision. Large objects usually tend to enter the inner canthus injuring the caruncle or the lacrimal drainage system and may become deeply buried within the orbit and in some cases tend to displace the globe.

The nature of the foreign body contributes to the severity of the response and considerably affects the decision of foreign body removal. Most metals are inert and in the absence of infection, they cause no disturbance to the eye and orbit. Copper is poorly tolerated and can induce purulent inflammation. Glass, stone, plastic, and bullets are often well tolerated and need no intervention unless they migrate to the surface and become extruded or palpable so that they can be easily removed. Organic foreign bodies are poorly tolerated and are usually associated with chronic inflammatory reaction and abscess formation.

CT is necessary to detect and localize the foreign body **(Figure 5)**. It can estimate its size and the extent of damage to the surrounding structures. The combination of axial and coronal scans can give three dimensional localization of the foreign body. CT resolution of metal foreign bodies is approximately 0.05 mm; of wood, 2.0 mm and of glass 0.75 to 2.0 mm according to the lead content. One millimeter sections in the scan are recommended to detect orbital foreign bodies. Absence of foreign body in the scan does not totally exclude its presence especially with the suggestive history and presence of symptoms.

Although MRI has no established role in foreign body detection, it should be remembered to avoid its use in cases of suspected metallic foreign bodies as they may be drawn out of their location with injury to the globe or adjacent orbital structures.

Most of inert foreign bodies do not require intervention, and the surgical removal decision should be consider the risk benefit. If the foreign body is to be removed, the surgical

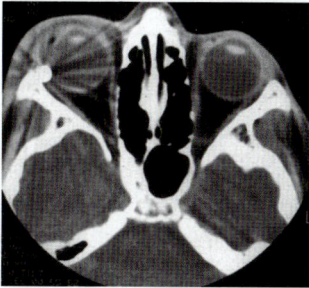

Figure 5: Axial CT scan showing an intraorbital metallic foreign body near the lateral orbital margin

approach is planned according to the site of the foreign body. The entrance wound should be explored in a manner that would not cause damage to orbital tissue. In case that such wound is not present or healed, anterior, medial or lateral orbitotomy can be used. If the foreign body is located at the orbital apex, a neurosurgical anterior craniotomy approach is required. If the foreign body is thought to be metallic, a surgical magnet can be used. Metal foreign body localizers can be used intraoperatively to confirm the radiographic information about the location of the foreign body.

Organic foreign bodies foreign bodies must be removed with great care as they usually fragment. This is followed by irrigation to remove the pus and small fragments. Pus is sent for culture and sensitivity for bacteria and fungi and appropriate treatment is given.

Complications associated with such procedure may be due to the surgery or the foreign body itself. The surgeon may fail to localize the foreign body, the foreign body may become fragmented or it may cause adjacent tissue damage, e.g. blood vessels, nerves and muscles leading to hemorrhage, diplopia or loss of vision.

FRACTURES

Orbital fractures can be generally divided to blow out fractures and fractures that involve the orbital rim

Orbital Floor and Blow-out Fractures

Blow-out fractures are the most common periorbital fracture seen in ophthalmic plastic surgical practice. A blow-out fracture by definition does not involve the inferior orbital rim. On the contrary, a floor fracture should involve the orbital rim. However, the findings and treatments are similar.

Pathogenesis

Two theories exist to explain the origin of orbital floor blow out fractures. The hydraulic theory by Smith and Regan postulated that when a blunt object (usually spherical and larger than the orbital base) hits the orbit, the globe and soft tissues are retropulsed suddenly increasing the intraorbital pressure. To relieve this pressure, the orbital floor "blows-out" into the maxillary sinus usually medial to the infraorbital canal where the bone is thinnest **(Figure 6)**. Sometime the medial wall gives way due to its fragility. This is considered a safety mechanism for the globe.

Fujino proposed a buckling force theory. When a blow strikes the inferior orbital rim, the rim is displaced posteriorly and the force is transmitted to the thin orbital floor that buckles and fractures into the maxillary sinus, then the inferior rim returns back to its normal position intact. In general, variable degrees of both mechanisms are supposed to be present in a given patient with a blow out fracture.

The fracture may be *linear* just parallel and medial to the inferior orbital groove, *trap door* that transiently separate at the groove, close spontaneously entrapping muscles and soft

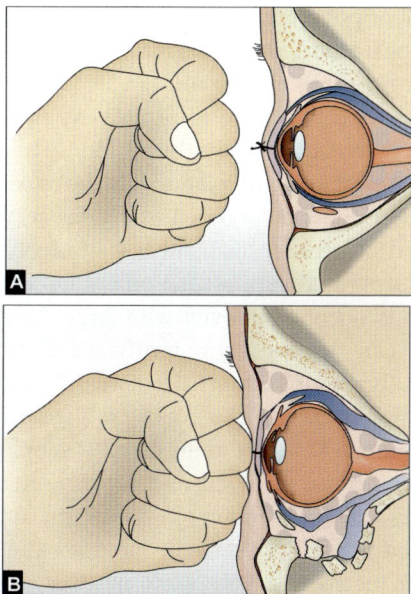

Figure 6: Left side shows a blunt trauma to the anterior orbit. Right side shows that the contents are compressed with increased intraorbital pressure so that the floor gives way

tissue and they are very common in children, *hinged fracture* along the inferior border of the ethmoid entering the maxillary sinus, *comminuted* or *combination* of all of the above. Non displaced and trap door type are more associated with diplopia while enophthalmos is more associated with hinged and comminuted types.

Clinical Presentation

Diagnosis of such fracture depends on suggestive history, periorbital ecchymosis and emphysema. Palpation of the inferior orbital rim may reveal a step off deformity, discontinuity or point tenderness. If the infraorbital canal is involved in the fracture, anesthesia may involve the ipsilateral cheek, upper lip, gums and nose.

Enophthalmos can be due to orbital expansion due to inferior displacement of the orbital floor. This could be accentuated by soft tissue herniation into the maxillary sinus mainly the periorbita, fat and connective tissue, damage to the Lockwood suspensory ligament as well as collapse of the fine fibrous septa that support the orbital fat and muscles. Globe ptosis is uncommon even with large floor fractures however, it can results from significant diminution of Lockwood's ligament support. Immediately after injury, enophthalmos can be masked by orbital hemorrhage and edema posterior and inferior to the globe. If enophthalmos is severe, a prominent superior sulcus deformity can be present.

Diplopia is a frequent finding in blow out fractures. This was attributed to inferior rectus or inferior oblique muscle entrapment in the fracture. Yet it was found that actual muscle entrapment is rare. Orbital fat entrapment is commoner and the fibrous septa that connect the fat and the periostium with the inferior rectus and oblique muscles tighten due to edema or intraorbital hemorrhage thus restricting ocular motility and felt as restriction on forced duction test. With time, these septa may stretch and relax improving the ocular motility and diplopia.

The patient usually suffers from vertical diplopia. The patient may have limited supraduction, infraduction or both. If the inferior rectus restriction is anterior to the equator, hypotropia results while if it is posterior to it, hypertropia results.

Injuries to the extraocular muscle or the motor nerves are additional causes for diplopia. Direct contusion or laceration of the muscle can be worsened by muscle hematoma. While the motor nerves can be damaged by hemorrhage within their sheath, stretched by orbital edema or hemorrhage or suffer from concussion.

Radiologic studies are helpful in establishing the diagnosis. Waters plain X-ray views provide an excellent view of the orbital floor, showing any bone disruption or herniation. Orbit CT especially the coronal cuts delineates the fracture and the bone soft tissue relationship **(Figures 7 and 8)**. However, the mere radiologic presence of a fracture is not an indication for surgical repair.

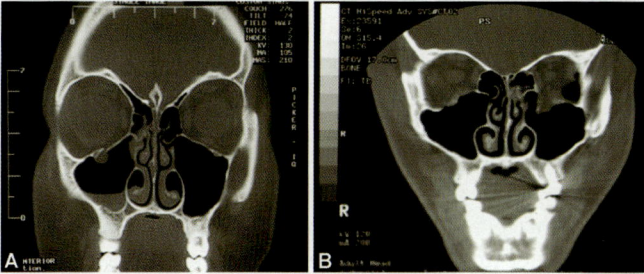

Figure 7: Left shows coronal CT scan with fracture floor and the tear drop appearance. There is a fluid level in the maxilla. Right shows a fractured mid floor with tissue herniation

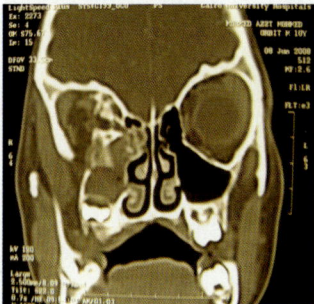

Figure 8: A combined floor and medial wall fracture

Management

Repair of the orbital floor fractures is mainly indicated in restricted ocular motility showing no improvement, diplopia especially within the central 30° field, enophthalmos of ≥ 3 mm or progressive, defects of more than 50% of the orbital floor that are almost always likely to cause enophthalmos as well as incarcerated muscle causing oculocardiac reflex on ocular motility and rare cases of globe ptosis.

Timing

No universally agreed guidelines exist for the repair of blow out fracture. If in doubt, the patient should be evaluated every 2-3 days during the first 2 weeks, diplopia fields and forced ductions are followed carefully for any change. During this time, hemorrhage and edema will resolve during the first week allowing more accurate assessment. As long as motility improves, the patient should be followed up. On the other hand, if surgery is to be done, the best time is not beyond 2 weeks. After this, adhesions between bone fragments, sinus mucosa and the orbital tissues render the repair quite difficult.

Procedure

Surgical repair of blow-out fractures comprises good exposure through incision, periosteal dissection and exposure of the fracture, release of the entrapped tissues as placement of an implant to prevent adhesions between the orbital tissues and nasal mucosa. The surgeon can proceed from an orbital (subciliary or fornix) approach or an antral (Caldwell- Luc) approach. The orbital approach is preferred as it is safer and more effective. In selected cases with large floor defects or with tenaciously herniated orbital contents, a combined orbital and antral approach can be used.

Implants

Many materials are available for repair of orbital wall fractures. They include:

Autogenous bone

Cancellous bone grafts cannot be used due to high absorption rate, 60-80% of the volume may be lost. Split thickness calvarial or membranous bones such as ribs, iliac crest or the cranium have less absorption rate; 15-30%. This material needs a second surgical site with incidence of morbidity such as hematoma, infection. Harvesting them needs proper and formal training. The graft is usually placed with the cortical side towards the recipient bone and it may need to be secured by micro or minilpates.

Alloplastic material

a. *Porous polyethylene:* It is porous integrated biocompatible implant with average pore size 200-240 microns. It is easy to mold manually or the help of heat yet it is structurally stable

b. *Silicone:* A nonporous material that is easy to fashion, inert, safe and effective with low rate of migration, infection and extrusion. It is preferred in cases of orbital volume augmentation.

c. *Methyl methacrylate polymer (cranioplastic):* It is mixed with copolymer to form a mixture that have a doughy consistency and can be placed to augment orbital volume. This material remains malleable for 3-5 minutes so that it can be shaped. If it hardens before molding is complete, a pneumatic drill is used to fashion it.

It is better to be avoided in patients with chronic sinusitis due to the reported incidence of systemic toxicity and late infection.

d. *Microplates*: They are used of there is no enough bone to support the implant. They are made of Titanium alloy. There are less corrosive than steel and produce less scatter on CT studies. They are not magnetic and can be safely imaged by MRI. They are used to reform the orbital rim, medial and lateral canthal angles as well as walls. The alloplastic implants are placed over them to augment the orbital volume.

e. Porous polyethylene implants with embedded titanium provide a new alternative to alloplastic implant materials for orbital reconstruction with a profile that combines several advantages of porous polyethylene and titanium implants.

f. Others like supramid and teflon.

g. Experimental work was done on bone morphogenetic protein (BMP) implant with and without platelet-rich plasma (PRP), which is supposed to promote fracture consolidation in the orbit fracture treatment with scarce inflammatory reaction, and may be a good alternative in orbit fracture reconstruction. Radiological studies suggested intramembranous and progressive cavitation and ossification without a reduction in implant size and with signs of calcium deposition; these events were confirmed by histological analysis.

Surgical Procedures

All are done under general anesthesia and forced duction test is performed initially to confirm the degree of tissue entrapment.

Incision

Variable incisions can be used to expose the inferior orbital rim as well as inferior part of the medial wall.

a. *Subciliary approach:* It is similar to that used in lower lid transcutaneous blepharoplasty. The lid is infiltrated with 1% lidocaine with 1:100:000 epinephrine and a horizontal incision 2mm below the lid margin is made. It should not extend too far laterally to avoid compromise of lymphatic drainage. A skin muscle flap is created and retracted inferiorly using Desmarres retractor. This approach is more associated with postoperative lower lid malpositions namely ectropion.

b. *Lower transconjunctival approach:* The inferior fornix is incised 4 mm below the lower edge of the tarsus. Lateral canthotomy and inferior cantholysis can be done to widen the exposed field. The conjunctiva, Müller's muscle and the capsulopalpebral fascia are severed and the plane between the orbicularis and the capsulopalpebral head is reached. Tissues are dissected till the inferior orbital rim is reached. A 4-0 silk tractional suture is passed through conjunctiva and lower lid retractors. This approach is preferred as it is simple, provides excellent exposure with no visible scar and it has minimal risk for post operative lid malpositions. However, there is a rare risk of entropion due to scarred posterior lamina.

c. *Antral (Caldwell-Luc) approach:* An incision is made in the gingival margin of the canine fossa. Periostium is elevated and separated from the anterior surface of the exposed maxilla. A periosteal elevator is used to create an osteotomy opening into the maxillary sinus. Bone fragments and blood are then evacuated from the sinus. In conjunction with orbital approach, the herniated tissues are gently reposited superior to the orbital floor. The maxillary sinus may then be packed with either petroleum gauze imbricated with antibiotic or a catheter balloon.

The other end of the gauze or catheter is brought out through an antrostomy to facilitate its removal. This approach has limited visualization, poor access for placement and securing the floor implant, poor hemostasis, higher infection rate, lack of permanent glob support and hazards of forcing bony fragments into the globe and optic nerve. That is why this approach is seldom used for fracture floor repair unless there is complete absence of orbital floor.

Exposure of the Orbital Floor

Dissection is carried out till the inferior orbital rim using blunt and sharp dissection keeping the orbital septum intact to avoid fat herniation. Then the periostium is opened 1.5 mm below the orbital rim and elevated from the orbital floor. With the help of periosteal elevator, the periostium is separated from the floor posteriorly; the fracture is localized and exposed, first the lateral border then the medial and posterior limits. The infraorbital bundle should be identified. Any unattached bone fragments should be removed.

Incarcerated tissues are freed from the fracture using hand on hand maneuver with the periosteal elevator and the metal suction tip or malleable retractors. This is easy in cases of recent fractures yet if the tissues are swollen, the extraction becomes difficult and the bone can be depressed into the maxillary antrum. In case of hinged fractures or in some selected cases, the fracture may be enlarged to achieve atraumatic release. Care should be taken to avoid undue bleeding and trauma to the nearby optic nerve.

Optic nerve should be checked every now and then by detecting the pupillary light reaction or dilating the pupil and noting the optic nerve perfusion by the ophthalmoscope.

Forced duction should be repeated to ensure that no more incarcerated tissues are present. Any bone fragments or blood should be aspirated from the maxillary antrum before the defect is covered.

A sterile alloplastic material is fashioned to cover the defect completely and overlapping the surrounding intact bone by 3-4 mm circumferentially. This sheet should not be too large or too thick. The edges are smoothened to avoid trauma to adjacent structures or erosion through the covering periostium. The alloplastic material should be soaked in antibiotic before it is inserted. The thickness of the plate usually range from 0.4-0.6 mm. Thicker implants are indicated in cases of significant enophthalmos and hypophthalmos yet they have the risk of limiting extraocular muscles. The more posterior the implant is placed, the more it reduces enophthalmos. The more anterior it is, the more it reduced hypophthalmos. The choice of the material depend on the nature of the fracture as well as the surgeon preference and training.

When the defect is large or multiple walls are involved, plates and screws are preferred; bone grafts may be a good choice in experienced hands. Titanium mesh may be used if the residual bone is not enough to support an implant. It is not enough by itself and it usually needs to be covered by bone or alloplastic material.

The implant can be fixated by either placing it behind the orbital rim and the mere periosteal closure will keep it in place or two small fixation holes are drilled in the infraoprbital rim just anterior to the defect as well as the anterior edge of the implant. Then the implant is secured to the orbital floor anteriorly by supramid 2-0 sutures.

Forced duction test is repeated. Coexistent medial wall fracture can be repaired at the same time. Hemostasis is secured and the periostium is closed over the implant. Lateral canthus is repaired in case of cantholysis and canthotomy. The opened layers are then closed anatomically.

Eye patch is better avoided and the patient should be watched for bleeding, pupillary reaction and visual acuity postoperatively. Systemic antibiotics, anti-inflammatory drugs as well as cold foments are proven useful.

Complications

Diplopia may persist or worsen after the surgery. This can occur due to fibrosis of the muscle, orbital fat or connective tissue septa either present prior to surgery or secondary to inflammation induced by the surgery. It can be due to unidentified nerve injury before surgery. Diplopia may worsen due to improperly placed implant or residual tissue entrapment. A muscle procedure is better deferred 6-12 months after surgery during which the diplopia may improve or the patient can wear prisms. If a surgery is to be done it is better to be with adjustable sutures.

Overcorrection may occur due to thick implant augmented by postoperative edema that usually resolves after a month. On the other hand *residual enophthalmos* may be present due to inadequate restoration of orbital volume, bone graft absorption, migrating implant or orbital fat atrophy. It can be mild requiring no further intervention. In some cases, minimal ipsilateral upper lid elevation using Fasenella Servat procedure or contralateral upper lid blepharoplasty to deepen the superior sulcus can be enough to camouflage the appearance. In more extensive cases, the implant may be exchanged for a thicker one.

The orbital implant may become infected. It may be oversized and extruding. In both conditions the implant should be removed and replaced with a proper sized one. If fibrous tissue sufficient to cover the defect has formed since the original surgery, the implant may not require any replacement. Chronic lid swelling with superior globe displacement may indicate the presence of a fluid filled cyst formed around the implant. The implant should be removed and the cyst excised.

Ectropion, lower lid retraction or chronic edema may result when the skin approach is used. Retraction can occur due to adhesions between the orbital septum and the inferior orbital rim. This can be corrected by recessing the lower lid retractors.

Persistent infraorbital nerve anesthesia may occur. It may be injured or just compressed by the implant. If the nerve is not cut, function usually returns within 1 year. Sometimes the implant can be exchanged with widening the foramen decompressing the nerve. In some cases, the patient may get tolerant to the numbness in this area.

Blindness may occur in 1: 1500 cases. It can be secondary to compression of the optic nerve by the implant, orbital edema or hemorrhage. This can be prevented by avoiding undue pressure on the globe during surgery, continuous optic nerve monitoring, screening patients for clotting abnormalities preoperatively, using intra and post operative steroids, complete hemostasis before wound closure, avoiding compressive ocular dressing postoperatively and continuous monitoring of the pupil and visual acuity.

It should be remembered that the optic nerve may be damaged from the original injury with delayed visual loss from edema and vascular occlusion and may appear coincidently with surgery and mistakenly blamed on the surgical procedure.

Naso-orbital and Medial Orbital Wall Fractures

These fractures result from a force delivered to the nasal bridge or medial orbital rim. These are the weakest in the midface bones and usually injured by the dashboard in cases of automobile accidents. They are commonly associated with fracture floor and contribute to the presenting enophthalmos.

In mild cases, the injury is limited to the nasal bone and the frontal process of the maxilla. In more severe cases, the lacrimal and ethmoid bones **(Figure 9)** may crack and splay laterally causing traumatic telecanthus, flattening and widening of the midface, rounding of the medial canthus, epistaxis, periorbital ecchymosis, subcutaneous emphysema (if the ethmoid is fractured), with bony nasolacrimal duct injury causing epiphora. The medial rectus is rarely entrapped in the fracture with less common horizontal gaze limitation.

CSF rhinorrhea suggests a cribriform plate fracture. Most of cases are managed conservatively. The patient is treated by bed rest, intravenous antibiotics and instructed not to blow the nose or smoke. If the condition persists, neurosurgical interference is required.

Hemorrhage may be severe if the anterior and or posterior ethmoidal arteries are injured. The bleeding usually stops promptly. However, nasal packing or direct ligation may be required. Any coexistent upper airway obstruction should be relieved.

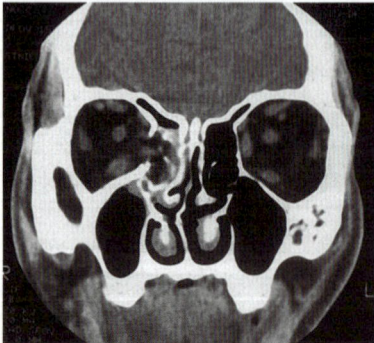

Figure 9: Medial wall fracture

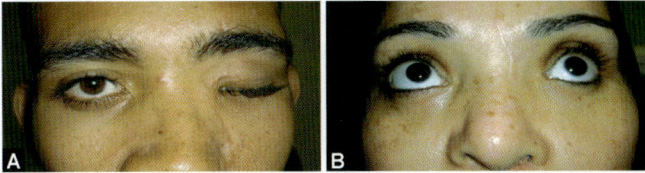

Figure 10: Cases of traumatic telecanthus. There is flattening of the nose, scar at the site of fracture. The case on the left side was associated with severe ptosis while both suffered from nasolacrimal duct obstruction

If the fracture extends to the lacrimal bone and ethmoid, traumatic telecanthus may result **(Figure 10)**. This usually requires repositioning of the bony fragments and transnasal wiring combined with canthal Y-V plasty. If there is enough bone support Y miniplate is inserted and used for the telecanthus repair.

If dacryostenosis is present, dacryocystorhinostomy may be required. Nasal bone fractures should be repaired by otolaryngeologist or plastic surgery. If associated with fracture floor, the floor should be repaired first with the implant the usually forms a platform for the medial wall implant

Transnasal Wiring: Surgical Technique

A. *If the contralateral nasal bone is intact*
Under general anethesia, a vertical incision is made nasal to the medial canthus. This may take a V-Y or C- U configuration if skin muscle advancement is also required in the reconstruction. The incision is carried to the fracture site adjacent to medial canthal tendon avoiding the lacrimal drainage system. The splayed bone at the posterior lacrimal crest is thinned using cutting burr. Either a 2-0 supramid suture or 27 gauge stainless steel wire is used to engage the superficial head of the tendon. If insufficient tendon remains, the supramid or wire may be positioned in the medial portion of the upper and lower tarsi.

On the intact side, a 15 mm vertical incision is made into the skin and subcutaneous tissues just anterior to the insertion of the superficial head of the medial canthal tendon. The periostium is opened vertically at the anterior lacrimal crest and reflected anteriorly. A 5 mm opening is made by a drill through the bone and nasal mucosa anterior to the attachment.

A Wright needle or 16 gauge trocar is passed from the surgically drilled opening (normal side) through the nasal septum, emerging at the fracture site. Some pressure is needed to penetrate the septum. Care should be taken to prevent momentum from carrying the needle immediately through the fracture site with the possibility of globe injury which lie in close proximity to the medial wall. Malleable retractors are placed to protect the globe

The supramid or wire suture are placed within the eyelet of the Wright needle or within the trocar after removing the stylet and this material becomes properly positioned as the needle/torcar is withdrawn. The two ends are tightened around 8mm metal bloster pin on the sound side and the traumatized canthus is quantitatively drawn medially as the supramid or wire is secured.

The deeper layers are closed with 5-0 Vicryl mattress suture, followed by skin closure with running 7-0 silk suture.If nasal pads are to be placed, this should be done before the trocar is removed. A second loop of wire is passed through the trocar after the transnasal wiring is completed but before the skin closure, the loop is cut leaving two free skin wires. The end of each is passed through one of two silicone pads. The wires from each side are twisted together over a dental roll to compress the skin in the canthal region. The nose pads and the skin sutures are left in place for 7-10 days, then the skin wires and pads are removed.

B. *If bilateral naso-orbital fractures*

If bilateral naso-orbital fractures, the bone may be insufficient on either side to support the reconstruction. In this condition, standard transnasal wiring technique takes place where two medial canthal incisions are made; bone penetration should be done at the posterior lacrimal crest level leaving intact bone anterior to this site to avoid forwards migration of the wire.

The trocar is passed and two looped 32 gauge stainless steel wires are passed; one loop with the ends of the other are tagged with the hemostat and they will become the skin wires, the other fixates the canthal tendons bilaterally. The medial canthal tendon is secured to the loop by 4-0 nonabsorbable suture. The two ends of the wire are twisted on themselves forming a second loop that is also secured to the medial canthal tendon on this side. The looped wire is tightened pulling the medial canthal angles towards the nasal septum. The skin wires are tied over nose pads to restore the concavity of tissues at the medial canthal area and removed in a similar time to the above.

C. *Lateral wall fractures*

The orbital plate of the zygoma is less able to absorb the trauma impact. It often fractures with orbital fat herniation into the temporal or malar regions. Lateral wall fractures are usually associated with fractures of the zygoma and corrected with replacement of the zygoma. Large defects usually need split cranial grafts with semi rigid fixation to the orbital rim.

D. *Trimalar (Tripod/ Tripartite) fractures*

It results form a lateral blow to the cheek resulting in a fracture of the zygomatic bone. Most commonly, the zygoma is fractured at its sutural junction with the frontal bone superiorly, the zygomatic arch laterally and maxilla medially. This can happen in different combinations. Trimalar fractures

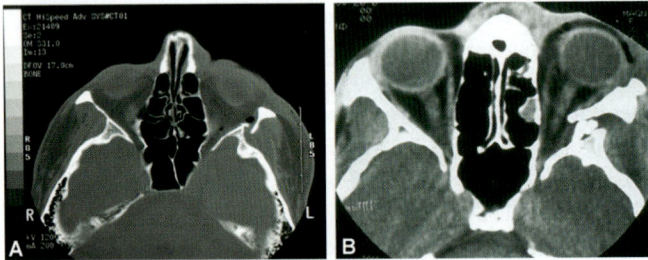

Figure 11: Axial scans showing varieties of zygoma complete fractures

may present with bone fragments either displaced or properly positioned. Non displaced zygoma fractures do not require surgery.

In cases of completely displaced fracture **(Figure 11)**, the bone fragment may be displaced posteriorly. This causes a step like deformity of the infraorbital rim at the zygomaticomaxillary suture, a flattened malar process and depression of the zygomaticofrontal suture superior to the lateral canthus. Hypothesia over the infraorbital nerve distribution is a common association. Difficulty to open the mouth can be present due to displaced fragment impinging on the temporalis muscle yet extraocular muscle imbalance is usually absent.

The incompletely displaced zygoma is hinged either at the frontal or maxillary attachment. If hinged to the frontal bone, there is usually no canthal displacement as the lateral canthal tendon and Lockwood ligament are still attached to the lateral orbital tuberculum. The main displacement is at the zygomaticomaxillary suture causing lower lid retraction inferolaterally and increased scleral show while the globe remains in its place. There is a step deformity at the inferior orbital rim and inferior rectus may be entrapped in the fracture site resulting in diplopia.

If the zygoma is hinged at the maxilla, the lateral tubercle is usually displaced inferiorly associated with outer canthus and globe displacement. There is a palpable gap in the lateral orbital wall. Sometimes the lateral orbital rim becomes displaced superiorly and posteriorly causing malar flattening associated with a bulge in the lateral orbital rim and the lateral canthal angle may be displaced superiorly. In either condition, there is no step deformity of the inferior orbital rim nor diplopia as there is no muscle entrapment.

Management: The fracture is reduced under general anesthesia and fixed in its place.

Surgical technique:
a. **Closed reduction:** that can be either done by:
- Towel clip that grasps the central portion of the fractured bone, elevating it into position until the fragment is felt to "pop" into place.
- An intraoral buccal sulcus incision where a blunt instrument is placed beneath the zygoma then upward and outward pressure is applied to restore the bone in place **(Figure 12)**.
- Gillis approach which is commonly used **(Figure 13)**. A 4 cm incision is placed at the temporal fossa hairline and carried down through the temporalis fascia and muscle to the periostium. A periosteal elevator is inserted beneath the temporalis fascia and gently passed downwards till a point below the zygoma. Leverage is applied to the elevator in an upward and outward direction reducing the fracture. The fragment can be guided by the surgeon's other hand.

In fresh fractures, the zygomatic bone once in place, it usually maintains its position. The temporalis fascia is closed with 4-0 vicryl while the subcutaneous layer is approximated by 5-0 vicryl in vertical mattress. The skin is finally closed by

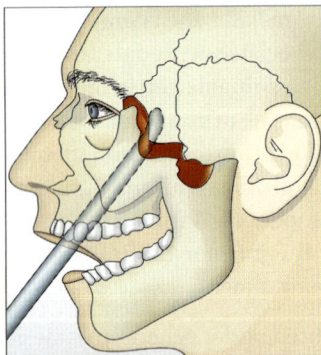

Figure 12: Lateral view for intraoral buccal approach

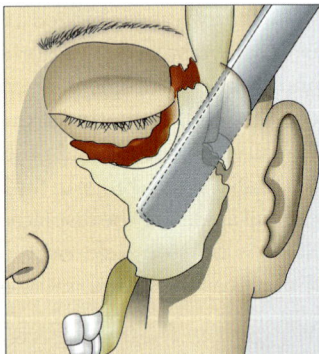

Figure 13: Gillis approach

6-0 silk sutures. If the zygoma is unstable, open and direct interosseus wiring is done.

b. **Open reduction:** A superolateral eye brow incision and a horizontal incision directly over the inferior orbital rim fracture site are fashioned. Dissection is carried to the fracture sites then a periosteal elevator is inserted via the inferior incision and the zygoma is rotated up into its position. All tissues entrapped within the fracture line should be released.

Specially designed miniplates and microplates are used to approximate the fractured bones. Small drill holes are placed on each side of the fractured zygomaticofrontral and zygmoaticomaxillary sutures while protecting orbital structures during drilling. The screws are advanced until the head is firmly supporting the plate.

Other methods of fixation include intramaxillary inflatable balloon and direct interosseus wiring where the bone fragments are united by 27 gauge wire that is tightened by wire twister without excessive tightening. It is effective in relatively stable fractures. The wire ends are cut leaving nearly

5 mm long and reposited in a drill hole or pressed flat against the bone to avoid injury to overlying structure.

If sufficient periostium remains, it should be closed by 5-0 interrupted vicryl sutures. Muscles and subcutaneous layers are also closed with 5-0 vicryl. Skin is closed by 6-0 silk sutures **(Figures 14)**.

If the malar flattening persists after reduction which usually occurs with comminuted fractures, the malar eminence can be augmented by alloplast or bone graft placed in a subperiosteal pocket via inferior fornix or Caldwell-Luc incision.

E. *Le Fort Fractures (Figure 15)*

Le Fort fractures involve the maxilla and are usually complex, asymmetric and incomplete. Pure Le Fort fractures are uncommon. Le Fort I is a low transverse maxillary fracture that does not extend to the orbit. The fragment of the maxilla containing the teeth is separated from the remainder of the facial bones. In severe cases, it may be free floating.

Le Fort II fractures are pyramidal, involving the maxilla, nasal bone and medial orbital floor. This fracture begins at the lower portion on the nasal bones, across the naso-orbital margin above the nasolacrimal canal through the medial orbital floor (sometimes associated with blow-out fracture) over the infraorbital rim through the inferior orbital canal involving the anterior and posterior walls of the maxillary sinus. This fracture crosses the posterior pillar of the upper jaw, the pyramidal and pterygoid processes, and pterygomandibular fissure ending at the medial orbital margin and lateral wall of the nose. This fracture may be partially displaced or free floating.

Le Fort III fractures create a craniofacial dysjunction involving both orbits, separating the maxilla from the skull; the facial skeleton is free floating attached to the cranium by

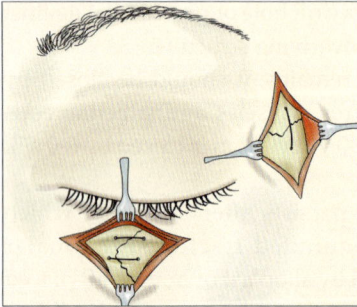

Figure 14: Incision and wiring in open reduction

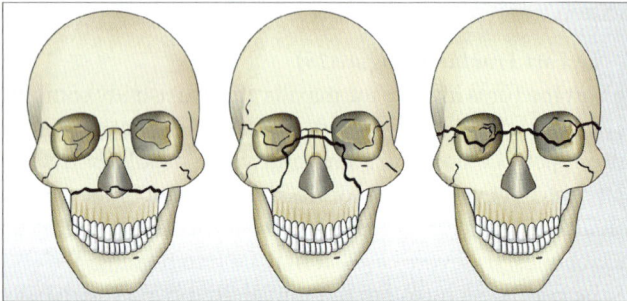

Figure 15: Le Fort fractures I, II and III respectively from left to right

only soft tissue. This fracture extends from the upper portion of the nasal bone, across the orbital margin near the frontomaxillary suture through the ethmoid bone passing posteriorly and inferiorly below the optic foramina to the inferior orbital fissure. It then separates into two segments; one extends upwards along the zygomaticosphenoid suture between the orbital roof and the lateral orbital wall crossing the lateral orbital rim at the zygomaticofrontal suture. The second portion extends inferiorly and posteriorly crossing the pterygoid process. The zygomatic arch is also involved.

Le Fort II and III may extend to the orbital apex affecting the optic nerve and reducing vision. Management of theses fractures require open reduction usually with arch bars. They may be associated with skull fracture thus requiring conjoint work with neurosurgery.

F. Orbital Roof Fractures (Figure 16)

Isolated roof fractures are uncommon due to the strength of the superior orbital rim. They can be seen with wounds inflicted by sharp objects, gun shots or in association with Le Fort III fractures.

It may be associated with brow and eyelid ecchymosis, forehead hypoesthesia, ptosis and diplopia. The latter is secondary to superior rectus or oblique affection as well as damage to the trochlea. Ptosis results from third nerve affection, direct muscle injury or muscle entrapment. The fracture may extend to the superior orbital fissure and optic canal with resultant damage to the optic, oculomotor, trochlear and abducent nerves. In rare occasions with large or depressed fracture it may present with globe displacement, secondary menigeocele or encephalocele with and pulsatile proptosis.

Superior orbital rim, frontal sinus and glabellar fractures either remain extracranial or communicate with the

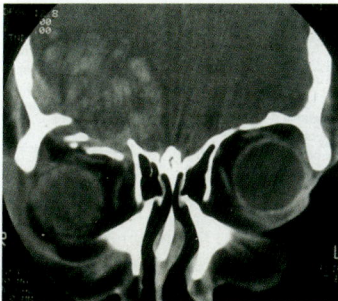

Figure 16: Coronal scan showing fracture roof of the orbit

intracranial compartment. If air is detected in the anterior cranial fossa in case of orbital roof fracture, this signifies a dural tear. Unless a significant displacement is found, superior orbital rim fractures don't need surgical reduction, displaced fractures of small size without involving the orbital roof and did not violate the intracranial space can be repositioned and wired under the microscope. All other superior rim or roof fractures should be evaluated and managed by a neurosurgeon.

G. Orbital blow-in fractures

Any of the four walls may be fractured and displaced towards the center reducing the orbital volume and causing edema, proptosis and optic nerve compression either directly or by secondary increase of intraorbital pressure. Diplopia and mechanical restriction of extraocular muscle movements as well as globe injuries can also be detected. The most common in fractured walls are the roof and the lateral wall **(Figure 17)**. Cases with optic neuropathy or marked proptosis causing exposure should be managed as soon as possible.

Role of Endoscopy in Management of Orbital Fractures

Endoscopic repair of orbital fractures could become a predictable and efficient treatment alternative to traditional

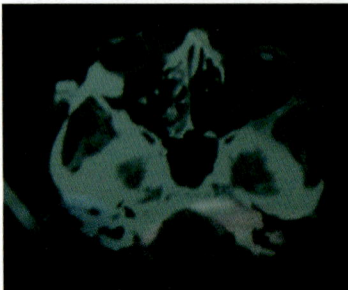

Figure 17: Fractured zygoma incarcerated behind the intact globe

method. It is can be used for repair of isolated floor or medial wall fractures not associated with orbital rim fractures. It has also been tested for repair of delayed cases with promising results. It offers a hidden incision, improved fracture visualization, and avoidance of postoperative eyelid malposition, however, specific knowledge of endoscopic anatomy is required.

Via an endoscopic endonasal approach, a wide middle meatal antrostomy in case of floor fractures or intransal ethmoidectomy in case of medial wall fracture is created. Adhesions between the protruded periorbita and the paranasal sinus mucosa are dissected and the bone fragments are removed. The orbital floor is supported by a saline filled balloon, which is connected with an infant feeding catheter and passed through the middle meatal antrostoma. After confirming the reduction of the orbital floor by postoperative CT, the catheter is ligated and cut in short to keep it in the nasal cavity. A silastic or Medpore implant sheet soaked in antibiotic solution can also be used for the floor or medial wall fracture repair. Temporary supporting of the orbital wall with a detachable temporary balloon, or a silastic sheet and Merocel packing was removed 4 weeks after surgery in the outpatient clinic **(Figure 18).**

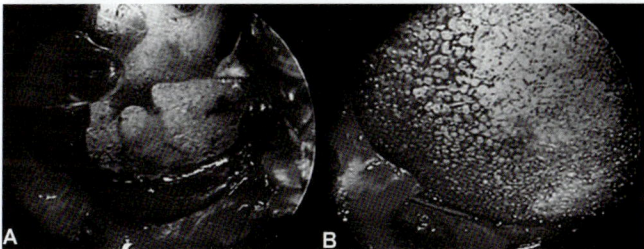

Figure 18: Endoscopic view of floor fracture
(A) Before surgery, (B) After repair

Management of Old Standing Orbital Trauma

The patient is evaluated in a manner similar to acute cases with more stress on the globe position, ocular motility, forced duction testing as well as diplopia fields. If globe reposition is indicated, it should be done before muscle or eyelid surgeries. Bony orbit may be restored by osteotomies and open reduction or volume augmentation.by placing an implant in the subperiosteal space. Soft tissues incarcerated in the sinus should be carefully removed however, fibrosis render this step difficult with more possibility of tissue injury. Adjustable suture technique is better used for muscle surgery in such cases. Sometimes, glasses with plus lenses can be prescribed for blind eyes to reduce the apparent enophthalmos.

Orbital Contour Deformity

This may arise from old trauma that was not or poorly repaired. If the defect is small, no further management will be needed. In case of large defects, subperiosteal custom-made implants are used. The extent of the deformity is defined by radiological studies and the ocularist takes mold of the affected region incorporating the defect. A positive impression is fashioned from the mold using the desired alloplastic material. This can be designed using special computer programs. Methyl methacrylate and proplast implants are usually effective.

Surgical technique: Under general anesthesia, one or two small incisions are placed adjacent to but not overlying the deformity in conformity with Langer's lines. The incision is carried down till the deformity using sharp and blunt dissection. If the periostium is intact, a periosteal pocket is created to receive the implant. Alloplastic materials soaked in antibiotic solution are mildly modified using scissors. The surrounding bone may be modified using a drill with fine burr head. The alloplastic material is placed within the periosteal socket and secured in place using 2-0 supramid sutures.

The wound is closed in two or three layers with interrupted sutures.

Late Hypophthalmos or Enophthalmos

Implantation of various materials in the subperiosteal space along the orbital floor can augment this area thus raising the globe and moving it anteriorly. Materials used for orbital floor fractures are used to correct globe malpositions yet they are thicker especially posterior. Beads and pellets forms of these materials can be used and they require smaller incisions. The floor exposure is very similar to the approaches described for orbital floor fracture repair. The periostium is incised elevated from the floor using periosteal elevator and malleable retractors. The implant is placed in the created space with the same precautions taken for floor fracture implants, i.e. pupil and forced duction test. Some authors inserted porous polyethylene (Medpor) particles diced about 1 × 1 cm diameter through a lateral canthal incision to orbital floor with successful results. The advantages of this technique are limited incision, decreased postoperative edema, volumetric adjustability, and applicability under local anesthesia.

Soft tissue fillers have been tried to correct enophthalmos, They include autologous fat, cross linked collagen (Zyplast) and self inflating hydrogel pellets. The latter should not be used in cases with visual potential as they may induce high pressures. Calcium hydroxyapatite gel (Radiesse) as well as hyaluronic acid can be injected to augment the volume in eyes with mild enophthalmos and intact vision. Hyaluronic acid was described to be injected intraconal.

The surgeon should always compare to the sound side for globe position, restoration of the supratarsal sulcus as well as alignment with the sound side. Correction of the condition may result in aggravating existing ptosis that requires surgical intervention.

Late Persistent Handicapping Diplopia

Muscle surgery is advocated after the motility and diplopia measurements are stabilized. Orbital floor surgery can improve it when it is performed up to 5 weeks post-trauma yet the extraocular muscle motility rarely improves after that. The surgery is individualized according to the degree of ocular imbalance. Adjustable sutures are preferred.

Most of patients suffer from diplopia on downgaze interfering with reading. If the eye can move up normally with normal forced duction test on upgaze. A reverse Knapp procedure is performed in which the medial and lateral recti are placed at or several millimeters behind the original inferior rectus insertion.

If the eye cannot move upwards normally with positive forced duction test, inferior rectus is recessed till the eye can be normally moved upwards during surgery. Then a modified reverse Knapp procedure is performed 3-6 months later; thus avoiding working on three muscles at the same time for fear of anterior segment ischemia.

Fadom operation can be done attaching the inferior rectus to the sclera in the sound eye. This decreases diplopia in down gaze yet it inhibits downwards movement and makes the patient tilt his/her head on reading.

Telecanthus

A Y-shaped miniplates can be used to correct telecanthus when there is enough bony support. In case of bone destruction, transnasal wiring is the procedure of choice.

Surgical technique: A medial orbitotomy incision is made just medial to the medial canthus and anterior to the lacrimal drainage system. Soft tissue and scar are debulked, any displaced bone fragments are either reduced or removed. A Y-shaped miniplate is attached to the nasal bone or frontal bone with screws keeping the long limb directed posteriorly. The medial canthal tendon is engaged by a wire on a free needle then passed through the corresponding hole of the plate mirroring the place of the posterior lacrimal crest. One of the previously placed screws is loosened and the wire is wrapped around its head.

The wire is tightened while the assistant keeps medial traction on the canthal tendon aiming at over correction. Then the ends of the wire are cut, twisted and bent back into the miniplate.

The tissues are closed in anatomical layers and finally the skin is closed using 6-0 silk sutures.

SUMMARY

Orbital and globe injuries are common in maxillofacial traumas. Proper and systematic assessment is mandatory to detect any subtle lesion and should be done as soon as life-saving measures are taken. Proper understanding of the anatomy, possible problems and their mechanisms is of utmost importance for proper management. Early reconstruction is desirable yet late repair is a challenge requiring many and staged procedures. The treatment is individualized according to the patient's condition. Proper assessment and planning is the key for obtaining good results.

BIBLIOGRAPHY

1. Barry C, Coyle M, Idrees Z, Dwyer MH, Kearns G. Ocular findings in patients with orbitozygomatic complex fractures: a retrospective study. J Oral Maxillofac Surg 2008 May;66(5):888-92.

2. Bilyk JR, Shore JW, Ward JB, Mckeown CA. Late orbital trauma: Diagnosis and treatment In oculoplastic surgery 3rd edition McCord CD, Tanenbaum M, Nunery WR (Eds) 1995 Raven press New York Chapter 18; pp 553- 80.

3. Coban YK, Kabalci SK. Surgical treatment of posttraumatic enophthalmos with diced medpor implants through mini-lateral canthoplasty incision J Craniofac Surg 2008 Mar;19(2):539-41.

4. Eppley BL, Dadvand B. Injectable soft tissue filers, clinical overview. Plast Reconstr Surg 2006;118: 98e-106e.

5. Farwell DG, Sires BS, Kriet JD, Stanley RB Jr. Endoscopic repair of orbital blowout fractures: use or misuse of a new approach? Arch Facial Plast Surg 2007 Nov-Dec;9(6):427-33.

6. Fernandes R, Fattahi T, Steinberg B, Schare H. Endoscopic repair of isolated orbital floor fracture with implant placement J Oral Maxillofac Surg 2007Aug;65(8):1449-53.

7. Ferraz FH, Schellini SA, Schellini RC, Pellizon CH, Hirai FE, Padovani CR. BMP implant associated with platelet-rich plasma in orbit fracture repair. Curr Eye Res 2008 Mar;33(3):293-301.

8. Frodel JL Jr. Computer-designed implants for fronto-orbital defect reconstruction. Facial Plast Surg 2008 Jan;24(1):22-34.

9. Garibaldi DC, Iliff NT, Grant MP, Merbs SL. Use of porous polyethylene with embedded titanium in orbital reconstruction: a review of 106 patients. Ophthal Plast Reconstr Surg 2007 Nov-Dec;23(6):439-44.

10. Gossman MD, Pollock RA. Acute orbital trauma. In Oculoplastic Surgery 3rd edition McCord CD, Tanenbaum M, Nunery WR (Eds) 1995 Raven press. New York Chapter 17; pp 515-51.

11. Hinohira Y, Yumoto E, Hyodo M, Shiraishi A. Reduction surgeries for delayed cases with isolated blowout fractures. Otolaryngol Head Neck Surg 2008 Feb;138(2):252-4.

12. Jeon SY, Kwon JH, Kim JP, Ahn SK, Park JJ, Hur DG, Seo SW. Endoscopic intranasal reduction of the orbit in isolated blowout fractures. Acta Otolaryngol Suppl 2007 Oct;(558):102-9.

13. Kaufman Y, Stal D, Cole P, Hollier L Jr. Orbitozygomatic fracture management. Plast Reconstr Surg 2008 Apr;121(4):1370-4.

14. Koltus BS, Dryden RM. Correction of anophthalmic enophthalmos with injectable hydroxyapatite (Radiesse). Ophthal Plast Reconstr Surg 2007; 23:313-4

15. Moore CC, Bromwich M, Roth K, Matic DB. Endoscopic anatomy of the orbital floor and maxillary sinus. J Craniofac Surg 2008 Jan;19(1):271-6.
16. Nesi FA, Walz KL (Eds). Orbital fractures and medial canthal reconstruction. Smith's practical techniques in ophthalmic plastic surgery. 2nd edition, Mosby St Louis, Missouri, 1994. Chapter 18; pp 227-37.
17. Putterman AM, Smith BC, Lisman RD. Blow out fractures. In Smith's Ophthalmic Plastic and Reconstructive Surgery, 2nd edition Nesi FA, Lisman RD, Levine MR (eds). Mosby St Louis, 1998, Chapter 8; pp 209-40.
18. Sargent LA. Nasoethmoid orbital fractures: diagnosis and treatment. Plast Reconstr Surg 2007 Dec;120 (7 Suppl 2):16S-31S.
19. Tay E, Oliver J. Intraorbital hyaluronic acid for enophthalmos. Letter to the editor. Ophthalmology 2008;115(6):1101.
20. Tenzel RR. Orbital and periorbital fractures. Textbook of Ophthalmlic Plastic and Reconstructive Surgery. Steven M, Podos, Yanoff M ed. 1st edition, 1993, Gower medical publications, New York Chapter 16 pp 322-37.
21. Tse R, Allen L, Matic D. The white-eyed medial blowout fracture. Plast Reconstr Surg 2007 Jan;119(1):277-86.

Preseptal Cellulitis and Orbital Cellulitis

22

Arif Adenwala, Mahesh Dalvi (India)

PRESEPTAL CELLULITIS

Definition

It is an inflammatory process involving the tissue anterior to the orbital septum.[4]

The orbital septum is fibrous sheet that extends from periosteum of the orbit as arcus marginalis and lies deep to orbicularis muscle.

In upper lid the septum fuses with levator aponeurosis. In lower eye lid the septum fuses with orbital retractor.

The orbital septum limits the spread of infection from preseptal space to the orbit.

Causes

Preseptal cellulitis is more common in children than orbital cellulitis. The causes can be divided in to 3 groups:[1, 3]

1. *Eyelid trauma:* Suppurative cellulitis may be seen secondary to lid trauma. Commonest organisms associated are *Streptococcus aureus* and *Streptococcus pyogenes*.
2. *Association with upper respiratory tract infection:* Organisms isolated are *Hemophillus influenza* and *streptococci*.
3. *Infection:* Periorbital edema develop from associated lid infection such as impetigo, herpes simplex, varicella or due to infected chalazion or dacryocystitis.

Pathogenesis[1,3,4]

Preseptal cellulitis can occur by several mechanisms:

A. Infection due to local trauma like insect bite.
B. Secondary to spread from contagious structure like conjunctivitis, hordoleum, dacryocystitis and impetigo.
C. Infection secondary to hematogenous spread during bacterimia due to nasopharyngeal pathology.

Clinical Features

- Usual clinical presentation is unilateral periorbital edema, pain and fever.
- Bilateral involvement is rare.
- Previous history of trauma or upper respiratory infection is seen.

On examination (Figure 1):

- There is presence of erythema, tenderness on the lids,
- Absence of proptosis or decreased extraocular movement (seen in orbital cellulitis)
- Presence of purulent discharge
- Bluish purple discoloration of eyelid

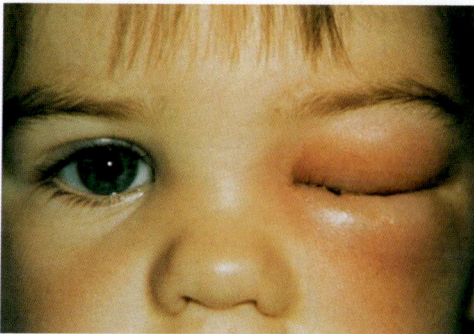

Figure 1: Preseptal cellulitis (*Courtesy:* Online Journal of Ophthalmology)

Management

Detailed History and complete clinical examination is must before going to further investigation.

Diagnosis[1,3]

Children with local cause for periorbital edema rarely need any further investigation.

- Complete blood count is done to rule out infection.
- If there is underlying lid trauma then culture of wound discharge is done.
- Blood culture is done if bacterimia or sepsis is concern.
- Lumbar puncture and examination of the cerebrospinal fluid is done to rule out meningeal involvement in cases where *H. Influenzae* type b is suspected.
- Cultures are taken from nose, throat, conjunctiva and aspirates of the periorbital edema in cases upper respiratory tract infection. X-ray paranasal sinuses is also done.
- CT scan of the orbit is performed to rule out orbital and subperiosteal involvement and cavernous sinus thrombosis.
- MRI is the study of choice to rule out cavernous sinus thrombosis.

Treatment

Main aim of the treatment is to prevent further complication. Opinion from ENT surgeon and pediatrician is important before starting the treatment.

In trauma related cases gram-positive coverage with cephalexin, augmentin clindamycin is given.

In absence of trauma, broad spectrum cephalosporins like ceftriaxone are used or depending on the culture report appropriate drugs are given:

Older children can be managed as out patient using oral broad spectrum antibiotics. Broad spectrum or newer cephalosporins can be administered.

Surgical treatment is hardly required. About 10% of the children will require surgical drainage of the lid abscess or para nasal sinus.

Complication[1,3]

1. CNS Infection like meningitis, epidural abscess, subdural empyema and brain abscess.
2. Orbital involvement leading to orbital cellulitis or orbital abscess.
3. Cavernous sinus thrombosis.
4. Toxic shock syndrome.
5. Eschar formation leading to scarring.

Prognosis

With appropriate and prompt treatment the prognosis is good.

ORBITAL CELLULITIS

Orbital cellulitis is an uncommon but important entity which can give rise to serious systemic and ocular complication.

Orbital cellulitis is an infection of the soft tissue of the orbit posterior to the orbital septum. Proper and prompt diagnosis and management is very important for treating the patients with orbital cellulitis.

Pathophysiology

Orbital cellulitis occurs in following three conditions:[1,2,4]

1. Extension of infection from periorbital structures mainly paranasal sinuses and from face, globe and lacrimal sac.
2. Direct inoculation from trauma and surgery.
3. Hematogenous spread from bacteremia.

Medial orbital wall is thin and is perforated by numerous blood vessels and nerves and also by other defects like Zuckerkandl dehiscence.

This defect in walls allows for easy communication of infectious material between ethmoidal air cells and subperiosteal space in the medial aspect of the orbit leading to formation of subperiosteal abscess.

Posterior in the orbit, the fascia between rectus muscles is thin and incomplete allowing easy extension between extra-conal and intraconal orbital space.

Infectious material can also be introduced in the orbit directly from accidental or surgical trauma.

Ethmoidal sinusitis is the most common cause of orbital cellulitis and aerobic non-spore forming bacteria is the most frequently responsible organism.

Clinical Features

Important significant sign is presence of proptosis and ophthalmoplegia **(Figure 2)**.

Other signs are:
• Conjunctival chemosis

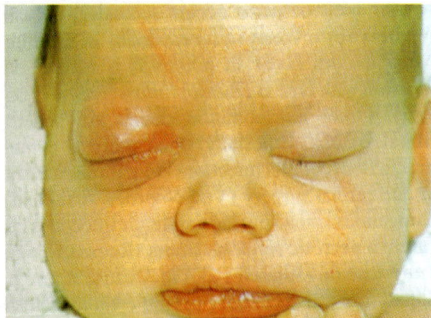

Figure 2: Orbital cellulitis (*Courtesy:* Anthony Moore: Paediatric Ophthalmology, David Taylor)

- Decreased vision
- Increased intraocular pressure
- Pain on eye movement.

It can also be accompanied with lid edema, rhinorrhea and increasing malaise.

Causes[1,2,4]

- It is commonly seen secondary to ethmoidal sinusitis mainly in children more than 5 years old in almost 90% cases.
- Bacterial infection like type B *Hemophillus influenzae*, *Staphylococcus aureus*, *Streptococcus pyogenes*, *Strep. pneumoniae* and anaerobes like *Bacteroides* species.
- Penetrating orbital trauma mainly incases of retained foreign body.
- Secondary to surgical procedures including orbital decompression, DCR, eyelid surgery, strabismus surgery, retinal surgery, etc.
- Fungi: Most common organisms are *Mucor* and *Aspergillus*.
  Aspergillus gives rise to chronic proptosis and decreased visual acuity.
  Mucor mycosis can lead to orbital apex syndrome.

Complication[1,4]

1. *Ocular:* includes exposure keratopathy, raised intracranial pressure, CRAO/CRVO, endophthalmitis, optic neuropathy.
2. *Intracranial:* Meningitis, brain abscess and cavernous sinus thrombosis. Cavernous sinus thrombosis is important complication and should be suspected in cases of bilateral orbital cellulitis, rapidly involving proptosis and presence of congestion of facial, conjunctival and retinal veins.

3. *Subperiosteal abscess:* It is located along the medial orbital wall. It is seriously entity having potential progression plus intra cranial extension.

Diagnosis:[1,4]

- Complete blood count: Leucocytosis with count more than 15,000 with shift to left is seen in most of the cases.
- Blood cultures prior to administration of antibiotics.
- Grams stain to identify the type of organism.
- Needle aspiration from the orbit is contraindicated.
- X-ray paranasal sinus for diagnosis of ethmoidal sinusitis.
- Dental examination to rule out any dental infection.
- High resolution CT scan is very diagnostic modality to conform the diagnosis and extent of the disease. It is used in detecting subperiosteal and orbital abscess which can be missed in normal X-ray.
- MRI is helpful in defining the orbital abscess and evaluation of cavernous sinus disease.
- Orbital ultrasound can also detect orbital abscess but is less reliable.
- Lumbar puncture is indicated in patients with meningeal signs to rule out meningitis

Treatment[4]

1. *Hospital admission:* Opinion from the pediatrician and ENT surgeon is important before starting with the management.
2. *Administration of broad spectrum antibiotics:* Ceftazidime 1 gm is given IM 8 hourly and metronidazole in dose of 500 mg every 8 hourly.

Alternative IV vancomycin can also be used. Antibiotic treatment is continued until the patient is apyrexial for 4 days.

Optic nerve function is monitored every 4 hourly for pupillary reaction, visual acuity, color vision.

Surgery is usually indicated:[4]
- Unresponsive to antibiotics
- Decreasing visual acuity
- Orbital/subperiosteal abscess. It is important to drain the infected sinuses as well as the orbits.

REFERENCES

1. Anthony Moore – Paediatric Ophthalmology, 13, 107-13. Preseptal and Orbital Cellulitis.
2. E- medicine Orbital Cellulitis
3. E-medicine Preseptal Cellulitis
4. Jack J Kanski – Clinical ophthalmology – Orbital Infections.17;567-70.
5. Londer L, Nelson DL. Orbital cellulitis due to Hemophillus influenza Arch Ophthalmology 1974;91:89-98.
6. Schranm VL, Myers EN. Orbital complication of Acute Sinusitis Otolaryngol 1978;86:221-30.
7. Wallers E, Wallers H, Hiles D. Acute Orbital Cellulitis, Arch ophthalmology 1976;94:785-8.
8. Goldberg F, Berne AS. Differentiation of Orbital Cellulitis from Preseptal cellulitis by Computed Tomography Paediatrics 1978:62:1000-9.
9. Barkins RM, Todd JK. Periorbital cellulitis in children. Paediatrics. 1978: 62:390-2.
10. Smith TF, O'Day et al. Clinical implications of preseptal cellulitis in childhood.

CARBUNCLE

Introduction

Acute suppurative inflammation of multiple meibomian glands along with the blockage of their ducts, results in eyelid abscess or carbuncle.

Clinical Features

- Intense pain
- Maximum tenderness can be elicited at a number of points on the swelling
- Swelling is usually away from the eyelid margin
- Multiple pus points are usually seen on the cutaneous surface **(Figures 1 and 2)**.

Differential Diagnosis

- Hordeolum externum
- Hordeolum internum
- Molluscum contagiosum
- Malignancy, etc.

Treatment

- Hot compresses are useful in the cellulitis stage.

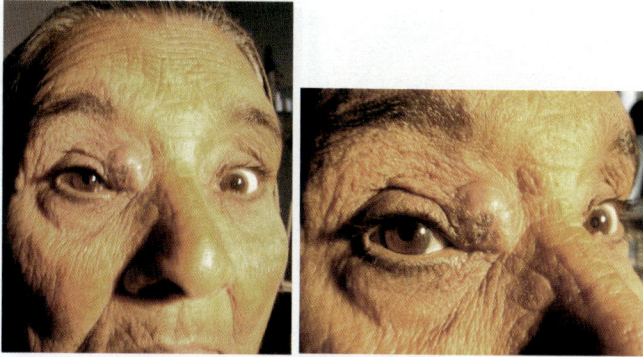

Figures 1 and 2: Carbuncle upper eyelid

- Systemic antibiotics and anti inflammatory medicines are advised.
- Pus is evacuated in the later stages through a transcutaneous incision parallel to the lid margin.

Prognosis

- Good, if managed in time.

CARUNCULAR ABSCESS

Introduction

The caruncle consists of a mass of fibrous tissue similar to that of the tarsal cartilages, in which are imbedded follicles secreting a fluid similar in nature to that of the meibomian glands. This fluid comes out through twelve to fifteen excretory orifices on its surface, which is covered by the conjunctiva.

The healthy caruncle is yellowish-red in color, slightly tuberculated on the surface, which, in addition to the excretory orifices, is beset with very delicate scarcely visible hair.

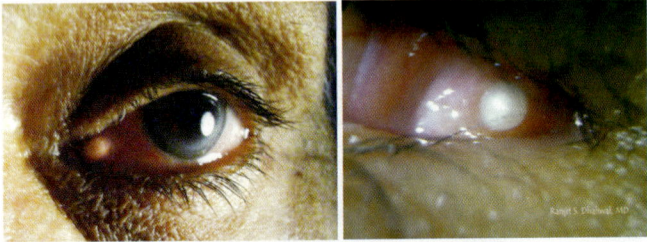

Figures 3 and 4: Caruncular abscess

The caruncular abscess is similar to that of the meibomian glands **(Figures 3 and 4)**.

Clinical Features

Similar to catarrhal inflammation of the caruncle and semi-lunar fold, but as suppuration takes place

- Pain becomes throbbing in nature, and
- Redness and swelling of the surrounding tissues increases, until
- It presents as a yellow point between the caruncle and the semi-lunar fold, which
- Bursts out, resulting in the evacuation of the abscess and
- Finally atrophy of the caruncle **(Figures 3 and 4)**.

Differential Diagnosis

- Caruncular growth
- FB embedded in the caruncle.

Treatment

- Oral broad spectrum antibiotics, along with
- Topical broad spectrum antibiotics in the form of eye drops or an eye ointment.
- Warm fomentation is applied on the medial canthus when suppuration is threatened.

- The abscess is opened with a sharp disposable needle or a lancet, once fluctuation is elicited or the yellow point presents.

Prognosis

- Good with medical treatment and surgical evacuation, if necessary.

CONCRETIONS (LITHIASIS)

Introduction

Concretions are yellowish white, hard, raised pin head sized lesions on palpebral conjunctiva. These are formed by accumulation of dead epithelial cell debris and inspissated mucous into the depressions called Henle's glands. They never become calcareous so the term concretion is a misnomer. The concretions get their name from the fact that these are hard and pointed and can scratch the cornea.

Clinical Features (Figure 5)

- Foreign body sensation
- Lacrimation, and
- Recurrent corneal abrasions.

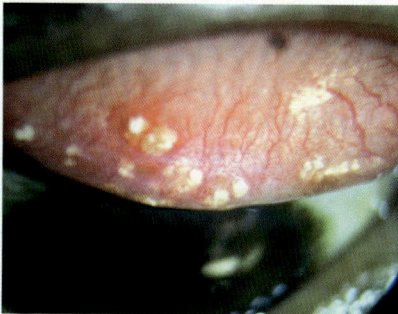

Figure 5: Concretions (Lithiasis)

Differential Diagnosis

- Concretions may occur in the elderly, or in
- Chronic inflammatory conditions like:
  - Vernal conjunctivitis,
  - Atopic keratoconjunctivitis,
  - Post-trachomatous degeneration, etc.

Treatment

Concretions are removed with a 26 G hypodermic needle after anaesthetizing the conjunctival sac.

Prognosis

Prognosis following removal is good, but recurrences do occur.

ECTROPION OF LOWER PUNCTA

Introduction

- Lacrimal puncta are small round or oval openings of the lacrimal canaliculi, approximately 0.3 mm in diameter and are situated at the edge of the medial end of each eyelid, in line with the openings of the meibomian glands.
- Upper punctum is situated 6 mm temporal to the inner canthus, while the lower punctum is 6.5 mm away.
- Each punctum is positioned astride a slight elevation called the lacrimal papilla, and is not visible in health, as it faces the bulbar conjunctiva, and dips into the pool of the tears, which collects in the inner canthus and is called Lacus lacrimalis **(Figures 6 and 7)**.

Clinical Features

- Chief complaint of the patient is excessive watering from the eyes.

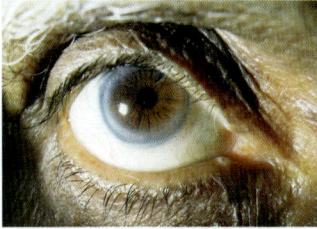

Figure 6: Ectropion lower punctum OD

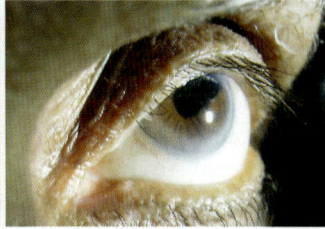

Figure 7: Ectropion lower punctum OS

- In old age the lacrimal papilla and the puncta become more prominent and rotate out, due to the laxity of tissues due to senile changes **(Figures 6 and 7)**.
- As the puncta do not dip into the lacus lacrimalis, this pool of the tears is not siphoned by the lacrimal passages and overflows onto the cheeks.

Differential Diagnosis

- Senile ectropion of the lower eyelids.
- Chronic conjunctivitis.
- Chronic blepharitis.

Treatment

- Three–snip operation to open up the lower lacrimal canaliculus onto the tarsal conjunctival surface.
- Conjunctivodacryocystorhinostomy may have to be resorted to in unrelenting cases.

Prognosis

- Fair to good chances of recovery of functions.

EYELASH IN THE CANALICULUS

Introduction

- Foreign bodies in the conjunctival 'cul-de-sac' are common, and cause great discomfort and irritation, till the time these are removed.
- Foreign bodies in the canaliculi are rare and not of much significance if these do not produce a blockage.
- Eyelash in the canaliculus is both, conspicuous to the examiner and irritating to the patient, as it protrudes out through the punctum and wipes over the conjunctiva with each movement of the eyelid **(Figures 8 to 10)**.

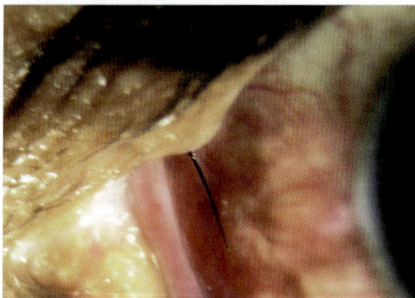

Figure 8: Eyelash in the canaliculus protruding through the punctum

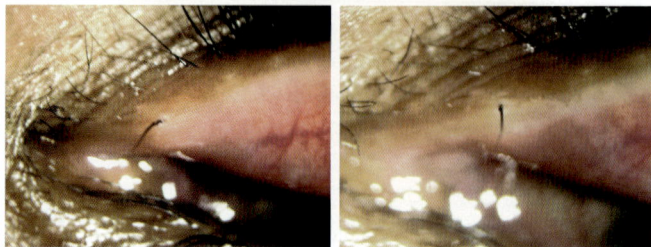

Figures 9 and 10: Eyelash in the upper canaliculus protruding through the punctum.

Etiology

- 11 to 13 eyelashes are shed daily, from each eye, and go into the conjunctival sac only if the patient happens to rub the eye. The flow of the tears takes these to the punctum, where once engaged, the siphon created and further rubbing of the eye, draws it into the canaliculus.
- The proximal end of the eyelash is the first to go through the punctum, because of its rigid nature in contrast to the limp distal end.

Treatment

Removal with an epilation forceps.

FOREIGN BODY IN SULCUS SUBTARSALIS

Introduction

No examination of the eye is complete, without everting the upper eyelid, for, the sulcus subtarsalis is an ideal place to stick to, for all foreign bodies in the conjunctival sac **(Figure 11)**.

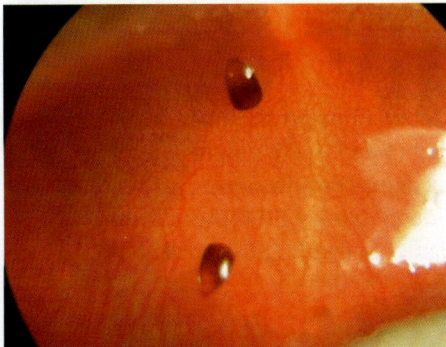

Figure 11: Foreign body in the sulcus subtarsalis

Etiology

- Unprotected driving of two wheelers, especially at dusk, when the insects fly towards the vehicular lights.
- Unprotected harvesting and threshing of crops.
- Unprotected working in front of lathes and grinders.

Clinical Features

Pain, lacrimation, photophobia and conjunctival discharge.

Treatment

Removal with a sterile 26 G hypodermic needle after anesthetizing the conjunctival sac with a local anesthetic and instilling a broad spectrum antibiotic ointment into the sac.

GRAVES' OPHTHALMOPATHY (THYROTOXICOSIS)

Clinical Features (Figures 12 to 14)

Symptoms

- Exophthalmos
- Dry eyes.

Signs

1. Lid signs
   - Retraction of upper lid (**Dalrymple's sign**) **(Figure 12)**
   - Lid lag (**Von Graefe's sign**)
   - Lid oedema (**Enroth sign**)
   - Infrequent blinking (**Stellwag's sign**)
   - Difficulty in everting the upper lid (**Gifford's sign**)
2. Ocular motility defects
   - Weakness of convergence (**Mobius sign**)
3. Conjunctival chemosis.
4. Proptosis.

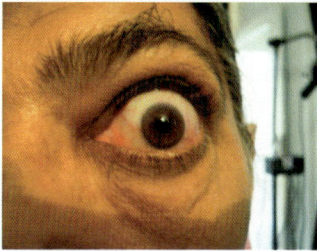

Figure 12: Exophthalmos: Dalrymple's sign

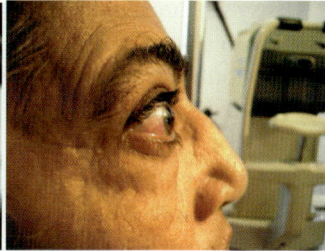

Figure 13: Exophthalmos: Right eye

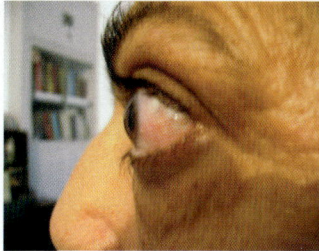

Figure 14: Exophthalmos: Left eye

5. Exposure keratitis.
6. Optic neuropathy.

Differential Diagnosis

1. Thyroid disorders.
2. Chronic nongranulomatous intraorbital lesions (pseudotumor).
3. Primary intraorbital tumors.
4. Secondary intraorbital tumours, etc. should be looked for.

Investigations

1. Positional tonometry.

2. Thyroid function tests.
3. B scan of the orbits.
4. Computerized tomography of the orbits.

Treatment

1. Treatment of the thyroid status.
2. Topical medical management
   - Lubricant eyedrops or tears substitutes to treat dryness.
   - Guanethedine 5% eyedrops to releive the spasm of the Muller's muscle.
3. Systemic steroids and radiotherapy to reduce the orbital oedema and inflammation.
4. Prismatic glasses to relieve diplopia.
5. Surgical management
   - Lateral tarsorrhaphy.
   - Extraocular muscle surgery.
   - Surgical management of the orbit.
   - Blepharoplasty
   - Cosmetic surgery for persistent lid retraction.

Prognosis

Depends upon the maintenance of the thyroid functions.

TRACHOMA

Introduction

- Trachoma is chronic keratoconjunctivitis, affecting primarily the superficial layers of conjunctiva and cornea.
- It is still one of the leading causes of preventable blindness, world over.
- Trachoma is not commonly seen in the developed countries, but only UK and some parts of Europe are entirely free from the endemic disease.

Etiology

- **Causative organism**
  - *Chlamydia trachomatis*, a Bedsonian organism belonging to the psittacosis—lymphogranuloma—trachoma (PLT) group.
- **Predisposing factors**
  - Contracted in early childhood, though can effect at any age
  - Female patients out number males.
  - No race is immune to this disease.
  - Areas having dry and dusty climate are more prone.
  - Poor and outdoor workers are affected more commonly.
- **Source of infection**
  - Main source is the conjunctival discharge of the patient.
- **Mode of spread**
  - Direct
  - Vector transmission or
  - Contaminated materials in clinics and homes.

Clinical Features

Symptoms

In the absence of secondary infection:
- Mild foreign body sensation is felt in the eyes
- Watering
- Stickiness of the eyelids and
- Very little mucoid discharge.

Signs

- Congestion of upper tarsal and fornicial conjunctiva.
- Chronic follicular conjunctivitis, classically more marked on the upper tarsal plate, though these may be present on the conjunctiva at other sites also.

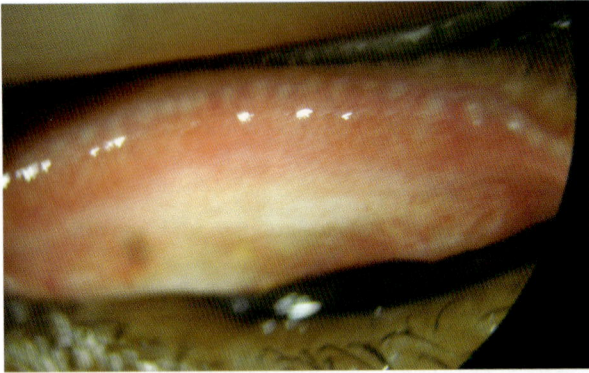

Figure 15: White line of Arlt

- Follicles lead to progressive scarring of the upper conjunctiva, producing a few linear scars or often a transverse band in the sulcus subtarsalis called **white line of Arlt (Figure 15)**.
- When marked scarring occurs, it leads to **entropion**, **trichiasis**, and **secondary ocular surface breakdown**, including **corneal ulceration**.
- Primary corneal involvement, which occurs along with the conjunctivitis, includes:
  - Epithelial keratitis
  - Marginal and central corneal infiltrates and
  - Superficial vascularization, which is more pronounced in the upper half of the cornea – as a fibrovascular pannus.
- Follicle formation at the limbus regresses to sharply defined depressions called **Herbert's pits**, at the base of the pannus **(Figure 16)**.
- **Concretions** may be formed due to accumulation of dead epithelial cells and inspissated mucus in the ducts of Henle.

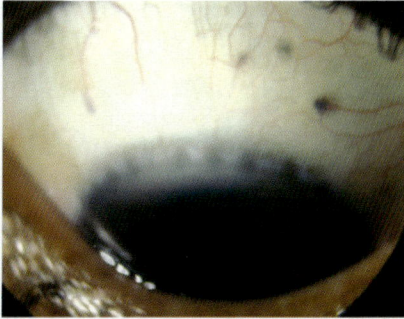

Figure 16: Herbert's pits

Grading of Trachoma

MacCallan classified the conjunctival changes occurring in trachoma, as follows:

1. **Trachoma I**
   - Immature follicles on the upper tarsal conjunctiva, including the central area, but there is no scarring.
2. **Trachoma II**
   - Mature (necrotic or soft) follicles on the upper tarsal conjunctiva, obscuring the tarsal vessels, but there is still no scarring.
3. **Trachoma III**
   - Follicles are present on the tarsus and definite scarring of conjunctiva is present.
4. **Trachoma IV**
   - There are no follicles on the tarsal plate, but definite scarring of the conjunctiva is present.

Differential Diagnosis

- Acute adenoviral follicular conjunctivitis (Epidemic kerato-conjunctivitis).
- Palpebral spring catarrh.

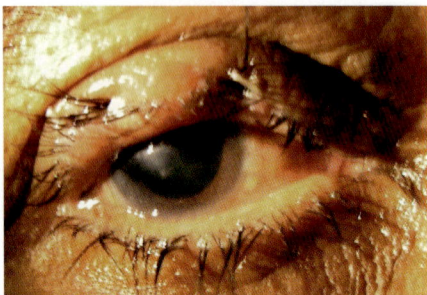

Figure 17: Surgery for entropion (a sequel to trachoma)

Treatment

1. Oral tetracycline or erythromycin, 250 mg thrice a day. Clinical response is slow and prolonged treatment is required. Tetracycline and erythromycin is preferred over oral sulphonamides, as they have lesser side effects as compared to the later.
2. Topical tetracycline or erythromycin ointments, twice a day for over to months.
3. Concretions are removed with a hypodermic needle under topical anesthesia.
4. Trichiasis is treated by epilation, electrolysis or cryolysis.
5. Entropion is surgically corrected **(Figure 17)**.
6. Xerosis is alleviated by artificial tear drops.

Prognosis

- Bad, unless prophylactic measures are taken and once it has started, unless it is treated aggressively.

HERPES ZOSTER OPHTHALMICUS

Introduction

- People over age 70 have a much greater chance of HZO infection.

- Those who are immunocompromised due to lymphoma, AIDS, Lyme disease, etc. are at an increased risk.
- Ocular involvement varies greatly and is often confusing in the early stages.
- Extreme care should be taken in differentiating this condition from herpes simplex virus (HSV), particularly when cornea is involved. One important fact is that the dendritic keratitis occuring in HZO is infiltrative, while the HSV dendrites are ulcerative.

Symptoms

Herpes zoster ophthalmicus (HZO) presents with
- nondescript facial pain
- fever and
- general malaise.
- The pain is very severe during the inflammatory stage.

Signs (Figures 18)

- 3 to 5 days later, a vesicular skin rash appears along the distribution of the fifth cranial nerve, and stays to one side of the vertical midline.

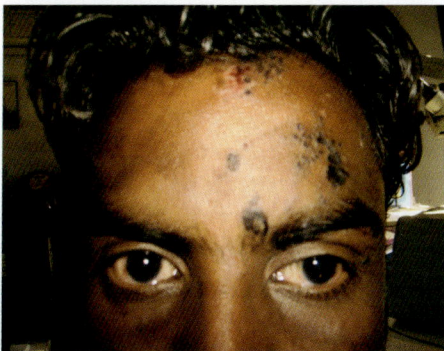

Figure 18: Herpes zoster ophthalmicus

- Fluid is discharged from the vesicles and scab appears after about a week.
- **Ocular involvement** may incorporate
  - follicular conjunctivitis
  - epithelial and/or interstitial keratitis
  - dendritic keratitis
  - uveitis
  - scleritis or episcleritis
  - chorioretinitis
  - optic neuropathy, and
  - neurogenic motility disorders as well (especially thr 4th cranial nerve palsy).
  - If vesicles appear at the tip of the nose (Hutchinson's sign), there is 75% likelihood of ocular sequelae.

Pathophysiology

- HZO occurs with the invasion of the trigeminal ganglion, by the HZ virus.
- This is a varicella-type virus and is referred to as "chicken pox" in children and "shingles" in adults.
- The virus remains dormant in trigeminal nerve cells, and any reduction in the immune system can reactivate it even years later.
- The virus spreads along the neurons of the ophthalmic (1st) and less frequently the maxillary (2nd) division of the trigeminal nerve.
- Vesicular eruptions occur at the terminal ends of sensory innervation, causing extreme pain.
- Nasociliary branch involvement most likely causes ocular inflammation, affecting typically the tissues of the anterior segment and the cornea.
- Other cranial nerves may also be involved, causing optic neuropathy (2nd cranial nerve) or even isolated cranial nerve palsies (3rd, 4th or 6th cranial nerves).

Treatment

1. Systemic component of the disease—
   - Is treated with oral Acyclovir, 600 to 800 mg, five times a day, for 7 to 10 days, starting the moment the condition is diagnosed.
   - Famciclovir 500 mg three times a day has been shown to be as effective in treating herpes zoster ophthalmicus as acyclovir 800 mg fives times per day.
   - To avoid post-herpetic neuralgia and to achieve maximum benefit from oral antiviral medication, start therapy within 72 hours of vesicular eruption. Otherwise, the patient may develop post-herpetic neuralgia and the oral antiviral therapy does not help.
   - Oral steroids may also be used to alleviate pain and associated facial edema. 40 to 60 mg of prednisone is given daily, tapered slowly over the next 10 days.
   - An antibiotic-steroid ointment may be applied to the affected areas twice daily, to treat the skin lesions.
2. Ocular management of the disease depends on the severity and tissues involved—
   - In severe cases having uveitis or keratitis, use cycloplegia (homatropine 5% tid).
   - After ruling out herpes simplex, we may also use topical steroids.
   - In a compromised eye, prophylaxis with a broad-spectrum antibiotic is a good idea.
   - Palliative treatment consisting of cool compresses, and oral analgesics in extreme cases, can be comforting.
3. Possibility of more complex ocular sequelae (chorioretinitis, optic neuropathy, cranial nerve palsies, uveitic glaucoma) must also be kept in mind, and apt management strategies planned, in these cases.

Update on Lasers in Oculoplasty

24

Sunil Moreker, Mayur Moreker (India)

INTRODUCTION

According to the American Society for Aesthetic Plastic Surgery, in the year 2000 over 5.7 million cosmetic surgical and nonsurgical procedures were performed in the United States which was a 25% increase above the total number performed in 1999. The most popular of these procedures was botulinum toxin injection, followed by chemical peels and microdermabrasion.[1] In the past one decade lasers have revolutionized treatment of common oculoplastic problems. The more recent applications of lasers as reported in recent literature in oculoplastic conditions are highlighted here.

ADVANCES IN PRINCIPLES OF PHYSICS AND APPLICATION OF THE LASER IN PLASTIC SURGERY

Newer principles help it be a new tool for skin rejuvenation.[2]
a. Decreased collateral thermal injury
b. Higher absorption by tissue water
c. Controlled ablation.

In recent lasers the theory of selective photothermolysis is used in pulsed lasers, and advances have taken place in the science of laser: tissue interactions. Particular advances in skin cooling, hair removal, intense pulsed light, and uses for aesthetic and nonaesthetic skin problems have made life simpler. Advances in skin cooling have allowed for wider use in all Fitzpatrick skin types without concomitant adverse reaction.[4]

TYPES OF LASERS

a. **Conventional CO_2 laser:** These infrared lasers have helps the oculoplastic surgeons in terms of good hemostasis, facilitating high precision surgery and controlled tissue ablation

b. **CO_2 laser-scanned continuous-wave or pulsed delivery systems:** Newer generation of carbon dioxide (CO_2) lasers have sparked the development of newer procedures for certain oculoplastic disorders. With the advent of scanned continuous-wave or pulsed delivery systems which have an added advantage in resurfacing procedures on the skin.[4]

c. **KTP 532 nm laser**

d. **Erb YAG laser**

e. **Ho:YAG**

f. **532 nm frequency doubled YAG laser**

g. **Nd:YAG laser-powered quartz laser scalpel.**

WORD OF CAUTION

The unique characteristics of the CO_2 laser mandate special attention to protection of the patient and surgical team, and careful preparation and training will help the prospective laser surgeon to successfully address the learning curve associated with this new technology.[4]

CONDITIONS

Treatments include[5,7] conditions involving:

a. Excessive blood vessels (e.g. port-wine stains),
b. Pigment (e.g. tattoos),
c. Inflammatory lesions (e.g. psoriasis),
d. Scars,
e. Excess hair,
f. Tumors, and
g. Wrinkles.

ADVANCES IN OCULOPLASTY[8]

a. Combining laser resurfacing with other aesthetic procedures, such as lower blepharoplasty and facelifting.
b. Laser assisted lacrimal surgery with the adjunctive use of mitomycin C.
c. Treatment of capillary hemangiomata with a tunable dye laser.
d. Advances in laser skin resurfacing, such as the combination of carbon dioxide and erbium:yttrium-aluminum-garnet lasers to achieve improved results
e. Lacrimal surgery[9] -Nd:YAG, Ho:YAG, Er:YAG lasers and the Nd:YAG laser-powered quartz laser scalpel.

FUNDAMENTAL RISKS

Fundamental risks that laser surgery entails are hypo- and hyper pigmentation and scar formation.[10]

AVOIDING POSTOPERATIVE COMPLICATIONS

Laser surgery for oculoplastic or dermatological indications—whether incisional work, removal of pigmented or vascular lesions, removal of hair, or resurfacing—necessitates that the practitioner have appropriate training in and understanding of not only the techniques but also of their advantages and disadvantages. To wisely choose the correct laser for a given problem, it has been pointed out that one must be aware of both the spectrum of disorders for which each laser is suited and the potential side effects.[11] New approaches to such operations include combining more than one type of laser or combining traditional cutting blades and lasers in an effort to reduce side effects and improve outcome.[12]

EVIDENCE OF TREATMENTS

Treatment of Port-wine Stain with KTP 532 nm Laser

Lesions of port-wine stain type are the most commonly occurring vascular malformations of the skin occurring in 0.3% of the population. Other therapies like cryosurgery, dermabrasion, radiation therapy or surgery and skin grafting produce unsatisfactory results. Introduction of highly selective lasers made port wine stains amenable to treatment-effectively and safely.

Latlowski et al[6] in a prospective analysis of treatment of Port-wine stains in 155 patients performed laser with at least 4-week intervals and on the basis of subjective scoring system comparing simultaneously shown pictures of the patients taken prior to and after the last procedure, classified them according to the outcome into a 4-degree scale: excellent outcome—75-100% improvement, with 100% perceived as eradication of the lesion; good—50-74% improvement; fair—25-49% improvement and poor—less than 25% improvement, including no observable improvement. In 81% of the lesions treatment with KTP 532 nm laser they found significant improvement which was reported satisfactory by the patient. Excellent outcome of treatment was seen in 31% of patients (31%), good in 27%, fair in 23%. In their series the port wine stains which failed to treatment were most commonly located on the limbs. They did not report any episodes of scarring or persistent pigmentary changes in any of the patients.

Use of the KTP Laser in the Treatment of Rosacea and Solar Lentigines

Treatment regimens rosacea and solar lentigines range from avoidance of causative factors to the use of topical agents or other modalities that target the superficial layers of the skin. Lasers offer the physician and patient the ability to target specific chromophores in the skin. Advances in laser technology led to the implementation of targeting certain characteristic pigments of abnormal areas with minimal damage to surrounding normal tissue. Rosacea and solar lentigines have characteristic cells that are targeted by a potassium-titanyl-phosphate (KTP) laser. The lesions are different in their origins but share the ability to be treated successfully with the KTP laser.[13]

Comparison of Lasers

Lieb et al[14] compared the erbium-YAG laser and the CO_2 laser to conventional eyelid surgery with a scalpel in 58 patients using the erbium-YAG laser and on 32 using the CO_2 laser, surgeries being benign tumor excisions and removal, xanthelasma removal, lower and upper eyelid blepharoplasties, and skin resurfacing in the area of the lower eyelid. They found that **wound healing with the CO_2 laser was significantly slower** because of its larger thermal necrosis zone, but the **hemostasis with the CO_2 laser made removal of deeper lesions easier.** Advantages are the wide application spectrum for incisional and ablative surgery. The erbium-YAG laser is an excellent for ablating superficial benign lesions, including that in the area of the lid margin and close to the lacrimal puncta without scars. The application spectrums of the erbium-YAG and CO_2 lasers complement one another. The erbium-YAG laser is superior for esthetic skin resurfacing and ablation of superficial lesions, and the CO_2 laser allows hemorrhage-free noncontact incisional surgery **(Figures 1A to C)**.

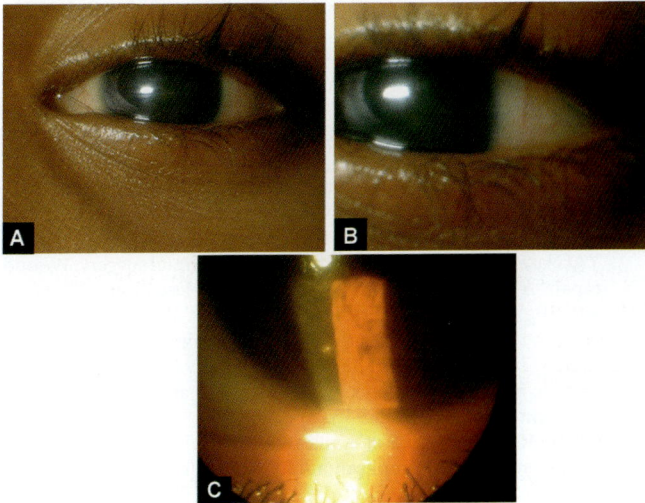

Figures 1A to C: (A) Pre-laser for trichiasis (B) Post-laser for trichiasis (C) Immediate post-laser trichiasis

CONCLUSION

Lasers can now be considered an important addition to the armamentarium of the oculoplastic surgeon.

REFERENCES

1. Morgenstern KE, Foster JA. Advances in cosmetic oculoplastic surgery.Curr Opin Ophthalmol 2002 Oct;13(5):324-30.

2. Pages JC, Gailloud-Matthieu MC, Egloff DV. Principles of physics and application of the laser in plastic surgery. Rev Med Suisse Romande 1999 Sep;119(9):739-42.

3. Nottingham LK, Ries WR. Update on lasers in facial plastic surgery. Curr Opin Otolaryngol Head Neck Surg 2004 Aug;12(4):323-6.

4. Goldbaum AM, Woog JJ. The CO_2 laser in oculoplastic surgery. Surv Ophthalmol 1997 Nov-Dec;42(3):255-67.

5. Laser treatment for skin problems. Drug Ther Bull 2004 Oct;42(10):73-6.

6. Latlowski IT, Wysocki MS, Siewiera IP. Own clinical experience in treatment of port-wine stain with KTP 532 nm laserWiad Lek 2005;58(7-8):391-6.

7. DiBernardo BE, Cacciarelli A. Cutaneous lasers.Clin Plast Surg 2005 Apr;32(2):141-50.

8. Choo PH. Lasers in oculoplastics.Curr Opin Ophthalmol 2001 Oct;12(5):357-61.

9. Fankhauser F, Kwasniewska S. Applications of the neodymium: YAG laser in plastic surgery of the face and lacrimal surgery. Wound repair. A review Ophthalmologica 2002 Nov-Dec;216(6):381-98.

10. Kimmig W. Laser surgery in dermatology. Risks and chances Hautarzt 2003 Jul;54(7):583-93. Epub 2003 May 15.

11. Raulin C, Kimmig W, Werner S. Laser therapy in dermatology and esthetic medicine. Side effects, complications and treatment errors Hautarzt 2000 Jul;51(7):463-73.

12. Tayani R, Rubin PA. Laser applications in oculoplastic surgery and their postoperative complications. Int Ophthalmol Clin 2000 Winter ;40(1):13-26.

13. Bassichis BA, Swamy R, Dayan SH. Use of the KTP laser in the treatment of rosacea and solar lentigines. Facial Plast Surg 2004 Feb;20(1):77-83.

14. Lieb WE, Klink T, Munnich S. CO_2 and erbium YAG laser in eyelid surgery. A comparison.Ophthalmologe 2000 Dec; 97(12):835-41.

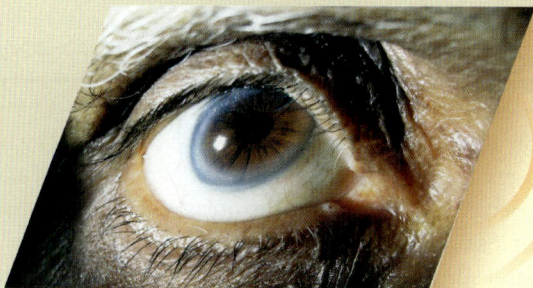

Recent Advances

Aesthetic Ophthalmoplastic with CO_2 Laser

25

Claudio Lucchini (Italy)

INTRODUCTION

Through experience, I have found that the laser CO_2 works well in aesthetic eyelid surgery. I believe it should be used in a conservative way by preserving the elimination of skin and never exceeding in the quantity of fat removed. This way the risk of a skull aspect can be avoided as a patient ages.

Laser surgery requires much expertise. It is very important to have perfect knowledge of the anatomy of the lids, which is very complex.

Transcojunctival blepharoplasty of the lower lid is my first surgery choice, CO_2 laser works very well and it is possible to have a complete lipectomy of the bags. Orbital septum is not violated, the orbicularis muscle is preserved and the skin is not cut or removed. These factors in the skin-muscle flap technique are responsible for the retraction of the lower lid and ectropion after blepharoplasty.

Recovery time is shorter, with less edema, no stitches, no pain, less retraction of the lid, no scleral show and no changes in the shape of the lower lid.

Although the transconjunctival technique does place the inferior oblique muscle and lid itself at risk, with careful technique, complications are unusual.

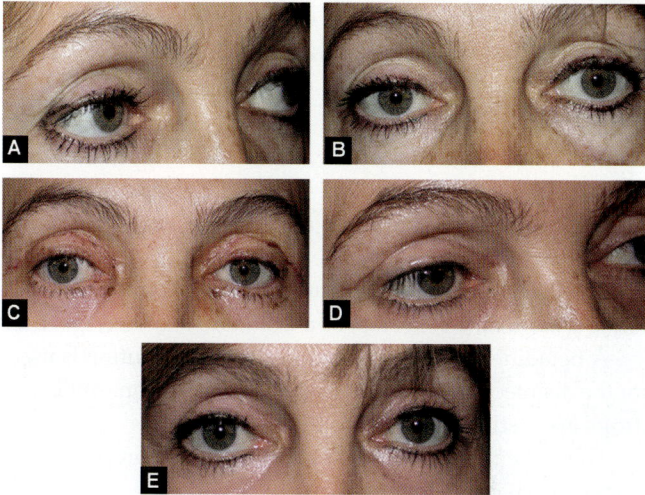

Figures 1A to E: (A and B) (Preop), (C) 7 days post-laser blepharoplasty 4 lids and skin resurfacing, (D) One month postoperative, (E) One month postoperative

To avoid skin laxity, the inferior lids could be treated with laser skin resurfacing **(Figures 1A to E).**

TECHNIQUE OF LASER BLEPHAROPLASTY

When using the CO$_2$ pulsed laser, the machine must be set correctly, depending upon the model. The surgeon must also check some important things in the surgery room before starting the operation.

Laser Safety

To avoid fire hazards the oxygen source must be turned off. Use wet towels near the surgery field, use an appropriate smoke evacuator, do not use volatile skin preparations or anaesthetics and use patient corneas metallic protectors. Remember that CO_2 laser can easy perforate the globe.

Preoperative Marking

I prefer to mark the preoperative area of the upper lid while the patient is still awake and in an upright position. The inferior lids are also marked if a transconjunctival approach and a skin laser resurfacing are scheduled.

The principles of marking are no different from the technique used with a cold steel or a Colorado needle **(Figure 2).**

A betadine solution or other not volatile solution is used for the disinfection of the lids and periocular region. Antibiotic drops are instilled.

The patient is draped and wet towels are prepared, the smoke evacuator is put in place.

Laser is set on pulse mode at a range of 5 or 6 watts and tested on a wet tongue blade; the beam must not penetrate the wood.

I suggest the use of pulse mode to any surgeon approaching laser blepharoplasty; it is far safer than CW mode.

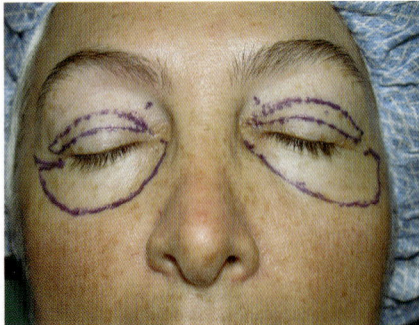

Figure 2: Preoperative marking

CW mode better controls bleeding but needs an expert surgeon who moves the laser beam precisely and quickly to avoid tissues heating and burning.

Anesthesia

Use lidocaine with epinephrine (1:200,000) with 1 cc of sodium bicarbonate per 10 cc. of lidocaine to avoid a burning sensation during injection.

Another syringe of 10 cc of lidocaine without epinephrine is prepared to use during surgery if necessary during lipectomy. Avoid using epinephrine in this step; it could induce a vessels constriction of the optical nerve with dangerous ischemic effects.

The cornea is anesthetized with 2 drops of 4% tetracaine and the metal scleral shield is lubricated with cellulose gel and placed on the cornea. The surgeon can then proceed to infiltrate the upper and lower lids. It is best to use the least volume of anesthetic possible and than perform a delicate massage to induce the penetration and spread of the anesthetic into the tissues.

Intravenous sedation analgesia is performed and controlled by the anesthesiologist.

The patient should be monitored with pulse oximetry and electrocardiography and should be given supplemental oxygen.

Upper Lid Laser Blepharoplasty

The laser incision follows the marks with constant, precise and rapid movements. Hesitation on any area could result in tissues being burnt.

This procedure requires extreme technical capacity and it is not for every surgeon.

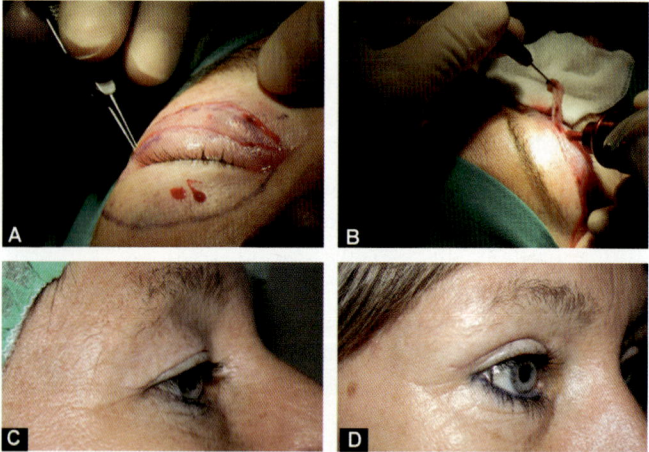

Figures 3A to D: (A) Right upper lid Incision of the skin and orbicularis. (B) Right upper lid Laser excision of the skin muscle flap. (C) Before. (D) After upper lids laser blepharoplasty

Check that the cut is complete and no bridges of tissue are present. Raise the lateral part of the flap with forceps and use scissors for the first 2 cm. of skin-muscle flap dissection, than continue dissecting with the laser beam **(Figures 3A and B).**

When the dissection is completed to the corner, remember to protect nasal skin by using a Jaeger bone plate or wet gauze pad to avoid accidental burns.

Bleeding must be controlled. The laser is defocused and used to coagulate any blood vessels.

With gentle pressure on the globe, the septum is incised in the medial and central part and fat is exposed.

Fat is gently grasped with forceps and placed on the zed plate, before the cutting laser beam is defocused to coagulate the vessels and refocused to cut the fat. Never pull up on the fat, it may cause severe bleeding.

If a large vessel is present I prefer to use an electric cautery and than cut with laser.

Explore the medial fat pad at completion to be sure that there is no bleeding. Any residual fat could be removed at this time.

Place a wet gauze on the upper lid and proceed to the other lid.

I close the wound starting from the nasal part using an itradermal suture with nylon 5-0.

The tail of the wound is suturated with 3 separated stitches, because in this area the obicularis muscle has a strong contraction and it would open the wound **(Figures 3C and D).**

Lower Lid Laser Blepharoplasty

Transconjunctival lower lid laser blepharoplasty is my standard lower lid technique. I use it for young patients as well as for more mature patients; where there is present a slight excess of skin and/or fat. Operating and recovery time is shorter.

The benefits of the transconjunctival approach are primarily that it avoids surgical violation of the orbital septum, there is less aggressive lipectomy, there are no stitches, the skin is untouched and the risk of scleral show or ectropion are avoided.

This is not an easy technique; it needs a long period of training, good control of the laser beam and a perfect knowledge of the anatomy.

The metal scleral shield is put on the cornea, the lower lids are anesthetized, a 5-0 silk suture is passed at the middle of the lid at the level of the grey line into the tarsal plate and used for retracting the lower lid anteriorly on a cotton tip to better expose the fornix.

A 5-0 silk suture is passed in the middle section of the conjunctival fornix used to retract the lower part of the lid.

The incision will be made for all the length of the lid, stopping before the lacrimal punctom, 4 or 5 mm below the lid margin. The incision will pass through to the end part of the vertically oriented blood vessels of the conjunctiva. At this point you reach the lid retractor muscles, where an incision made inferiorly, deep in the fornix, would result in excessive bleeding, poor exposure of fat, and possible injury to the inferior oblique muscle.

Set the laser in CW mode, start with 5 watts, if bleeding is present, increase to 5,5 or 6 watts.

First pass to incise the conjunctiva, then pass to cut through the capsulopalpebral fascia and lid retractors muscles.

Forceps are then used to separate the tissues and expose the orbital septum. Simultaneously the assistant produces a gentle pressure on the globe to bulge the fat pads. Before cutting any structure try to obtain maximum visibility of the field using a metal Desmarres retractor.

Incise the septum over the nasal, central and lateral fat pads, and ballot the globe to bring the fat pad forward (**Figures 4A to D**).

Nasal and central fat pads generally prolapse quite easily. Make an accurate coagulation of any large vessels present in the nasal fat pad. Caution should be used if the inferior oblique muscle is visible along the inferior and lateral edge of the nasal fat pad.

The lateral fat pad is more difficult to mobilize because it is adherent to the lower eyelid retractors and covered by an often thick septum that is densely adherent to the inferior lateral rim. Even when properly mobilized, a deeper further fat may only become apparent after first removing the existing lateral fat and the globe.

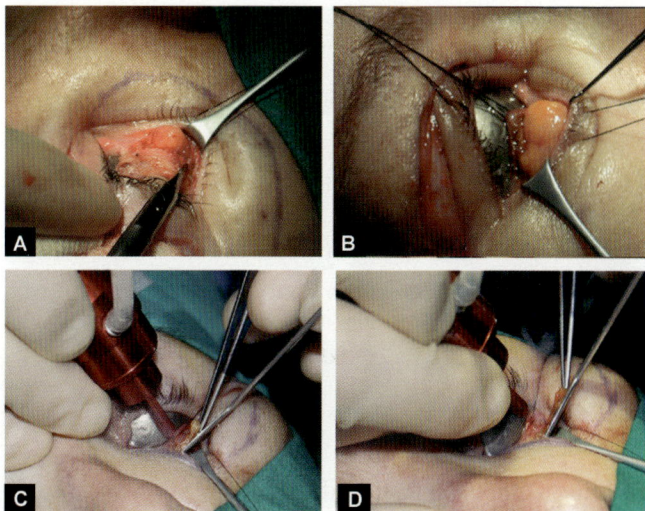

Figures 4A to D: (A) Right inferior lid. The central fat pad. (B) Right inferior lid Central fat pad prolapse. (C) Left inferior lid laser lipectomy. (D) Laser lipectomy

Reposition the eyelid and ballot to look for any residual bulging fat, and check for any bleeding.

At the end of the surgery instil drops of antibiotic or use antibiotic ointment, which is applied to the inferior fornix **(Figures 5A to D)**.

Postoperative Recovery

1. Use icepacks for 5 days.
2. Use oral and topical antibiotics for 7 days.
3. Heed written instructions that include the warning signs of retrobulbar hemorrhage.
4. Avoid heavy lifting
5. Elevate the head of the bad, while sleeping, for 1 week.
6. Avoid contact lenses for 10 days
   Patients are generally seen one week following surgery.

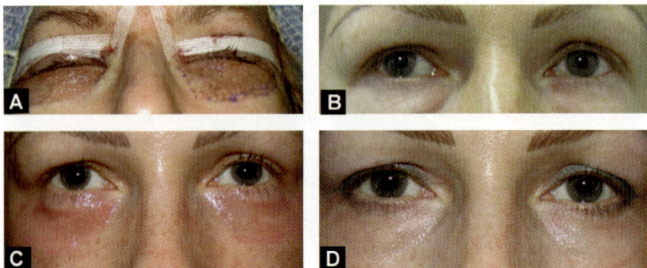

Figures 5A to D: (A) Postoperative medications. (B) Before. (C) 7 days after lower lids laser transconjunctival blepharoplasty and erbium skin resurfacing. (D) 1 month after surgery

Laser Blepharoplasty of the Lower Lid with Skin-muscle Flap

Patients with excess fat and skin require a skin-muscle procedure.

Preoperative safety precautions are the same as described previously in the section on laser transcojunctival blepharoplasty.

One 5-0 silk suture is passed through the gray line into the tarsal plate and used as a retraction suture.

The incision line is marked approximately 1mm below the cilia from the medial canthus towards the lateral canthus.

Start from the lateral area to incise through to the orbicularis layer to fashion a myocutaneous flap. The assistant places two double hooks on the inferior cut border and holds the lower lid to expose to the surgeon the aereola plane between the orbicularis muscle and the underlying orbital septum.

When this layer is evident, a gentle pressure on the globe allows any fat to protrude forward. With the laser beam, incise the septum and remove prolapsed fat from the central, nasal and lateral pads.

If necessary a lateral canthoplasty procedure is performed.

The tip of the myocutaneus flap is stretched to determine how much the lateral portion of the flap overlaps the underlying incision. If necessary, carefully excise the excess of tissue.

Closure of the skin flap is performed using 6-0 nylon sutures.

BIBLIOGRAPHY

1. Aiache AE, Coll. The suborbicularis oculi fat pad: an anatomic and clinical study 1995;95(1):37-42.
2. Bames H Baggy. Eyelids Plast Reconstr Surg 1958;22:264.
3. Boo-Chai K. Blefaroplastia nas palpebras orientais. In Avelar MA: Anestesia loco-regional em Cirurgia Estetica. Heditora Hipocrates, 1993:pp 116-20.
4. C.Lucchini, Coll "Laser Chirurgia Estetica delle Palpebre e del Viso" Dogma Edizioni 2001;45-57.
5. Castanares S. Blepharoplasty for herniated intraorbital fat. Anatomic bases for a new approach. Plast Reconstr Surg 1951;8:46.
6. De Miranda JC, Coll. Blefaroplastia. In Avelar MA: Anestesia loco-regional em Cirurgia Estetica. Heditora Hipocrates 1993:109-15.
7. Freund RM, Coll. Correlation between brow lift outcomes and aesthetic ideal for eyebrow height and shape in females Plast Reconstr Surg 1996;97(7):1343-8.
8. Lessa S, Coll. A Simple Canthopexy. Rev Soc Bras Cir Plast 1999;14 (1):59-70.
9. Loeb R "Esclera Aparente". In Loeb R Cirurgia Estetica das Palpebras. Sao Paulo (ed) 1988:17-32.
10. Loeb R. Cirurgia Estetica das Palpebras. Sao Paulo (ed) 1988.
11. Loeb R. Ectropios, hematomas e outras complicaçoes. In Loeb R. Cirurgia Estetica das Palpebras. Sao Paulo (ed) 1988:163-86.
12. Loeb R. Saliencias tegumentais, adiposas, musculares e ossea. In Loeb R. Cirurgia Estetica das Palpebras. Sao Paulo (ed) 1988 pp 33-94.
13. May JW, Coll. Retro-Orbicularis Oculus Fat (ROOF). Resection in aesthetic blepharoplasty: a 6 years study in 63 patients 1990;86(4):682-89.
14. Monasterio OF, Coll. Lateral Canthoplasty to change the eye slant. Plast Reconstr Surg 1985;75(1):1-10.

15. Pitanguy I, Coll. Atlas de Cirurgia Palpebral. Revinter (ed) 1994.
16. Pitanguy I. Anatomia. In Pitanguy I and Coll Atlas de Cirurgia Palpebral Revinter (ed) 1994 pp 21-32.
17. Rees TD. Blepharoplasty and Facialplasty. In McCarthy JG Plastic Surgery Volume 3 Saunders (ed) 1990 pp 2320-414.
18. Watanabe K. Ocidentalizaçao das palpebras. In Avelar MA: Anestesia loco-regional em Cirurgia Estetica. Heditora Hipocrates, 1993;121-4.
19. Wesstfall CT, ShoreJW, Nunery WR, et al. Operative complications of the of the transconjunctival inferior fornix approach. Ophtalmology 1992;98:1525-8.

ABLATIVE LASERS SKIN RESURFACING

The changes of aging in facial skin, like wrinkles, atrophy of the skin, superficial irregularities, actinic damage, hyperpigmentation, dermal thickening and hyperkeratosis are not correctable by skin-tightening procedures alone.

Introduction

With the development of short-pulsed, high peak power or rapidly scanned CO_2 lasers and erbium: yttrium- aluminium-garnet (Er:Yag), very good results can be obtained in reducing wrinkles in the periocular region using the skin resurfacing technique, with minimal thermal damage.

Principles of Laser Skin Resurfacing

CO_2 laser (10.600 nm) is strongly absorbed by water. Water is present in more than 80% of the skin's volume.

Ninety percent of CO_2 laser light energy is absorbed within 20 to 50 μm

The absorption of this laser energy causes rapid heating and ultimately the vaporization of intracellular water with resulting tissue ablation.

It is very important to stop the laser action when papillary dermis is achieved, to avoid further, deeper damage to the tissue.

The effect of the CO₂ laser is immediately noticeable by thermal shrinkage and the stimulation of a long-term healing response characterized by the formation of new sub epidermal collagen and elastin fibers.

The tightening of the dermis creates wrinkle reduction.

To reduce the thermal damage zone the laser pulse duration must be shorter than 0.5 to 1 ms; this is called the thermal relaxation time. The energy fluency per pulse necessary to vaporized tissue is approximately 5J/ cm².

Several CO₂ lasers have been developed that can achieve tissue vaporization 20 to 30 μm. of depth with residual thermal damage zones of 25 -70 μm.

Never forget that the lid's skin thickness is about 60 μm, the thinnest layer of skin on the human body!

The Erbium laser emits a light with a wavelength of 2940 nm; the absorption of this wavelength in water is 12 to 18-fold that of the CO₂ laser. This increase of energy from the Er:YAG laser within the superficial layers of tissue produces a thermal damage zone of less than 10 μm. The minimum energy fluency per pulse necessary to vaporized tissue is approximately 1.6 J/cm². The thermal damage zone does not increase with additional passages of the Erbium laser, making this laser an extremely precise ablative tool **(Table 1 and Figure 6)**.

Preoperative Evaluation

Laser skin resurfacing performed only in the periorbital region is much safer than a full face treatment.

In any case, it is suggested to follow some basic rules when selecting patients.

Avoid treating patients with a history of immune system compromise, autoimmune diseases, keloid formation, Fitzpatrik class IV, or primary Herpes simplex.

Table 1: Comparison of CO_2 and Erbium laser

	CO_2	Er:YAG
Ablation fluence	4-5 J/cm²	1.6 J/cm²
Wavelength	10.6 µm	2.94 µm
Thermal damage	70-150 µm	10-50 µm
Tissue penetration	30 µm	1 µm
Collagen shrinkage	++++	+

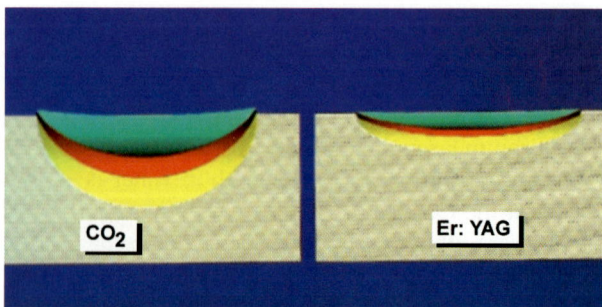

Figure 6: Erbium laser a precise ablative tool

Isoretinoin (Accutane) treatment or deep peeling in the recent past may impair follicle and sweat gland activity, thus generating a delayed or absent re-epithelialization after resurfacing.

Lower eye lid laxity may predispose a patient to ectropion.

Wound Healing

Generally re-epithelialzation is completed within 7 days for Er:YAG and 10 days for CO_2 laser.

Erythema takes 2-3 weeks to resolve after Erbium laser or 5-6 weeks after one pass in delicate resurfacing mode (Feathertouch, Ultra Pulse 5000 C).

Anesthesia

CO$_2$ resurfacing may be performed with a local or regional anaesthetic.

Topical anesthetic cream (Emla®) applied 45 minutes before the Erbium laser resurfacing is normally sufficient.

Laser Safety

Regard the paragraph in Laser Blepharoplastic

Laser Treatment Strategy

In my personal experience, I have found that using ablative resurfacing to complete laser transconjunctival blepharoplasty reduces the laxity of the lid's skin and enhances the cosmetic effect on the non dynamic wrinkles.

In some patients only laser skin resurfacing is indicated to reduce the aging effects on the periorbital area.

In young patients I prefer to use Erbium laser as apposed to the CO$_2$ laser, which I use when the wrinkles are deeper and skin laxity is present.

I prefer not to be aggressive on the crow's feet or glabellar region for two reasons:

There is a longer time of recovery and erythema, and I can obtain excellent result with botulin toxine.

Laser Treatment Technique

A betadine solution or other not volatile solution is used for the disinfection of the lids and periocular region. Antibiotic drops are instilled.

The cornea is anesthetized with 2 drops of 4% tetracaine, the metal scleral shield is lubricated with cellulose gel and placed on the cornea, the surgeon marks the resurfacing area, and then the lower lids and periorbital region are infiltrated with lidocaine (CO$_2$ treatment).

CO_2 Laser Skin Resurfacing of Crow's Feet and Lower Lid Cheek Junction Area

Use a square, medium sized spot to treat the marked area. Pay attention not to damage lashes. Laser spots impacts must be perpendicular to the skin surface, on the peripheral contour, just on the pen marks. I impact the laser spots with an angle of 45° to reduce the step between treated and non treated area.

With just one pass of the pulsed CO_2 laser, epidermal debris is not wiped away, therefore reducing the healing process. Spots overlapping is allowed in order of 10% **(Figure 7).**

Erbium Laser Skin Resurfacing of Crow's Feet and Lower Lid Cheek Junction Area

Use a square medium size spot to treat the marked area, pay close attention not to damage the lashes. Laser spot impacts must be perpendicular on the skin surface, set the laser: fluence 14.2, spot 3.0 mm, energy 1.0 mJ, frequency 8Hz; 5 passes are generally needed to arrive to the papillary dermal. Stop, in any case, when bleeding starts **(Figure 8).**

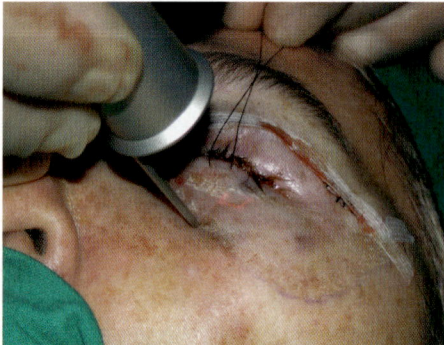

Figure 7: Laser CO_2 skin resurfacing after laser blepharoplasty

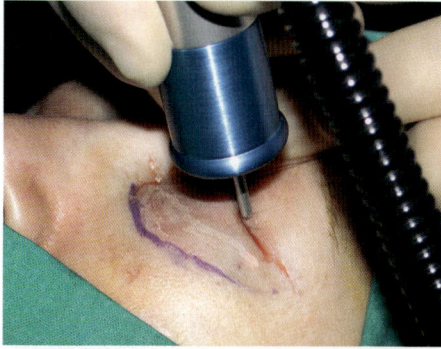

Figure 8: Laser skin resurfacing Er. YAG after laser transconjunctival blepharoplasty

Postoperative Wound Care

Vaseline is applied 4 or 5 times a day until re-epithelialization is completed. The patient is asked to apply a wet compress, 4 times a day, with a solution of 1 tablespoon of white vinegar in 1 cup of water.

Oral antibiotic is prescribed for one week.

Steroid cream is applied nightly for 3 days. A mix of Vaseline with steroid cream (1:3) is applied 4 times a day for 5 days.

Then a hydrant cream with a sunscreen of 15 SPF is used. If the patient is exposed to the sun, a 100% SPF (total sun block) is recommended to avoid hyper- pigmentation. This regime is followed for three months.

Postoperative Complications

Following these rules, it is unlikely that complications will arise during or after surgery.

Prolonged erythema, lasting more than 3 months, is possible but can be resolved with topical steroid therapy.

Hyperpigmentation can be resolved with the application of topical bleaching agents.

BIBLIOGRAPHY

1. Alster Tina S. Cutaneous resurfacing with CO_2 and erbium: YAG lasers: preoperative,intraoperative and postoperative considerations. Plastic and reconstructive surgery 1999;103(2):619-32.
2. Alster TS, West TB. Ultrapulse CO_2 laser ablation of xanthelasma. J.American Academy of Dermatology 1996;34:848-49.
3. C.Lucchini, Coll. "Laser Chirurgia Estetica delle Palpebre e del Viso" Dogma Edizioni 2001;pp 45-57.
4. Collawn SS, Boissy RE, Vasconez LO. Skin ultrastructure after CO_2 laser resurfacing. Plast Reconstr Surg 1998;102:509-15.
5. Dover JS, Hruza GJ. Laser skin resurfacing. Semin Cutan Med Surg 1996;15:177-88.
6. Fitzpatrich RE. Facial resurfacing with the pulsed CO_2 laser. Facial Plast Surg Clin 1996;4:231-40.
7. Fitzpatrick RE, Williams B, Goldman MP. Preoperative anesthesia and postoperative considerations in laser resurfacing. Semin Cutan Med Surg 1996;15:170-76.
8. Fitzpatrick Richard E. Laser resurfacing of rhytides. Dermatologic Clinics 1997;15(3):431-47.
9. Fulton JE. Complication of laser resurfacing. Dermatol Surg 1997; 24:91-9.
10. Geronemus RG, Alster TS, Brandt FS, Dover JS, Fitzpatrick RE. Tabletalk: Common questions about laser resurfacing . Dermatol Surg 1999;24:121-30.
11. Goodman GJ. Combining laser resurfacing and ancillary procedures. Dermatol Surg 1998;24:75-8.
12. Ho C, Nguyen Q, Lowe NJ, Griffin ME, Lask G. Laser resurfacing in pigmented skin . Dermatol Surg 1995;21:1035-7.
13. Hruza GJ. Skin resurfacing with lasers. Fitzpatrick 's J Clin Dermatol 1996; 3:38-9.
14. Lewis AB, Alster TS. Laser resurfacing: persistent erythema and post-inflammatory hyperpigmentation. J Geriatr Dermatol 1996; 4: 75-6.

Endoscopic Dacryocystorhinostomy— Recent Advances 26

Sunil Moreker, Sneha Kataria, M.V Kirtane, Gauri Mankekar (India)

INTRODUCTION

Dacryocystorhinostomy or DCR is done for nasolacrimal duct obstruction via either an external approach or an endoscopic approach.

HISTORY

The first reported dacryocystectomy was performed by Celsus in 50 AD followed by Galenas of Pergamos. Anel first irrigated the lacrimal duct and Bowman reported the technique of probing. Toti, an Italian performed the first external dacryocystorhinostomy for obstruction. In 1895, Caldwell first reported the endonasal approach and Rice in 1990 was the first to report good results with the same.

ANATOMY AND PHYSIOLOGY [1]

The lacrimal apparatus includes superior and inferior punctum, the superior and inferior canaliculi, the sac and the nasolacrimal duct, that opens into the inferior meatus. The lacrimal pump functions due to the lid movement which causes the puncta to acquire tears into the lacrimal sac. When the eyes open a negative pressure is created in the lacrimal sac and causes the valves in the canaliculi to open and suck in tears and when the eyes close positive pressure open the valve at the nasolacrimal duct to push the tears down further into the nose.

The anterior portion of the middle turbinate is an anatomical landmark for the lacrimal apparatus. The lacrimal fossa has the anterior lacrimal crest, which consists of the frontal process of the maxillary bone and the posterior lacrimal crest is made up of the lacrimal bone.

EVALUATION OF EPIPHORA

Watering from eyes can be due to a variety of reasons like the blockage of the nasolacrimal duct, over secretion of tears or foreign body in the eye, etc.

Epiphora is excess tearing due to insufficient drainage and can be differentiated from pseudo-epiphora, which is reflux tearing due to the main gland oversecreting.

The causes for Epiphora can be broadly divided into anatomical or physiological causes. Anatomical causes can be complete or partial obstruction of the nasolacrimal duct (NLD) or canaliculi. Where as a physiological obstruction is due to a functional problem even though the anatomy of the NLD is normal, which could be due to lacrimal pump failure or punctal eversion.

Causes of the Nasolacrimal Duct Obstruction

A. Dacryocystitis due to nasal allergy, septal deviation and sinusitis.
B. Lacrimal stones.
C. Inflammations like tuberculosis, leprosy
D. Non infectious inflammations like sarcoid
E. Tumors—malignant epithelial neoplasms
F. Lacrimal sac cysts

G. Trauma

H. Radiation therapy

EXAMINATION

Punctum

Pouting puncti, stenosis, canaliculitis and ectropion punctum or entropion punctum **(Figures 1A and B).**

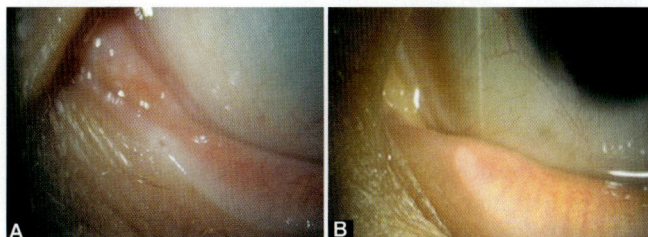

Figures 1A and B

Sac Syringing

Syringing is a primary procedure done as part of the evaluation of epiphora. A drop of anesthetic is instilled in the conjunctival sac and then irrigated with normal saline. A punctum dilator can be used before inserting the cannula if the punctum is too small. Before the test the patient is told that the saline may pass into the nose and throat and asked to inform the clinician if he/she feels it in the throat. Syringing is usually done through the lower punctum as it is easily accessible but can be done through both puncta. If the saline passes through the NLD and reaches the throat it is patent and there is no anatomical obstruction. A patent syringing can indicate a physiological cause for obstruction. If the saline regurgitates through the opposite punctum, then there is a block at the common canaliculus or upper sac. If the saline regurgitates through the same punctum, then the punctum which is being tested is blocked. There can also be a partial block in the NLD where the patient feels a small amount of saline in the throat and some of it regurgitates. Probing can be performed after syringing to determine where the block is. On probing if you reach a hard stop it means that the common canaliculus is patent. But if you reach a soft stop then obstruction of the common canaliculus can be suspected hard versus a soft stop.

The Jones Test

The test is done by instilling fluorescein in the conjunctival sac and visualizing it in the nose after a period of five minutes. If dye not seen in the nose after five minutes, then a secondary test is done, by irrigating the duct. If after irrigating the duct no dye is found in the nose, the dye has never really reached the lacrimal sac to begin with and it's a partial obstruction. If dye is seen by irrigation, it is likely to be pump failure.

Dacryocystogram

For the dacryocystogram, the patient is in supine position and the contents of the sac should be first emptied by massage and irrigated thoroughly with saline to remove any residual mucoid material. After placing a topical anesthetic in the conjunctival sac, the radiopaque dye is then injected in the lacrimal sac through a tube in the punctum. Radiographs are taken as soon as the dye is injected. They are usually obtained in the posteroanterior view and lateral view.

Indications for DCG

- Complete obstructions of the lacrimal system: If you reach a soft stop during syringing suggesting a complete obstruction, DCG will determine if the obstruction is in the canaliculus or the sac.

- Incomplete obstructions: in incomplete obstructions it will give us the exact location of the blockage.
- Tumors of the lacrimal sac are assessed with DCG.
- Previous lacrimal sac surgery.

A DCG can cause little discomfort to the patient and does not allow any physiological assessment of the lacrimal sac. A preoperative radiograph DCG can be placed on the view box in the operating room. This could be helpful while performing the operation **(Figure 2)**.

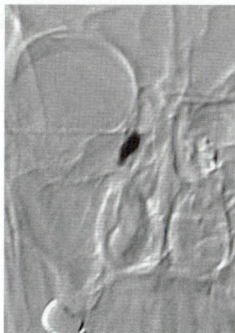

Figure 2

Dacryoscintigraphy with Radiolabeled Materials
Lacrimal Dacryoscintigraphy (LDS)

LDS is a form of nuclear imaging of the lacrimal sac. A drop of radionuclide is instilled in the palpebral aperture or conjunctival sac. Radiographic images are taken to follow the radionuclide through the lacrimal system. The patient is advised to blink normally and the images are taken every 10 seconds for the first 2-3 minutes and then every 5 minutes for a total of 20 minutes.

Indications for LDS

- Complaint of epiphora even with patent syringing: if syringing is patent it could indicate a functional black like lacrimal pump failure, even though the anatomy of the lacrimal system is normal.
- Patients with Lid Laxity: LDS can determine if the lid laxity is the cause for lacrimal pump failure.
- Assessment of Punctal occlusion: LDS can determine the efficacy of punctal occlusion.

LDS causes less discomfort for the patient, as there is not tube to be inserted. Studies have shown that LDS is a marginally superior technique to DCG. LDS gives us physiologic or functional information about the lacrimal sac, but no anatomic details.[2] Thus, LDS needs to be done in conjunction with a DCG or syringing and cannot be the only diagnostic procedure. LDS has also been shown to be more sensitive in detecting abnormalities in the upper lacrimal system.

All three procedures; syringing, DCG and LDS have to be performed complementary to each other and cannot indicate the cause for epiphora alone **(Figure 3)**.

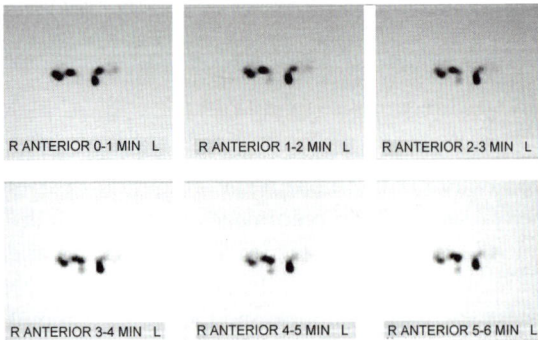

R ANTERIOR 0-1 MIN L   R ANTERIOR 1-2 MIN L   R ANTERIOR 2-3 MIN L

R ANTERIOR 3-4 MIN L   R ANTERIOR 4-5 MIN L   R ANTERIOR 5-6 MIN L

Figure 3

Extrinsic Tumors

CT scan[2] to exclude extrinsic tumors, lacrimal sac mucoceles, the state of the sinuses and dacryoliths for you.

ENDOSCOPIC DCR

First described by McDonogh in 1989. The anterior portion of the middle turbinate is used as a landmark. A mucosal flap is elevated, exposing the lacrimal fossa. This bone is drilled out, that is the frontal process of the maxillary bone and some of the lacrimal bone, exposing the nasal lacrimal sac. A probe is used to tent the sac, and the sac is incised to create a ostium so that tears can drain from the canaliculus directly into the nose through the middle turbinate and bypass any obstruction in the nasolacrimal duct. This ostium is kept open with a tube stent with a silicone tube placed through the puncta into the sac and out the nose. The tubes are retained for six months.

Advantages of the Endoscopic DCR

A. There is no external scar.
B. It preserves the lacrimal pump system.
C. Any intranasal pathology that might have caused failure of the first procedure can be corrected, including adhesions, enlarged middle turbinate and septal deviation **(Figure 4)**.
D. Negative pressure was detected during blinking and forced blinking in all normal subjects and in most patients who had successfully undergone DCR. In contrast, positive pressure was detected in cases with epiphora and patients in whom DCR had failed. Negative pressure was higher after endoscopic than external DCR. During the Valsalva maneuver there were no pressure changes in normal cases and patients with epiphora. In contrast, positive pressure was detected after all of the successful procedures (being

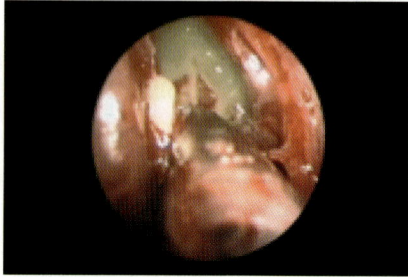

Figure 4

higher after external than endoscopic DCR) and in most of the patients in whom external DCR failed. In normal subjects, negative pressure is created during blinking. In cases with epiphora due to NLD obstruction, the lacrimal pump is affected but its function is restored after successful DCR. The suction power of the pump mechanism is more effective after endoscopic than external (Acta Oto-Laryngologica, Volume 123, Issue 2 February 2003; pp 325-9).

Disadvantages

A. No Mucosal flaps made -Mucosal flaps have been found to decrease recurrence rates in the external procedures.
B. A smaller rhinostomy is performed in Endo DCR than in the external procedure
C. No suturing of flaps.

Complications

A. Closure of the ostium
B. Intranasal adhesions
C. Canalicular laceration
D. Pyogenic granuloma

E. CSF leak

F. Orbital hemorrhage can occur from the interior ethmoid artery during the endoscopic procedure

Comparison of External and Endo-DCR

Hartikainen et al[3,4] did a prospective study comparing endoscopic to external DCR of 64 patients followed up for one year. He found a patency rate of 75% in the endoscopic cases versus 91% externally. This did not, however, reach a statistically significant difference. After revision procedures, there was a 97% success rate in both groups.

Lasers in DCR[5-8]

A. Massaro[5] used an Argon laser

B. Holmium-Yag[8] laser has advantages of fiberoptic delivery, effective bone ablation, soft tissue coagulation and shallow depth of penetration, which makes it safer.

C. KTP laser

Adjuvants in DCR

Mitomycin-C[9,10] an alkylating agent has been found useful by Camara et al[11] improving success rate for endoscopic DCRs from 89 to 99% with no complications.

RECENT MODIFICATIONS

A. The new technique involved creation of a **large bony ostium and mucosal flaps**[12] to create an anastomosis between the lacrimal sac mucosa and nasal mucosa.

B. **Mechanical endonasal dacryocystorhinostomy (MENDCR)**[13] creation of a large ostium as well as mucosal flaps improves the efficacy of this endonasal technique.

C. **Modified endoscopic dacryocystorhinostomy with posterior lacrimal sac flap**[14] for nasolacrimal duct obstruction. The new technique involved the creation of a large posterior flap at the medial lacrimal sac wall, reflecting it posteriorly, followed by removal of the remaining small anterior flap

D. **Moreker Kirtane Suturing of Endoscopic nasal and sac flaps in Endonasal DCR-**the authors follow a technique of suturing of the nasal and sac flaps in endoscopic DCR (video enclosed)

E. **Moreker Mankekar technique of Tissue glue for apposing flaps-**The authors follow a technique of holding the nasal and sac flaps with tissue fibronectin glue (video enclosed)

REFERENCES

1. Yung MW, Logan BM. The anatomy of the lacrimal bone at the lateral wall of the nose: its significance to the lacrimal surgeon. Clin Otolaryngol 1999;24:262-65.
2. Francis IC, Kappagoda MB, Cole IE, Bank L, Dunn GD. Computed tomography of the lacrimal drainage system: retrospective study of 107 cases of dacryostenosis. Ophthal Plast Reconstr Surg 1999;15:217-26.
3. Hartikainen J, Grenman R, Puuka P, Seppa H. Prospective randomized comparison of external dacryocystorhinostomy and endonasal laser dacryocystorhinostomy. Ophthalmology 1998;105:1106-13.
4. Hartikainen J, Antila J, Varpula M, Puuka P, Seppa H, Grenman R. Prospective randomized comparison of endonasal endoscopic dacryocystorhinostomy and external dacryocystorhinostomy. Laryngoscope 1998;108:1861-66.
5. Massaro BM, Gonnering RS, Harris GI. Endonasal laser dacryocystorhinostomy: a new approach to nasolacrimal duct obstruction. Arch Ophthalmol 1990;108:1172-6.1989;103: 585-7.
6. Metson R, Woog JJ, Puliafito CA. Endoscopic laser dacryocystorhinostomy. Laryngoscope 1994;104:269-274.

7. Meullner K, Bodner E, Mannor GE, Wolf G, Hoffman T, Luxenberger W. Endolacrimal laser assisted lacrimal surgery. Br J Ophthomol 2000;84:16-8.

8. Sadiq SA, Hugkulstone CE, Jones NS, Downes RN. Endoscopic holmiun:YAG laser dacryocystorhinostomy. Eye 1996;10:43-6.

9. Szubin L, Papageorge A, Sacks E. Endonasal laser-assisted dacryocystorhinostomy. Am J Rhinol 1999;13:371-4

10. Weidenbecher M, Hoseman W, Buhr W. Endoscopic endonasal dacryocystorhinostomy: results in 56 patients. Ann Otol Rhinol Laryngol 1994;103:363-7.

11. Camara JG, Bengzon AU, Henson RD. The safety and efficacy of mitomycin C in endonasal endoscopic laser-assisted dacryocysto-rhinostomy. Ophthal Plast Reconstr Surg 2000;16:114-8.

12. Tsirbas A, Wormald PJ. Endonasal dacryocystorhinostomy with mucosal flaps. Am J Ophthalmol. 2003 Jan;135(1):76-83.

13. Tsirbas A, Wormald PJ. Mechanical endonasal dacryocysto-rhinostomy with mucosal flaps.Br J Ophthalmol. 2003 Jan;87(1):43-7.

14. Yuen KS, Lam LY, Tse MW, Chan DD, Wong BW, Chan WM. Modified endoscopic dacryocystorhinostomy with posterior lacrimal sac flap for nasolacrimal duct obstruction. Hong Kong Med J. 2004 Dec;10(6):394-400.

Special Oculoplasty Surgical Procedures 27

Daljit Singh (India)

PLICATION OF ORBICULARIS OCULI FOR PTOSIS

The surgery involves the exposure of the orbicularis oculi muscle, by making a skin flap that starts from near the upper orbital margin downwards. The orbicularis oculi fibers near the lid margin are joined to the proximal orbicularis fibers with the help of 80 microns stainless steel sutures.

Steps of Operation

Exposure of the Orbicularis Oculi Muscle

A skin-deep curved incision with its convexity towards the orbital margin is made. The central highest point of the convexity is about 5 to 7 mm from the orbital margin. The incision line slopes gently towards the either end. The ends are kept away from the lid margin by at least 7-8 mm **(Figures 1 and 2)**.

The skin is carefully separated from the underlying orbicularis oculi muscle close to the incision line. It is then progressively undermined and separated, right up to the lid margin. During the process of undermining and separation of the skin, the tip of the blunt curved corneal scissors is kept directed towards the skin, so that the orbicularis muscle is not excessively injured or carried along with the skin. A clean dissection in the right plane minimizes oozing of the blood.

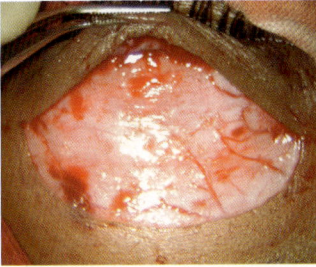

Figure 1: Exposure of the orbicularis oculi muscle

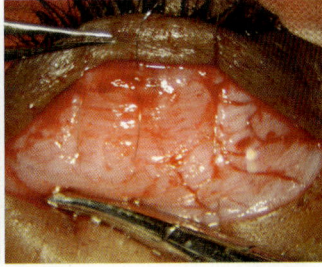

Figure 2: 80 microns vanadium steel sutures have been passed through the orbicularis oculi muscle at three places

Sometimes, a few bleeding points will need to be cauterized with a bipolar or a radio-cautery.

The reflection of the skin flap is best done with a 6 X head worn magnification. It gives a degree of freedom of movement that is not possible with an operating microscope. One can look under the skin flap and carry out the dissection with confidence. Bright illumination for 5-6 cm. operation area is obtained from the operating microscope. This light trans-illuminates the skin and helps to identify and separate the orbicularis fibers from the skin. In addition a hand held light is required to sometimes directly illuminate under the skin flap for better visualization **(Figure 3)**.

The making of the skin flap exposes the arches of orbicularis oculi fibers. They are circularly disposed, dark pink in appearance and a number of blood vessels of various sizes are seen coursing over them **(Figure 4)**.

Plication of the Orbicularis Muscle

Vanadium steel 80 micron wire attached to an atraumatic needle is used for plication. The first suture is applied in the middle. The needle is passed under a 2 mm strip of the

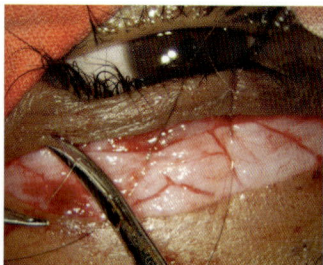

Figure 3: Steel sutures have been tied, bringing the upper and the lower orbicularis oculi fibers together

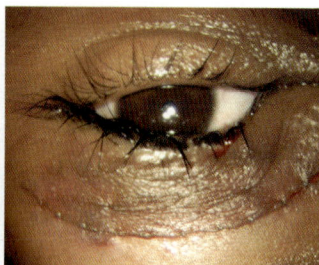

Figure 4: The skin flap has been closed with superficial 80 microns sutures

orbicularis close to the lid margin. The same needle then lifts a 2 mm strip of the orbicularis muscle towards the orbital margin. The selection of the proximal site varies according to the degree of ptosis. It is closer to the superior orbital margin in cases of severe ptosis. When the central suture is tied the lid margin is seen to rise. The cornea gets exposed. At this stage the cornea is covered with a thick layer of visco-elastic material like methyl cellulose. A reef-knot is used. The ends of the suture are cut close to the knot with a stout scissors. A single suture produces an angulation in the lid margin. To produce a natural looking lift to whole of the lid, one or two sutures are applied on either side of the central suture.

At the end of plication, the following can be noted:

1. The lid margin rises to expose the cornea. If the patient looks straight ahead, the lid margin may appear in the vicinity of the upper limbus.

2. The reflected skin flap looks much bigger than the raw area that needs to be closed.

3. The upper lid margin may in some cases, show a tendency to stand away from the eyeball.

Managing the Palpebral Skin Flap

The loose skin flap is fixed as follows:

a. The under-surface of the skin is sutured to the plicated orbicularis muscle at three points with single throw 80 micron vanadium steel sutures. This prevents the skin from hanging down.

b. A 2-3 mm strip of the skin is excised.

c. The skin flap is closed with 10-12 single throw superficially applied 80 micron vanadium steel sutures.

Bandaging the Eye

The upper lid is gently pushed down to close the eye. When pressure is released the eyelid moves up, revealing the elasticity of movement. No Frost suture is required. The eyelid is carefully closed, taped and pad and bandage is applied.

The result of orbicularis oculi plication are shown in the following picture. There is lid lag on looking downwards, but there is no lagophthalmos. The eye can be closed easily **(Figure 5)**.

SUTURELESS CONJUNCTIVAL ROUTE PLICATION OF LEVATOR MUSCLE FOR PTOSIS

Introduction

The ability of the Fugo blade to incise and blunt-dissect in a bloodless manner, encouraged me to explore the possibility of searching the levator muscle, through fornix incisions and to advance it to the anterior surface of the tarsal plate. Thus developed a novel technique for ptosis repair.

The indications for ptosis surgery are a mild moderate or severe degree of ptosis. It can be performed on both infantile and adult ptosis. Most cases are uniocular. When it is bilateral, I prefer to do one eye at a time. It is not indicated for paralytic ptosis.

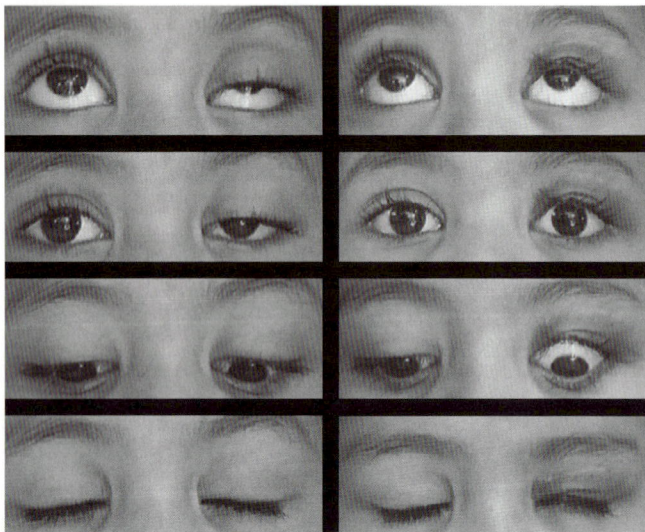

Figure 5 : Preoperative and 2 days postoperative appearances in a 9 years old child, who had severe unilateral ptosis with poor levator function

Anesthesia

During surgery, the lid has to be double everted, so that there is considerable pull on the lid. At the time of searching, holding and bringing out the levator there is pull on the muscle. To do all this, I prefer general anesthesia.

Surgical Technique

1. The lid is double everted with Desmarre lid retractor.
2. Thick nylon stay sutures are passed at the upper edge of the tarsal plate, one in the middle and one on either side at a distance of about 6 mm. The weight of the artery forceps holding them keeps the lid everted.

3. The conjunctiva over the double everted tarsus is ballooned with lignocaine.

4. Three conjunctival vertical incisions about 10 mm long are made in line with the stay sutures. The incision is made with a 100 microns Fugo blade tip. When this tip crosses a large subconjunctival vessel, there is bleeding. To prevent this, all the visible blood vessels in the proposed line of incision are ablated/closed with a 300 micron tip at low energy. Alternatively, the incision may be started and completed with the 300 micron tip only. This leaves a minor gap in the conjunctiva, which is of no consequence for the surgical result **(Figure 6)**.

5. The fornix ends of the conjunctival incisions are undermined towards the orbit.

6. The structure directly under the incised conjunctiva is Muller muscle. Muller muscle takes its origin from under the levator muscle. If this muscle is pulled anteriorly, we can easily catch the levator muscle in its aponeurosis. While the Muller muscle is red, the levator muscle looks pearly white.

The amount of levator muscle pulled anteriorly depends upon the severity of ptosis. The greater the ptosis, more the anterior pull of levator needed.

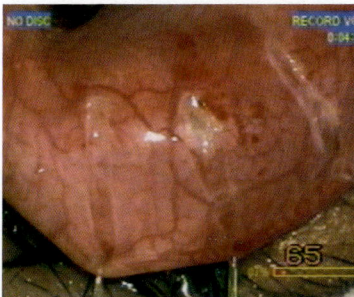

Figure 6: The conjunctiva has been ballooned and three incisions have been made with 300 micron Fugo blade tip

7. Vanadium steel suture, 80 microns size, is passed through the levator muscle caught at the end of each conjunctival incision. The sutures are secured with mini clamps **(Figure 7)**.

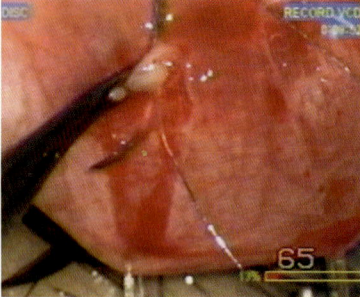

Figure 7: Levator muscle has been brought out and 80 micron vanadium steel suture has been passed through it

8. Now the anterior surface of the tarsal plate is exposed with the help of 300 microns blunt Fugo blade probe. The exposure is done at the three proximal ends of the conjunctival incisions. Exposure of tarsal plate occurs as we ablate Muller muscle and the underlying stretched aponeurosis of levator muscle. The ablation begins close to the nylon stay sutures, which provide us a clue of the depth at which Fugo blade is working. The most important point is not to ablate the tarsal plate, only expose it. Exposure of the tarsal plate with Fugo blade is usually bloodless. If a large vessel is in the way, it shall bleed. The very same Fugo blade tip is touched to the bleeding spot to stop the bleeding. The exposure process is accomplished with Fugo blade without charring of the tissues. This in turn prevents postoperative reaction and edema **(Figure 8)**.

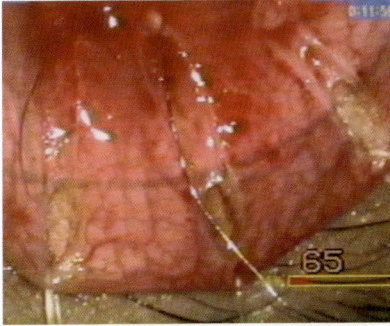

Figure 8: Three areas on the anterior surface of the tarsal plate have been exposed with 300 microns tip of Fugo blade, in line with the nylon stay sutures

9. The levator holding steel sutures are then passed through the exposed/prepared anterior surface of the tarsal plate. The needle is entered through partial thickness of tarsal plate about 3 to 3.5 mm from the upper edge of the tarsal plate, and is made to come out about 1.5 mm from the edge **(Figure 9)**.

10. The levator is attached to the tarsal plate with a reef knot to the steel sutures. Excessive force is not used lest the tarsal plate get cheese wired **(Figure 10)**.

11. Stay sutures are removed. The lid is returned to its normal position.

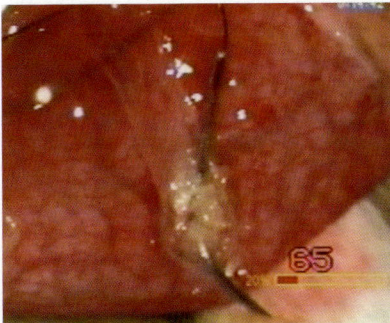

Figure 9: The suture has been passed through half thickness of the tarsal plate

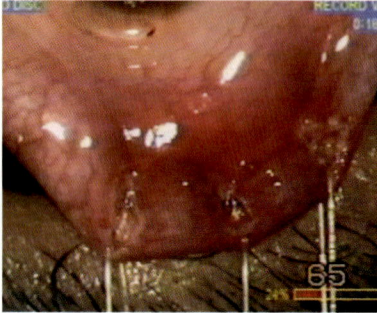

Figure 10: All the three sutures have been tied and cut. We are looking at the anterior surface of the tarsal plate. When the lid is returned back this surface is away from the cornea

12. The lids are temporarily tied together with a thick nylon suture for 24 hours for adults and 48 hours for the children.

It will be noted that Fugo Blade is needed for the crucial steps of incising the conjunctiva and exposure of the anterior surface of the tarsal plate.

Postoperative Management

Steroid-antibiotic eye ointment three times a day for 15 days. Artificial tear drops 7-8 times a day and making sure that the patient is able to close the lid. A pad and bandage at night time for the first few days.

There is little or no inflammatory reaction after the surgery. A part of the credit goes to the Fugo Blade that ablates without charring and collateral damage and a part goes to the simplicity and atraumatic nature of the surgical technique.

It is important to watch the lid margin, if there is any in turning. In turning can happen if the levator is attached far too anteriorly from the superior edge of the tarsal plate. In a very severe ptosis case, when an excess of levator has to be pulled out, the same situation can happen. The tarsal plate moves up, while the other tissues of the lid tend to hang over

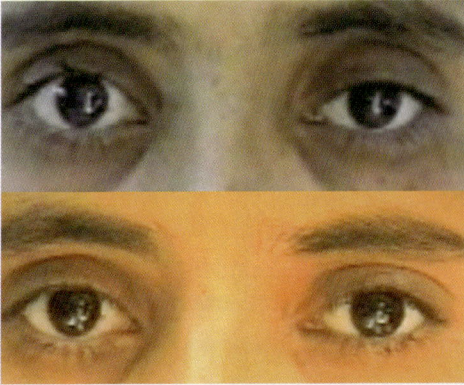

Figure 11: Slight ptosis, before and six months after surgery

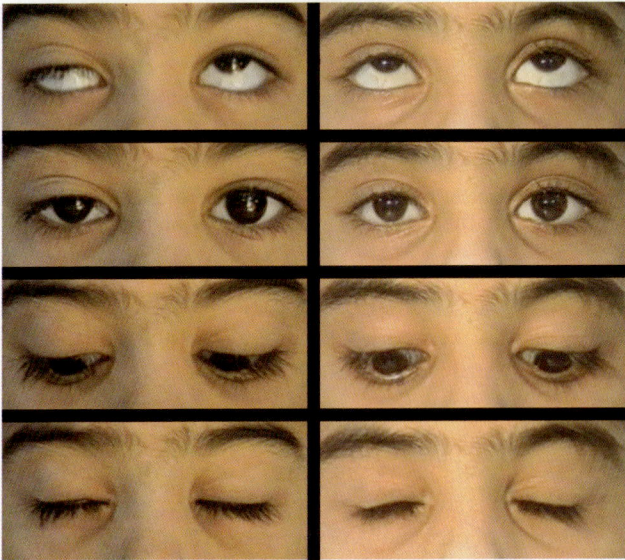

Figure 12: Ptosis with poor levator function. Pediatric patient, age 7, who was operated at the age of 3. The slight inequality shall be corrected by orbicularis plication later on, if the patient so desires

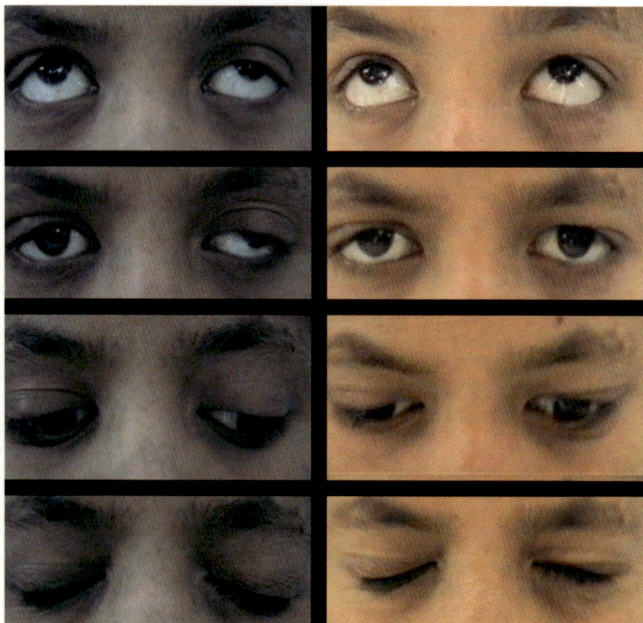

Figure 13: Unilateral severe ptosis with good levator function, in a 13 years old patient. The postoperative appearances are one year after the operation

the lid margin. Temporary sutures lifting the skin prevent the cilia from striking the cornea. A bandage lens may be kept for a few days if needed.

We have done over 180 operations during the past 4 years. More than 90% of the cases have a satisfactory outcome. When the correction is short of expectations, I do additional surgery of "plication of orbicularis oculi muscle", about 6 months or more after the primary operation **(Figures 11 to 13).**

BIBLIOGRAPHY

1. Singh D. Orbicularis Plication for Ptosis. Ann Ophthalmol 2006;28;3: 185-93.
2. Singh D, Kaur A, Singh K, Singh SK, Singh RSJ. Sutureless Levator Plication by Conjunctival Route. Ann Ophthalmol 2006;38,4:285-95.

Guided Sling Surgery: Jacob-Agarwal Technique of Frontalis Suspension with Single Stab Incision

28

Amar Agarwal , Soosan Jacob, Dhiya Ashok Kumar (India)

Ptosis management is a real problem. There are various techniques for treating it. A new surgical technique for acquired and congenital ptosis with poor levator function in which Seiff silicone suspension set is used in frontalis sling procedure is described. Here the entire length of the silicone set is guided in the muscle plane through a single stab incision of 2 mm. The advantage of the procedure includes less surgical time, no multiple incisions, no postoperative scars or edema and early recovery. Six eyes of 5 patients underwent the technique for congenital ptosis with poor levator function. The postoperative outcome was comparable with conventional frontalis sling surgery. Thus it provides good cosmesis while retaining the usual advantages of standard sling procedures.

INTRODUCTION

Frontalis muscle suspension procedure[1-3] is the gold standard for the treatment of congenital ptosis with poor levator function. It creates a linkage between the frontalis muscle and the tarsus of the upper eyelid, which allows for a better eyelid position in primary gaze. There have been various modifications[4-6] of performing the sling procedures in the recent past. Different sling materials[7-9] namely from autologous facia lata to several suture materials have been tried. Our technique differs from the conventional procedures by use of a single stab incision in making the pentagon or triangle and guiding the silicone sling in the muscle plane with one external incision while suspending the frontalis muscle.

SURGICAL TECHNIQUE

The upper eyelid is infiltrated with lidocaine 2% with 1:100,000 epinephrine. In children and adolescent patients, surgery is performed with general anesthesia. Under aseptic precaution, the eye is cleaned and draped. The pentagon shape is marked over the skin with a marker **(Figure 1A).** Amount of upper lid elevation needed is again decided on table. Single supra eyebrow stab incision of about 2 mm is put on the superior mark of the pentagon about 5 mm from the eyebrow **(Figure 1B)**. Sterile Seiff silicone frontalis suspension set dipped in antibiotic solution is then taken. It has a long silicone tube with stainless hollow rods on both ends with moderately sharp ends. The silicone sling of the set measures about 23.5 mm on each side and the rod measures about 6.3 cm. The overall diameter of the tube is 0.9 mm. One end of the tube is advanced through the stab incision in the muscle plane **(Figure 1C)** and guided along the incision sites marked. When the corner of the pentagon is reached, it is then turned downwards along the marks made on the overlying skin. Care is taken so that the surgeon maintains the muscle plane all throughout the procedure. If crumbling of tissue is observed while advancing the rod, it indicates that the plane of the tissue in which the rod is positioned is not uniform. Surgeon's left hand index finger **(Figure 1D)** can be used to palpate while the rod is advanced underneath. When the lid margin is

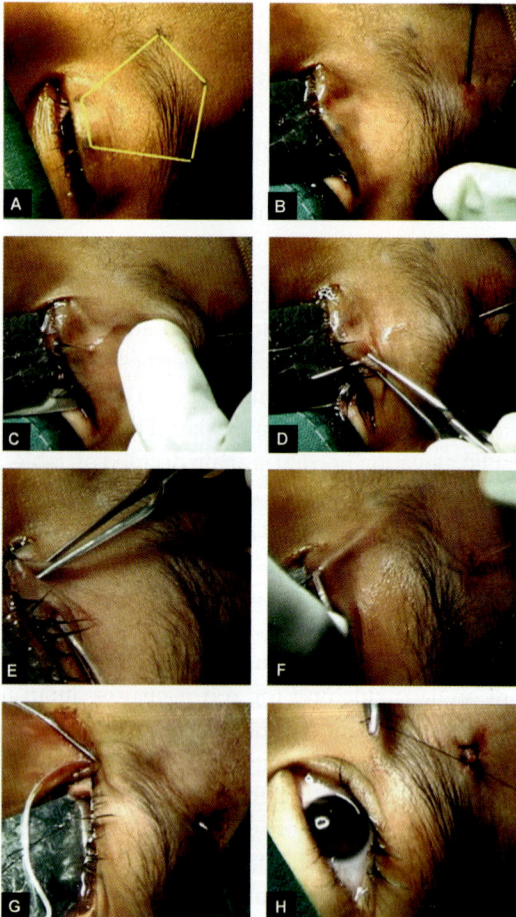

Figures 1A to H: Single pentagon (A) is marked on the skin. Seiff suspension set is passed through the supra brow incision (B) and advanced through the stab incision in the muscle plane (C, D). Then turned laterally (E, F), brought to the other end of the pentagon and finally through the same superior stab incision (G, H). Skin of the supra brow incision closed with a nonabsorbable suture

reached, the needle end is palpated and again turned laterally **(Figures 1E and F)** and brought to the other end of the pentagon. Finally it is brought back through the same superior stab incision **(Figures 1G and H)** and exteriorized. Lid margin is adjusted according to the amount of correction. When the two ends of the silicone rods are tied, automatically the upper lid margin is positioned. Minimum 4 knots are placed and the knots are buried below the subcutaneous layer. A stay suture is placed with 6-0 vicryl or any non absorbable suture to secure the silicone knot in position. If needed, one can also hitch the silicone tube knot to the underlying periosteum. The single supra brow stab incision is closed with silk suture.

DISCUSSION

The advantage of the technique is that with minimal skin incisions and less surgical time, the clinical outcome of conventional frontalis sling procedure is obtained. Postoperative lid edema, pain and suture related complications due to multiple sutures can be avoided. The technique can be performed in all eyes with ptosis and poor levator function which necessitates frontalis sling. The stab incision used is only about a 2 mm. The surgeon if faces difficulty while changing the direction of the rod; the rod is curved to pass it smoothly along the lid curvature. It is advantageous over the conventional procedure that involves five stab incisions which creates more bleeding and edema in the postoperative period. Though mild immediate postoperative edema was encountered in our technique, it was observed to resolve spontaneously within 24 hours. There have been reports in the past on minimum incision[10] and incision less sling procedures.[11] Our technique differs from their procedure[10] by being permanent and use of silicone rod instead of non absorbable suture[9]. Though silicone material[12-14] for frontalis sling suspension has been tried successfully, our method of guided sling procedure with silicone sling has not been reported. Skin of infant is prone to early scar formation and moreover forehead scars caused by frontalis suspension procedures can be a cosmetic problem in future as the child grows. We believe our technique will provide better aesthetic and functional results in such patients with poor levator function and requiring better cosmetic results. In our 6 months postoperative follow up, the results are comparable with conventional technique. However long duration follow up and comparative study with conventional technique in large study population might be required to evaluate the long-term prognosis. Simple learning curve, good cosmesis, less number of sutures with better functional results while retaining the usual advantages of standard sling procedures are the unique features of our technique.

REFERENCES

1. Wagner RS, Mauriello JA, Nelson LB, et al. Treatment of congenital ptosis with frontalis suspension: a comparison of suspensory materials.Ophthalmology 1984 Mar;91(3):245.
2. Unilateral Frontalis Sling for the Surgical Correction of Unilateral Poor-Function Ptosis Ophthalmic Plastic and Reconstructive Surgery 21(6):412-6.
3. Clauser L, Tieghi R, Galie M. Palpebral ptosis: clinical classification, differential diagnosis, and surgical guidelines: an overview. J Craniofac Surg 2006 Mar;17(2):246-54.
4. Goldberger S, Conn H, Lemor M. Double rhomboid silicone rod frontalis suspension. Ophthal Plast Reconstr Surg 1991;7:48-53.
5. Dailey R, Wilson DJ, Wobig JL. Transconjunctival frontalis suspension (TCFS). Ophthal Plast Reconstr Surg 1991;7: 289-97.
6. Advances in the diagnosis and treatment of ptosis. Curr Opinion Ophthal 2005 Dec;16(6):351-5.

7. Wasserman B, Sprunger DT, Helveston EM. Comparison of materials used in frontalis suspension. Arch Ophthalmol 2001;119:687-91.

8. Ben Simon GJ, Macedo AA, Schwarcz RM, et al. Frontalis suspension for upper eyelid ptosis: evaluation of different surgical designs and suture material. Am J Ophthalmol 2005 Nov;140 (5):877-85.

9. Yagci A, Egrilmez S. Comparison of cosmetic results in frontalis sling operations: the eyelid crease incision versus the supralash stab incision. *JAAPOS* 2003 Jul-Aug;40(4):213-6.

10. Betharia M. Frontalis sling: a modified simple technique. *Br J Ophthalmol* 1985 Jun;69(6):443-5.

11. Yip CC, Goldberg RA, Cook TL, McCann JD. Incision-less frontalis suspension. *Br J Ophthalmol* 2004;88:585-6.

12. Carter S, Meecham WJ, Steiff SR. Silicone frontalis slings for the correction of blepharoptosis: indications and efficacy. Ophthalmology 1996;103:623-30.

13. Brun D, Hatt M. Ptosis operations with silicone suspension at the eyebrow 1991 Dec;199 (6):457-60.

14. Bernardini F, de Conciliis C, Devoto MP. Frontalis suspension sling using a silicone rod in patients affected by myogenic blepharoptosis. Orbit 2002; 21:195-8.

Modified Corrugated Intracystic Implant for Chronic Dacryocystitis: A Journey to Innovation

29

Anil M Shah (India)

INTRODUCTION

I started my private practice at Nandurbar, which is located in backward area of Maharashtra. Actually it is small tribal area. I was the first ophthalmologist surrounding 50 km area. Therefore from the first day, I started getting patients. I started my practice with two cataract set, one DCR set, one enucleation set and a refraction set. That time I was doing intracapsular cataract surgery. Then, I purchased second hand microscope and started doing extracapsular cataract surgery. It was my first IOL after 1 year of my practice. That time I used to do dacryocystectomy (DCT) and dacryocystorhinostomy (DCR). But one day I heard one comment from my one of my colleague that "To do DCT is a crime". Because of that thought I became alert and from that time I stopped doing DCT and all my surgeries were DCR.

Usually ophthalmologist who is performing cataract and IOL are always habitual in working blood less field. I was getting handsome money from IOL. With that practice many of them were reluctant of doing DCR. In spite of my good practice for cataract and IOL I was regularly doing DCR regularly.

DCR SURGERY

Performing DCR required a big courage and disturbing night sleep. DCR is most unpredictable surgery with success rate varied from patient to patient. DCR surgery is performed in chronically inflamed and vascularizes area. So there is always uncontrolled bleeding which cannot be stopped by any means other than repeated packing and pressure. In spite of doing all these measures when the pack is removed the bleeding again starts. Bleeding also occurs with each removal of lacrimal bone by nibbler and bleeding also suddenly increases when nasal mucosa is incised. I have seen many surgeon and even my self, taking lot of struggle for getting one suture to the the nasal mucosa and lacrimal sac. The surgery is performed in a very narrow and deep area which required lot of surgical skill. The patient's nasal packing is done which is not easily accepted by patient. I have seen many patient canceling their surgery when nasal packing is tried.

In spite of all these difficulties and struggle I was performing DCR surgery successfully for more than one decade. But two patients made me stop doing this surgery. One patient had profuse nasal bleeding and he was about to die but with the help of my ENT surgeon, physician and anesthetist we could save his life. For six months I stopped doing this surgery. But after six month I again started surgery and second patient had profuse bilateral nasal bleeding due to sudden rise in blood pressure after 24 hours. After that event I thought seriously and stopped doing DCR that was my last DCR surgery. For next 2 years many patient came to me but some how I gave many reasons and cancelled their surgery. But my underlying conscious was not allowing me to keep quite.

Intracystic Implant

That time I came across with one article for intracystic implant by Dr Pawar and I was immediately attracted to the technique. I have gone through the details and then I tried these implant to many of my patients.

Nowaday the surgery has changed. The time required for surgery is reduced. On table bleeding was less and controlled. Implantation of tube was easy. On table petancy was obtained. The surgery was safe and simplified. No nasal packing was required. No intraoperative and postoperatively bleeding. I became very much happy and then I started doing surgery regularly.

For more than 2 years I performed many surgeries and I was telling my friend about these surgeries. But during postoperatively I came across with problems. Few patients had extrusion of implant through nasal cavity, few patients had block implant. But few patients had funny problem. Postoperatively patient had sac patent but still the patient had repeated complaints of watering. Even after 6 months patient had sac petency on table but their complaint persist. So the failure rate was more than what I thought.

Now again I got disturbed. What to do now?

Endonasal Surgery

By that time the popularity of endonasal surgery increased and then I have decided to refer all these patients to ENT surgeon. A surgery which was primarily bread and butter of the ophthalmologist was becoming right of ENT surgeon. But what can we do?

Laser DCR

During that period laser DCR came. I attended one workshop. The surgery was simple and I decided to go for it. I was little reluctant to buy it due it is high to cost. During that period one of my ENT surgeons visited my clinic and while discussing with him, he commented that for functioning any DCR surgery minimum 3 mm opening is required and this is not possible with laser DCR. Actually he was promoting endolaser DCR Then I contacted to endolaser surgeon and they said that repeated surgery is required and so they were also not happy.

A Thought

Now what to do? My mind was constantly wondering. During that period my son, who was studying in 3rd M.B.B.S. came to home. I was going through his new surgical book and that time I read a comment that "All drainage implant that comes in contact with air must be corrugated (e.g. Breast abscess) and all drainage implant that do not come in contact with air must be tubular (e.g. Hydrocephalous)". With that statement I got the answer to the question, why intracystic implant was not working, because it was a tubular implant and was coming in contact in with air. With that thought in my mind I slept that night but I was unable to get sound sleep. Though, I stopped doing intracystic implant, in my mind there was something that can be done.

One Sunday evening I was sitting with my family. My mother in law came that morning to meet me. While talking with each other I suddenly got up and went down stare in my operation theater. I took small tube from saline set, made cut on both side and dipped in to the glass of water and to my surprise what I wanted had happened. Then I took intracystic implant and made similar cuts and I got the desired result. My idea worked and I got the solution to the problem. On the next patient I tried that idea and to my surprise it worked successfully. After that I tried this to so many patients and the results were fantastic.

The idea is "To convert tubular drainage into corrugated drain".

Then I presented a scientific paper at Maharashtra Ophthalmic Conference, Aurangbad for which I received the "Innovation Award"

Physics Principal (Figure 1)

The tubular implant when comes in contact with air function like a closed pipette. If the tip of the pipette is closed from above with the figure then the water column will not drain because, the atmospheric pressure is more than the pressure of water column in the tube. When the finger is removed the water column will drain out but a small drop of fluid at the bottom of will not drain. Even if you vigorously shake the tube that water will remain.

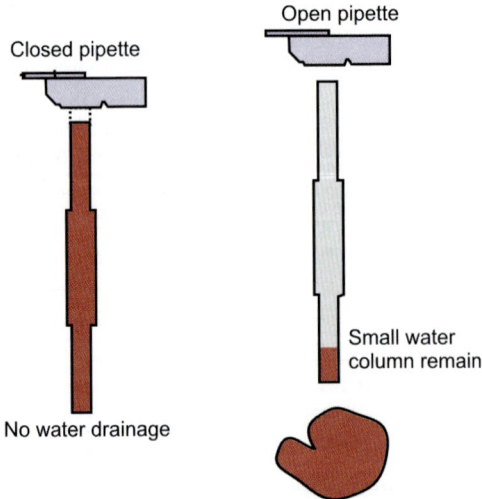

Figure 1: Closed and open pipettes

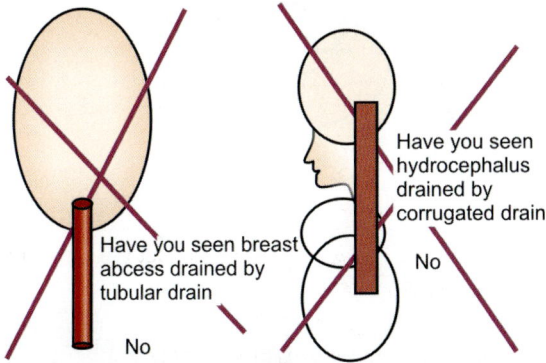

Figure 2: Breast abscess and hydrocephalus

Have you seen a tubular drainage for breast abscess or rectal abscess? No.

Have you seen a corrugated drain for hydrocephalus? No **(Figure 2)**

So the conclusion is:

Tubular intracystic implant behaves likes a closed pipette after the suturing of lacrimal sac. So water column remains in the tube but the drainage of fluid does not occur. To drain the fluid from the tube the implant must be corrugated **(Figure 3)**.

Theoretical Consideration

Functioning of Nasolacrimal Duct

The nasolacrimal tube is vertical tube. There is a valve at the lower end. The fluid forms a water column in to the nasolacrimal duct. With the inspiration fluid flow occurs because the intranasal atmospheric pressure goes below the pressure of water column in the nasolacrimal duct. With

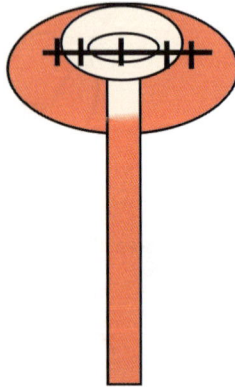

Figure 3: Tube function as closed pipette after sac suturing

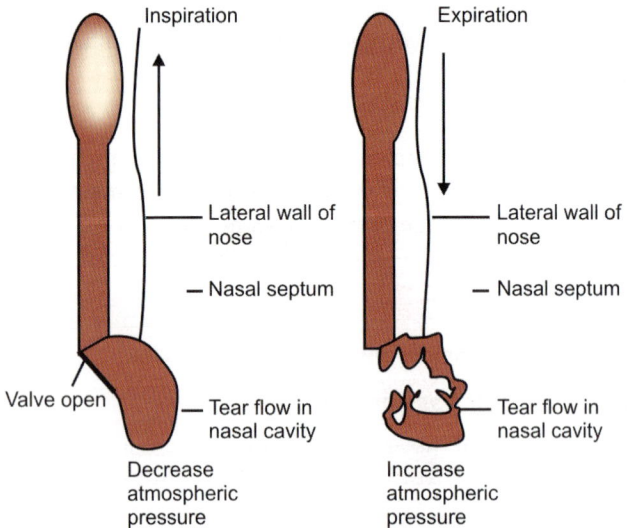

Figure 4: Physiology of nasolacrimal duct

expiration the intranasal atmospheric increases and the flow of fluid stops temporarily **(Figure 4).**

Functioning of DCR

In DCR, drainage works only when the intranasal atmospheric pressure is equal to the atmospheric pressure in to the lacrimal sac. Minimum 3 mm opening is sufficient for DCR to function **(Figure 5).**

Drawbacks of Conventional Implant

A thought came in my mind that by simply inserting the tube in to the lacrimal sac and draining the fluid into the nasal

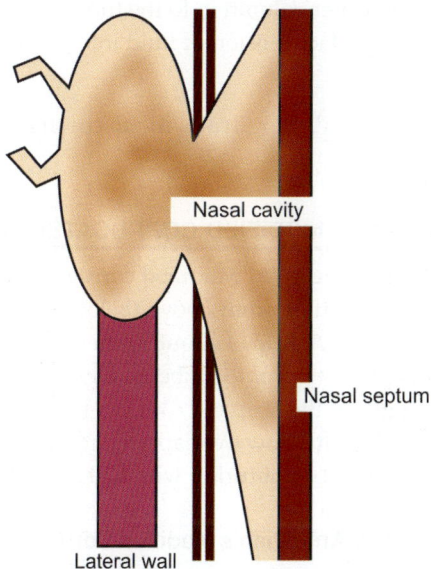

Figure 5: Drainage occurs when intranasal atmospheric pressure and sac pressure is balanced

cavity though appears logically correct but technically it do not work. If the thing is so simple then why it is not so popular? There are few drawbacks of conventional implant.

- It is a tubular so it does not obey the law of physics and the basic surgical principle
- On table – patency is false positive because the fluid is forcibly injected in to the tube above the atmospheric pressure.
- Postoperative – Patency is false positive because the fluid is injected in to the tube above the atmospheric pressure.
- So in spite of positive result the patient's complaints are persistent.

The aim is:
- To break the water column in to the tube.
- To break the surface tension of fluid into the tube.

The answer is:
To convert, the tubular drain in to corrugated drain **(Figure 6).**

PREPARATION OF MODIFIED CORRUGATED IMPLANT

To convert intracystic in to "Modified corrugated implant" a cut is made on the tube from above (below the collar) and from the lower end. A strip of about 3 mm width is removed on either side of the wall of the tube exactly opposite to each other. The length of the strip is 2/3rd the length of the tube from above and from below overlapping in the center. Tip of the implant is closed by suturing with 6/0 silk **(Figure 7).**

Advantages of Dr Anil Shah's Modified Corrugated Implant

- The vertical strip is removed from the tube breaks the water column and the surface tension of the fluid.

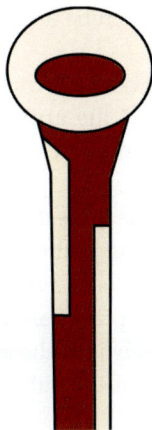

Lateral slit overlapping in the center

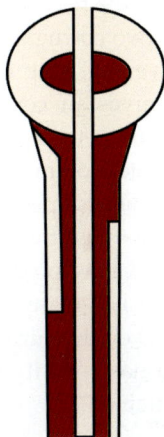

Two corrugated plate

Figure 6: Converting the tubular drain into corrugating drain

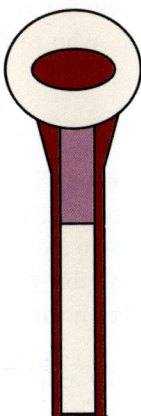

Cut from below

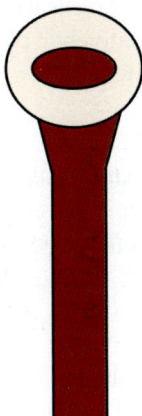

Central overlapping

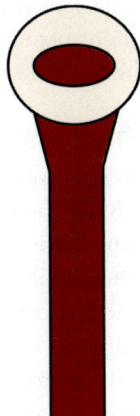

Cut from above

Figure 7: Anil Shah's modified corrugated intracystic implant

- Due to the removal of vertical strip, the tube is converted in to two corrugated plates.
- The vertical strip overlapping in the center forms a hole that gives air communication so that the atmospheric pressure in the nose and the sac is balanced. It also breaks the water column.
- If the tube is open at the end then, some time, the implant may not pass through nasal mucosa and tenting of nasal mucosa may occurs. But if the tip is closed with suture then it has many advantages. The implant can be fully loaded on the introducer. It can be easily introduced deep in to nasal cavity and the strength of the tube is also maintained.

Selection is

20 patients were operated in last 6 month between the age group of 30 to 70. Selected cases were of chronic dacryocystitis and mucocele. Failed DCR cases were excluded. All patients had sac patent postoperatively[15] patient, who came follow up over 6 month had patent sac.

Surgical Procedure

In this technique intracystic implant developed by Dr. M.D. Pawar has been used. The intracystic implant has been used as a method of treatment for epiphora due to the obstruction to the nasolacrimal duct. The aim behind this design is to make surgical procedure safer, quicker and improve the success rate.

The conventional implant is technically easier. Bleeding during surgery is reduced and no nasal packing is required. The surgery becomes OPD procedure.

I have tried conventional implant but my success rate was low. So I made few modifications on the implant and made a new "Modified Corrugated Intracystic Implant" and my success rate improved significantly.

Available

The implant is available in ETO sterilized blister peel open pack, ready to use on table. Implant is prepared as per design. The implant can also be re sterilized by autoclaving.

Material

Modified corrugated implant **(Figure 8).** Introducer **(Figure 9),** Perforator **(Figure 10)**, 5-0 Vicryl suture, and other surgical instrument for DCR.

Procedure

All the surgical procedures were done under local anesthesia similar to as used in conventional DCR. Sac is exposed. Identify medial palpebral ligament and exactly below make a vertical incision of about 3 mm on the anterior-lateral wall of the lacrimal sac.

Irrigate the sac with saline to remove blood and purulent material. Irrigate sac with 1;1000 adrenaline so as to avoid oozing during surgery **(Figure 11)**.

Stay suture to implant: A suture is passed from lower end medial edge of vertical incision. It is passed from outside to inside in to the lumen of sac. The needle is taken out of the lumen and passed through the two holes of the intracystic implant below the collar of implant. Again the suture is passed inside to out side the medial wall of the lacrimal sac from the upper end of the vertical incision. Cut the needle from the suture. This is a "U" shaped loop of suture holding the implant to the lacrimal sac. After introducing the implant in to the nasal cavity the thread of the suture is pulled out and a

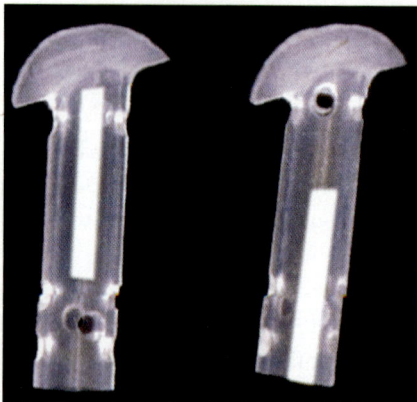

Figure 8: Dr Anil Shah modified corrgated intracystic implant

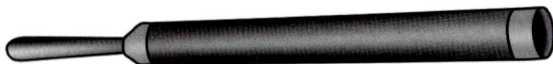

Figure 9: Introducer for implant

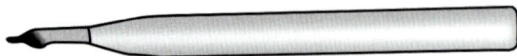

Figure 10: Perforator for fracturing lacrimal bone

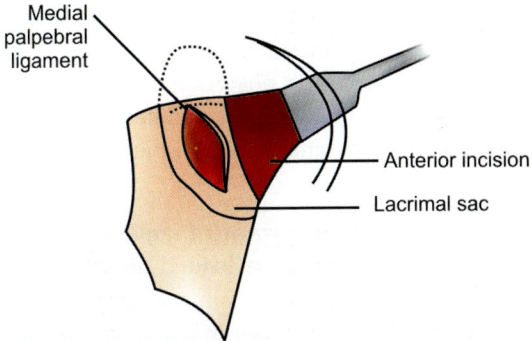

Figure 11: Vertical incision below medial palpebral ligament

knot is given on the medial wall of the lacrimal sac. This stay suture holds the implant in proper place postoperatively **(Figure 12)**.

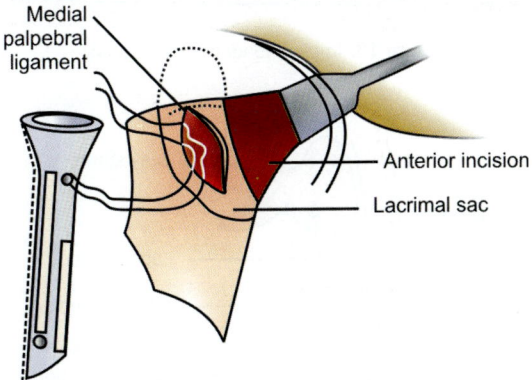

Figure 12: Stay suture to implant

Perforation: A perforator is passed through the posterior wall of the lacrimal sac, lacrimal bone and nasal mucosa. The instrument points towards posterior, medial and lower direction. Keep the perforator for few minute then rotate inside so that the fractured lacrimal bone is separated away. Take out the perforator.

Implantation of modified corrugated implant: An implant which is kept on stay suture is loaded on the introducer **(Figure 13).** Now the implant is introduced through the anterior opening the lacrimal sac in the sac in to the nasal cavity negotiating the posterior medial wall of the lacrimal sac and a newly fashioned ostium. It is placed in such way that it points towards posterior, medial and lower direction. The wider portion (collar) lies in the cavity of the sac and the other end lies in the middle meatus or lower meatus **(Figure 14).**

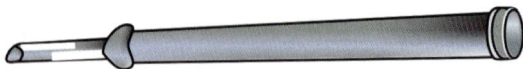

Figure 13: Implant loaded on introducer

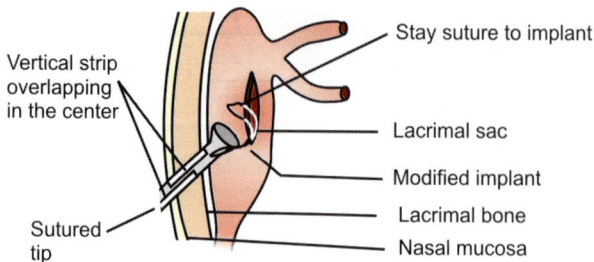

Figure 14: Implantation of modified implant

Checking patency: Saline is injected through the funnel of the implant. Observe the fluid draining into the nasal cavity. Observe the air bubble from the nostril via the implant. Once the patency is confirmed the knot of the stay sutured is tied.

Closure of sac: The sac and the surgical field is irrigated with saline and 1:1000 adrenaline. The sac is closed with interrupted 5-0 Vicryl suture. The muscle and the skin are sutured in layers. Sac syringing is do on table to check the patency.

Postoperative: Postoperative care is similar to that of DCR surgery. Decongestive nasal drops are used in the nostril of the operated eye for 3 times a day for 1 week. After 7 days skin suture are removed and sac syringing is done to check the patency of implant.

Complications

On table or postoperatively extrusion of implant is prevented due to stay suture applied to the implant. Blockage of implant is not seen postoperatively over a period of 6 months. Complications like blockage due to blood clot or granulation also decreased.

Sincere Effort

The lacrimal sac is situated on the boundary of ENT and ophthalmology. ENT surgeons are the lacrimal sac to their side.

Patient comes first to the ophthalmologist with the complaint of watering and it the duty and right of ophthalmologist to solve the problem.

This is my sincere effort to pull the lacrimal sac to the ophthalmologist side.

Management of Dysfunction of Meibomian Glands with Fugo Blade 30

Daljit Singh (India)

INTRODUCTION

Anterior blepharitis refers to inflammation of the eyelashes and follicles. Posterior blepharitis refers to meibomian gland orifices. Blepharitis often is associated with systemic diseases, such as rosacea, as well as ocular diseases such as dry eye syndromes, conjunctivitis and keratitis. Many patients give a history of a drug reaction or fever.

Patient with posterior blepharitis have ocular complaints of burning, watering, foreign body sensation, photophobia and decreased vision.

On examination, one may find crusting of the lashes and meibomium orifices and plugging and "pouting" of the meibomian orifices. Corneal findings can include punctuate epithelial erosions and corneal ulcers or pannus.

Posterior blepharitis is related to dysfunction of the meibomian glands. The meibomian secretions become waxlike and block the gland orifices. The diagnosis is made by visual inspection which demonstrates the plugging and "pouting" of the meibomian orifices. Testing patients for tear insufficiency may aid in the treatment.

MEDICAL TREATMENT

The medical treatment consists of 3 steps.
1. Warm moist soaks to lids.
2. Wash eyelid margin to clean the gland orifices.
3. Antibiotic ointment to lids.

If an adequate medial trial is not effective then Fugo Blade application may be useful. Both lids of one eye are treated at a time so that the patient can compare with the untreated one. The worst eye is treated first. Anesthesia consists of a topical anesthesia and anesthetic lid blocks **(Figure 1).**

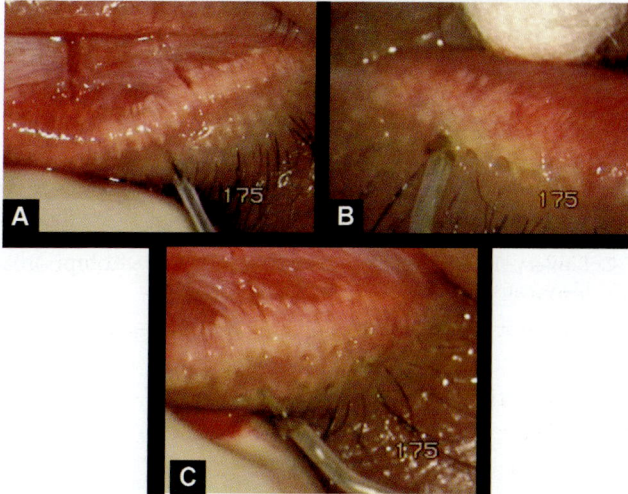

Figures 1A to C: Shows the pointed 300 microns Fugo blade and the heavily plugged meibomian glands. The activated tip penetrated for about 1 mm into the meibomian duct. All the plugs get removed in a matter of seconds

A pointed 300 microns tip of Fugo plasma blade is used at the lowest energy settings. The activated tip is placed into each of the plugs. During surgery the plugs melt as the tip enters the meibomian gland ducts for 1 mm distance. Due to the peculiar property of the plasma energy there is no burning or charring of the lid tissue.

Within 3-4 hours the patient's usual feeling in one of complete relief. Since the meibomian gland secretions are fatty, this floats over whatever tear fluid (natural or artificial) fluid exists in the conjunctival sac and over the cornea. Thus the evaporation of tears is reduced. Dry eye patients continue using artificial tears.

Another use of the Fugo blade is districhiasis. Districhiasis is a hair growing from the meibomian gland. For example, with SJ Syndrome the Fugo blade is used in an identical fashion to remove the cilia from the meibomian gland. Some hair may regrow and need to be retreated.

BIBLIOGRAPHY

1. Cohen EJ. Cornea and external disease in the new millennium. Arch. Ophthalmol. Jul 2000;118 (7): 979-81.
2. Lowery RS. www.emedicine.com/oph/topic81.htm adult blepharitis.

Fornix Reconstruction

31

Kirit Mody (India)

INTRODUCTION

Lower fornix reconstruction is difficult surgery for ophthalmologist, not familiar, with steps of surgery and it needs better postoperative care than other oculoplastic surgeries.

At time you may have to deal extensive reconstruction in cases of congenital anomaly and need amniotic membrane graft or if other eye is normal, the healthy conjunctiva.

In cases of small symblepharon, the surgery is simple and may need small graft from the same eye or other eye. While in socket surgery you need good bucal mucosa or amniotic membrane graft. The surgery is very gratifying and results are good for neat and precision surgeon.

SYMPTOMS AND SIGNS

The socket looks inflamed and congested associated with watering and discharge. The artificial eye looks slipping out from the socket or if retained it looks forward protruded artificial eye. Many times patient may not like to wear the eye and the purpose of cosmetic correction is wasted.

Patient who had anterior broad symblepharon may complains of inability to move the eye particularly in superior position. Inferior movement may be restricted but not absent.

In cases of Stevenson Johnson syndrome and similar diseases, there is extensive adhesions between eyelids and bulbar conjunctiva with change in character of conjunctiva and main complain is of severe dry eye and related symptoms.

In few patients only symptom is cosmetic appearance dye to localized fleshy looking symblepharon. The lower tear meniscus is disturbed and watering is main symptom.

ETIOLOGY

A. Congenital cryptophthalmos and ankyloblepharon or absence of fornix formation
B. Chronic inflammatory conditions leading gradual loss of lower fornix, while in cases of socket constant irritation by poorly manufactured eye, resulting in total absence of lower fornix..
C. Trauma is responsible in many cases whether it is due to mechanical, chemical agents like acid or alkali and radiation injury.
D. Stevenson Johnson syndrome, ocular pemphigus.

These above conditions neither do nor require any differential diagnosis as they are no diagnostic problems and any special investigations. In cases of severe dry eye the success of surgery is limited.

TREATMENT

One should be familiar with anatomy and dimension of conjunctival sac.

Like deapth of superior fornix is 13 mm, inferior fornix 9 mm, lateral fornix 5 mm, and medial fornix nil. The distance from the bottom or apex of fornix to orbit is superiorly 5 mm, inferiorly 6 mm, laterally 4 mm and medially nil.

While limbus to fornix distance superiorly and inferiorly 8-10 mm, laterally 14 mm and medially 7 mm.

Preoperative Evaluation

1. One should examine the fornix and measure how much shallow is the fornix, as it may be useful to dissect the amount of bucal mucosa required in cases of socket surgery. It is always necessary to have 25% extra tissue to compensate for shrinkage.
2. Evaluate the status of conjunctiva for active inflammation and existing fibrosis.

It is also necessary in cases of symblepharon to decide how much conjunctiva of symblepharon is available.

Look for any active infective diseases of eyelids, conjunctiva and cornea and treat them.

I have divided techniques in 2 parts, for small broad in width symblepharon and total reconstruction of lower fornix.

Partial Reconstruction

Technique

1. Local injection
2. Mark the area of diseased tissue
3. Inj. s/c local anesthetic with adrenaline to facilitate the incisions on conjunctiva.
4. Cut palpebral border of conjunctiva as it is to be used later on as tarsal conjunctiva.
5. Pass mattress sutures from free end of cut bulbar conjunctiva and through skin at desired level of fornix.
6. Fix mattress sutures over the skin.
7. Conjunctival graft over the bulbar area of defect with 8/0 vicryl.
8. Ointment and pressure dressing.

Wet field cautery, sponge swabs and viscoelastic material must.

Figure 1 shows dissection of symblepharon and attaching with bulbar part, if it is less vascularised and small mucosal graft for tarsal conjunctiva.

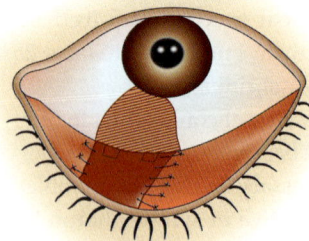

Figure 1: Conjunctival dissection of Symblepharon and graft placement.

One can use amniotic membrane or patient's conjunctiva for bulbar conjunctiva and vascularized part of symblepharon for tarsal conjunctiva DeO.

Lower Fornix Reconstruction

Following points will help surgeon in deciding how to perform better surgery.

Here I have discussed and out line the technique for lower fornix reconstruction in cases where artificial eye was not fitting properly due to absenc of lower fornix

- Degree of fornix shrinkage
- Amount of reconstruction
- Available tissue
- Amniotic membrane or mucosal graft
- Surgery may be done in stages
- Plastic or glass haptic confirmers with holes.

Technique

1. Incision in fornix near limbal side, as it may be posssible to have some conjunctival tissue to cover part of tarsal area or alternatively one can take incision on posterior lower lid boarder. Prefer as much as patients' own tissue if it is not severely diseased. Dissect and free boarder can be fixed with mattress sutures **(Figures 2 to 5)**.

2. Suture graft material with free boarder of conjunctiva or palpebral lid margin.

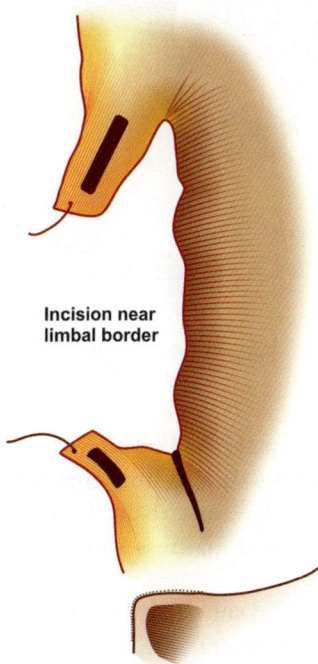

Incision near
limbal border

Incision near
lid margin

Figure 2: Socket surgery
incision near limbal border

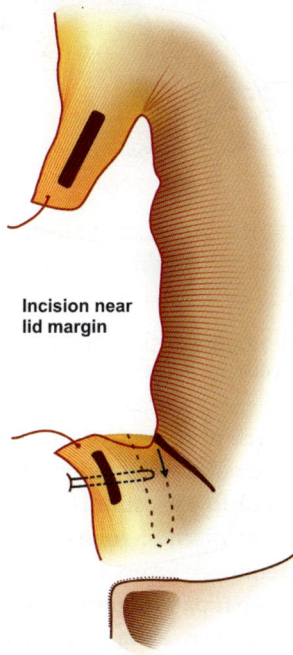

Figure 3: Incision near lid
margin

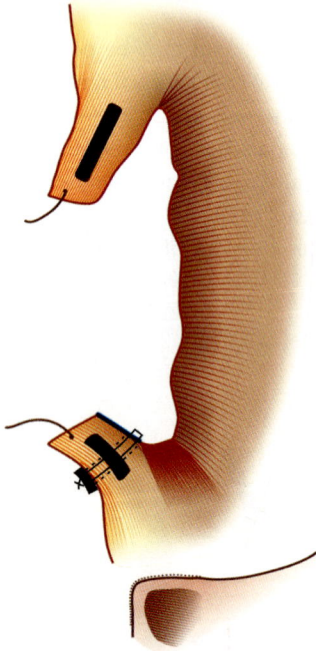

Figure 4: Suturing the conjunctiva over tarsal area

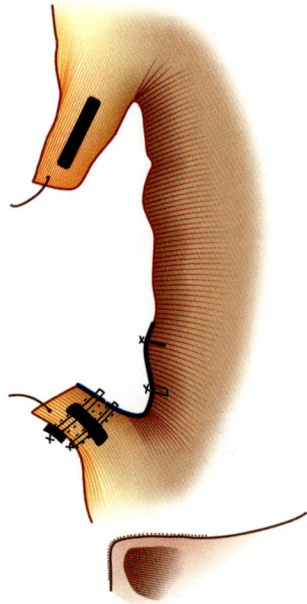

Figure 5: Suturing the mucosal graft

3. Place of silicone or silicon rod material at possible site of apex of fornix, and pass mattress sutures from silicon to graft to periostium of lower orbital rim to skin. Tie them with piece of rubber. Minimum 3 mattress sutures are required.

4. Bulbar part of graft fashioned and sutured. Always allow 20 to 25 % extra graft for shrinkage of tissue.

5. Larger graft may need additional mattress sutures passing from graft to superficial sclera.

6. Examine the fornix for additional sutures.

8. Dressings,
   • Surgeon should dress every day and inspect for infection
   • Glass rod
   • Gentle irrigation
   • Prosthesis **(Figures 6 to 10)**

This case is rare congenital anomaly–a variant of Cryptophthalmos–ankyloblepharon by ankylosis.

Eyelids were partially formed and fused with the eye ball. The visible bulbar conjunctiva was hypermic, chemosed,

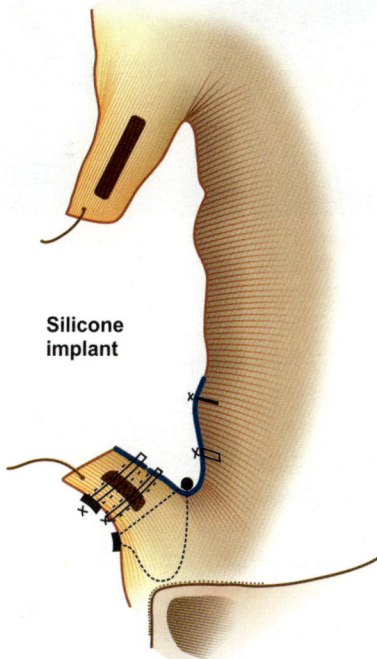

Figure 6: Placement of silicone rod in lower fornix

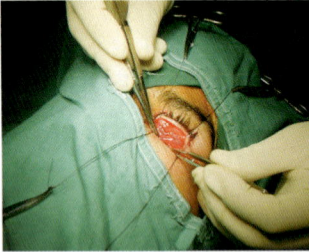

Figure 7: Conjunctiva Incision

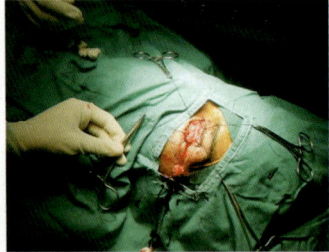

Figure 8: Conjunctival and mucosal graft suturing

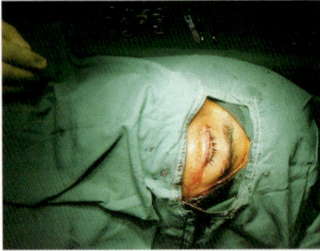

Figure 9: Fixing silicon rod in lower fornix with mattress sutures fix over the skin with rubber pieces

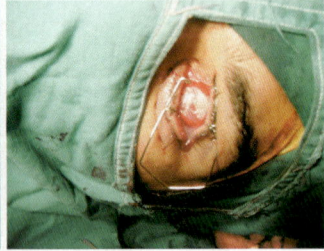

Figure 10: Placement of plastic shell or confirmer placed in socket

edematous and dry, the eye appeared on first impression as buphthalmic or exophthalmic eye.

The patient was operated jointly by ophthalmologist and plastic surgeon for reformation of fornix with amniotic member graft **(Figures 11 to 15).**

The results of fornix reconstruction is very rewarding surgery and one must prepare for good post operative care.

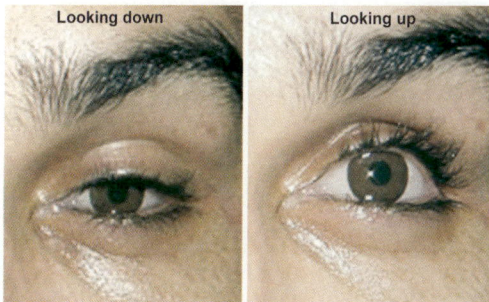

Figure 11: Patient looking up and looking down with artificial eye

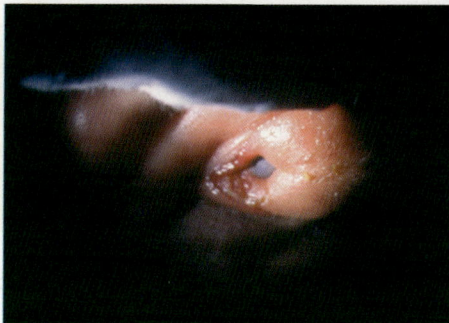

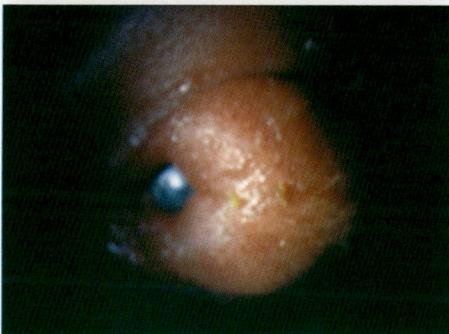

Figures 12 and 13: Cryptophthalmos—Ankyloblepharon by ankylosis before surgery

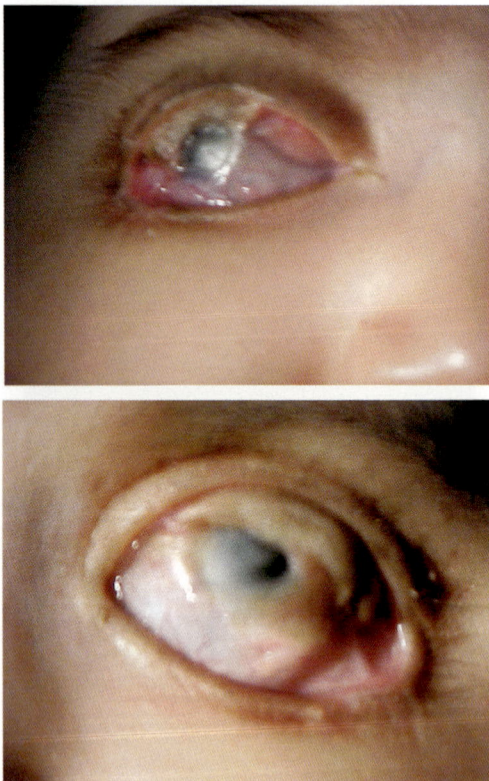

Figure 15: Cryptophthalmos—Ankyloblepharon by
ankylosis after surgery

Sebaceous Gland Carcinoma and Muir-Torre's Syndrome 32

Sunil Moreker, Sneha Kataria, Mayur Moreker, Murad Lala (India)

INTRODUCTION

Periocular sebaceous gland carcinomas (SGCs) occur in the eyelids either sporadically or as a phenotypic feature of Muir-Torre syndrome (MTS).

Muir-Torre syndrome is is currently considered a subtype of the more common hereditary nonpolyposis colorectal cancer syndrome, in which multiple primary malignancies occur together with sebaceous gland tumors.[1]

Lynch syndrome or hereditary non-polyposis colorectal cancer (HNPCC) is an autosomal-dominant disorder characterized by predisposition to colorectal cancer and extracolonic malignancies, frequent multiple primary tumors in the same patient, and early age of cancer onset.

EPIDEMIOLOGY[2]

Cutaneous SGC incidence rates (IRs) and IR ratios were examined in 9 US Surveillance, Epidemiology, and End Results Program registries (1973-2003) and 95% confidence intervals (95% CIs) calculated for subsequent cancers among 2-month survivors of SGC and for subsequent SGC after other primary cancers. This data showed that, nearly 90% cases are diagnosed among whites (IR, 0.11 per 100,000 person-years), with significantly lower IR were noted among blacks (IR, 0.04).

Eyelid SGC IRs showed no sex differences and stabilized in recent years. Survivors of SGC had a 43% (95% CI, 15%-76%) increased risk of subsequent cancer, and risk of SGC was elevated by 52% (95% CI, 24%-84%) among survivors of other cancers. Patterns suggestive of genetic predisposition included more than 20-fold risks for early-onset (diagnosed in patients aged less than 50 years) SGC associated with colon, pancreatic, ovarian, or uterine corpus cancers, whereas late-onset SGC (diagnosed in patients aged >/=50 years) predisposed to ureter cancer.[2]

GENETICS

Patients with MTS showed microsatellite instability(MSI) characteristic for hereditary nonpolyposis colorectal cancer (HNPCC), which is caused by autosomal dominant inherited DNA mismatch repair (MMR) defects. Mutational analyses of the MMR genes hMSH2 and hMLH1 have revealed different germline mutations in the hMSH2 gene. In some cases a truncating germline mutation is seen in the MMR gene hMLH1. The defect is thought to be the result of a mutation in mismatch repair genes and associated with microsatellite instability.[3, 4] It is caused by either a mismatch-repair (MMR) defect or inactivation of the fragile histidine triad (FHIT) gene which is associated with MTS-like signs, including SGC. The genetic alterations are associated with microsatellite instability (MSI) and inactivation of the FHIT gene. Loss-of-function mechanisms affecting the FHIT gene are identified as intragenic deletions eliminating the coding exons 5 and 6 on one hand, and complete biallelic methylation of the FHIT transcription regulatory region on the other hand. Either somatic inactivation of the FHIT gene associated with MSS or inactivation of the MMR system resulting in MSI contribute to the development of periocular SGCs in presumptive.[5]

Second Hit Theory

Microsatellite instability in tumor tissue develops after somatic inactivation of the corresponding second mismatch repair allele ("second hit"). sebaceous tumors from patients with genetically proven Muir-Torre syndrome the loss of heterozygosity most probably is not the preferred mode of somatic inactivation of the second MSH2 allele.

Duplication

In some cases duplication of exon 7 of the MSH2 gene in MTS is seen.[14]

Immunohistopathologic Correlation

MSI correlates with loss of MSH2 and MLH1 immunostaining.

Epithelial markers—CEA, EMA[30] **(Figure 1)**

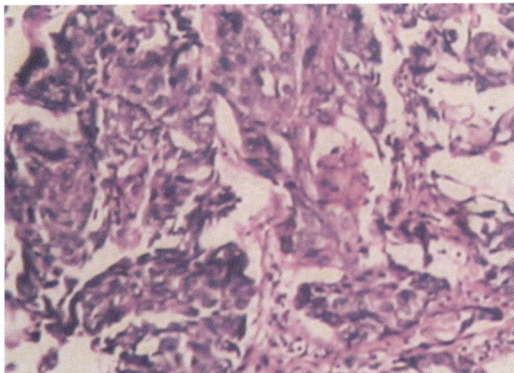

Figure 1

GENETICOPATHOLOGICO-CLINICAL CLASSIFICATION

Moreker-Kataria-Lala Classification of Sebaceous Gland Carcinomas

A. Lynch syndrome. No probable second hit.

B. Miur-Torre syndrome—Cystic sebaceous carcinoma-probable second hit—Cystic sebaceous tumors (CST) are well-circumscribed, large, deeply located dermal sebaceous proliferations with a cystic growth pattern. MLH1 and MSH2 gene mutations have an equivalent etiopathological role both for Lynch syndrome and for MTS.[7]

   1. The most common is a variant of hereditary non-polyposis colorectal cancer, which is characterised by defects in mismatch repair genes and early-onset tumors.

   2. The second type does not show deficiency in mismatch repair and its pathogenesis remains undefined.[18]

C. Sebaceous carcinoma in nevus sebaceus of Jadassohn

D. Pagetoid tumors lid.

E. Conjunctival and lid sebaceous carcinoma

F. Caruncle Sebaceous carcinoma.

G. Collision sebaceous and basal cell carcinomas of the eyelid or kissing tumors sebaceous and basal cell carcinoma.

PRESENTATIONS

Vary from a yellow-pink nodule with telangiectatic vessels on the left lower eyelid in some patient and a yellowish-red, pedunculated lesion with intrinsic vascularization on the right superior tarsal conjunctiva in another to a pagetoid spread or cystic in Muir-Torre syndrome **(Figures 2A and B)**.

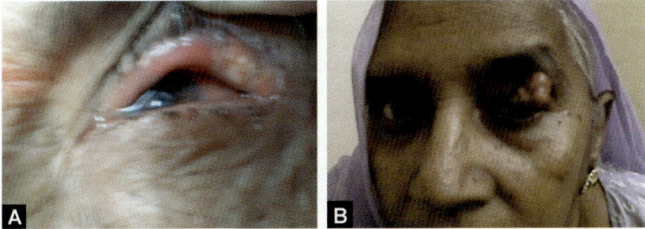

Figures 2A and B

ROLE OF FNAC

The neoplasm is known to masquerade as other benign and less malignant lesions, resulting in delay in diagnosis and relative high morbidity and mortality. Fine needle aspiration cytology (FNAC) of recurrent upper eyelid nodules treated elsewhere as chalazion is advocated by the chief author. Cytological smears suggestive of malignancy are subsequently subjected to histopathology and the role of FNAC in early diagnosis and subsequent appropriate surgical management of eyelid sebaceous gland carcinoma to prevent recurrence and metastasis cannot be underscored.

Sentinal Node Biopsy[20]

sentinel lymph node (SLN) are identified by using technetium Tc 99m sulfur colloid as a tracer. 33% have regional lymph node metastasis. The false-negative rate is higher than that reported for SLN biopsy at most other anatomic sites. Patients with negative findings from SLN biopsy still require careful long-term follow-up because they may develop regional or distant metastasis.

TREATMENT

Treatment According to Type[23]

Group A—Sebaceous gland carcinoma with conjunctival intraepithelial (pagetoid) invasion,

Orbital exenteration may be necessary in 36% in group A.

Group B—Sebaceous gland carcinoma without conjunctival intraepithelial invasion.

Historic data indicate a nearly 30% local recurrence rate with standard surgical excision. Excision by means of Mohs micrographic surgery is more efficacious.

ADJUVANTS

Topical Mitomycin[24]

Topical 0.04% mitomycin-C four times daily is administered for 1 week followed by 1 week off medication. The treatment cycles is repeated until resolution of the conjunctival malignancy is clinically evident.

Neoadjuvant Treatment [26,27]

Neoadjuvant chemotherapy, using a combination of carboplatin and 5-fluorouracil.

Eyelid-sparing orbital exenteration may be performed after 3 cycles of chemotherapy, followed by radiotherapy to the regional lymph nodes.

Radiotherapy[31-33]

> 55 Gy.

a. Tumor too large for resection.
b. Palliative and for secondaries.

But it is important to keep in mind that radiotherapy may induce malignancy in benign tumors.[28,31]

Reconstruction

A. **Cutler-Beard bridge flap**—Full-thickness eyelid defects are conventionally reconstructed by either a Hughes flap or a Cutler-Beard bridge flap.

B. **The Cutler-Beard bridge flap technique with use of donor sclera** for upper eyelid reconstruction

C. **The switch flap** is an alternative method and is not very widely practiced. The technique involves switching a full-thickness flap on a pedicle to fill a defect from lower lid to upper or vice versa. The pedicle is divided in three weeks. The recipient lid is reconstructed by direct closure and the donor lid by direct closure with or without cantholysis or sliding flap, or it is left to heal by second intention.

D. **Double-bridged flap reconstruction of the upper eyelid** that spares the eyelid margin can provide excellent functional and cosmetic results, particularly in cases of nonmarginal eyelid tumor excision

E. **Orbicularis oculi myocutaneous advancement flap for upper eyelid reconstruction**—Two-stage reconstruction of partial or total full-thickness upper eyelid defects. In the first stage, a single tarsoconjunctival flap from the donor lower eyelid reconstitutes the posterior lamella, and a full-thickness skin graft reconstructs the anterior lamella. The tarsoconjunctival flap is incised 1.5 to 2 mm from the lower eyelid margin rather than the 4 to 6 mm necessary to preserve the marginal artery in the Cutler-Beard procedure. In the second stage, 5 to 8 weeks later, the skin tarsoconjunctival flap is severed

F. **Hard palate mucoperiosteal graft** for posterior lamellar reconstruction of the upper eyelid

G. **Moreker's surgery of direct opposite lid split with lid sharing with semicircular flap (Figures 3A and B).**

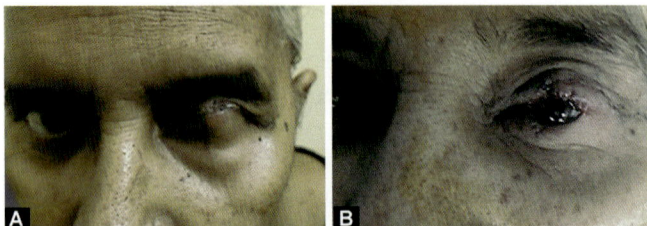

Figures 3A and B

In the Cutler-Beard procedure, the full-thickness lower lid is sutured by advancement into the upper eyelid defect. In our procedure which is different from this the upper lid is excised with wide margin with intraoperative frozen section support and then reconstructed with a semicircular flap opposite to the Tenzel's flap moved at the lateral canthus as seen in the photographs. The remaining gap is filled by a lid split of the lower lid and suturing of lower lid tarsus to the levator and the lower lid anterior lamella being sutured anteriorly to the residual skin orbicularis complex superiorly to keep the eyes closed for a period of 6 weeks. At the end of 6 weeks the lid is split to give excellent lid closure and upper lid function with good cosmetic results.

The evaluation of good reconstruction includes contour of lid, condition of wound, cornea and donor site were examined for infection, dehiscence, corneal ulcer, notching, trichiasis, and recurrence. The preoperative and postoperative photographs are also compared

MORTALITY

Tumor-related deaths occur in only in 6.7%, which is lower than previous reports and may be related to earlier detection or improved surgical excision.

Metastasis

- Risk of tumor-related metastases is similar in both groups
- Lung metastasis is known from meibomian gland carcinoma of eyelid.
- Metastatic adenocarcinoma to the retina has been reported in a patient with Muir-Torre syndrome.
- Radical neck dissection may be needed if neck nodes involved.

FACTORS ASSOCIATED WITH POOR PROGNOSIS[34]

1. Vascular, lymphatic, orbital invasion.
2. Both lid involvement and multi-centric origin.
3. Poor differentiation.
4. Duration of symptoms more than 6 months.
5. Tumor diameter more than 10 mm.
6. Highly infiltrative pattern and pagetoid invasion of epithelium.

Screening for MTS

The immunohistochemical testing for MSH-2, MSH-6, and MLH-1 is useful for rapid identification of an underlying mismatch repair defect and early diagnosis of MTS.[9]

59% of sebaceous neoplasia exhibit a mutation in at least one mismatch repair protein gene. The positive predictive value of each is as follows: MLH-1 88%, MSH-6 67% and MSH-2 55%.

FOLLOW UP GUIDELINES[13]

Evidence indicates that for individuals with or at risk of MTS or HNPCC, colonoscopy every 1-2 years beginning at age 20-25 or 10 years younger than the youngest age at diagnosis in the family can be strongly recommended. Additionally, most experts believe that an annual history and physical examination, including a complete skin examination and urinalysis, as well as periodic endometrial sampling and/or transvaginal ultrasound for women, are worthwhile screening tests for these high-risk patients.

RECENT ADVANCES

Switching from tacrolimus to sirolimus halts the appearance of new sebaceous neoplasms in Muir-Torre syndrome.

REFERENCES

1. Ramirez CC, Berman B. Cutaneous signs and syndromes associated with internal malignancies. Skinmed. 2005;4:84-90; quiz 91-82.

2. Dores GM, Curtis RE, Toro JR, Devesa SS, Fraumeni JF Jr. Incidence of cutaneous sebaceous carcinoma and risk of associated neoplasms :insight into Muir-Torre syndrome. Cancer. 2008 Oct 17.

3. Barana D, van van, Wijnen J, et al. Spectrum of genetic alterations in Muir-Torre syndrome is the same as in HNPCC. Am J Med Genet A. 2004;125:318-9.

4. Ponti G, Losi L, Di Gregorio C, et al. Identification of Muir-Torre syndrome among patients with sebaceous tumors and keratoacanthomas: role of clinical features, microsatellite instability, and immunohistochemistry. Cancer. 2005;103:1018-25.

5. Popnikolov NK, Gatalica Z, Colome-Grimmer MI, et al. Loss of mismatch repair proteins in sebaceous gland tumors. J Cutan Pathol. 2003;30:178-84.

6. Goldberg M, Rummelt C, Foja S, Holbach LM, Ballhausen WG. Different genetic pathways in the development of periocular sebaceous glandcarcinomas in presumptive Muir-Torre syndrome patients.Hum Mutat. 2006 Feb;27(2):155-62.

7. Tsalis K, Blouhos K, Vasiliadis K, Tsachalis T, Angelopoulos S, Betsis D. Sebaceous gland tumors and internal malignancy in the context of Muir-Torre syndrome. A case report and review of the literature. World J Surg Oncol. 2006 Feb 8;4:8.

8. Ponti G, Losi L, Pedroni M, Lucci-Cordisco E, Di Gregorio C, Pellacani G, Seidenari S. Value of MLH1 and MSH2 mutations in the appearance

of Muir-Torre syndrome phenotype in HNPCC patients presenting sebaceous gland tumors or keratoacanthomas. J Invest Dermatol. 2006 Oct;126(10):2302-7. Epub 2006 Jul 6.

9. Bertholom JL, Guyomard JL, Stock N, Dugast C, Martinel C, Chatel MA, Charlin JF. Sebaceous tumors of the eyelids in a patient with Muir-Torre syndrome J Fr Ophtalmol. 2006 Jun;29(6):654-8.

10. Marazza G, Masouyé I, Taylor S, Prins C, Gaudin T, Saurat JH, French LE. An illustrative case of Muir-Torre syndrome: contribution of immunohistochemical analysis in identifying indicator sebaceous lesions. Arch Dermatol. 2006 Aug;142(8):1039-42.

11. Jones B, Oh C, Mangold E, Egan CA Muir-Torre syndrome: Diagnostic and screening guidelines. Australas J Dermatol. 2006 Nov;47(4):266-9.

12. Levi Z, Hazazi R, Kedar-Barnes I, Hodak E, Gal E, Mor E, Niv Y, Winkler J. Switching from tacrolimus to sirolimus halts the appearance of new sebaceous neoplasms in Muir-Torre syndrome. Am J Transplant. 2007 Feb;7(2):476-9. Epub 2007 Jan 4.

13. Al-Shobaili HA, AlGhamdi KM, Al-Ghamdi WA. Cystic sebaceous carcinoma: is it a constant pathognomic marker for Muir-Torre syndrome? J Drugs Dermatol. 2007 May;6(5):540-3.

14. Lachiewicz AM, Wilkinson TM, Groben P, Ollila DW, Thomas NE. Muir-Torre syndrome. Am J Clin Dermatol. 2007;8(5):315-9.

15. Yanaba K, Nakagawa H, Takeda Y, Koyama N, Sugano K. Muir-Torre syndrome caused by partial duplication of MSH2 gene by Alu-mediated nonhomologous recombination. Br J Dermatol. 2008 Jan;158(1):150-6. Epub 2007 Oct 17.

16. Chhibber V, Dresser K, Mahalingam M. MSH-6: extending the reliability of immunohistochemistry as a screening tool in Muir-Torre syndrome. Mod Pathol. 2008 Feb;21(2):159-64. Epub 2007 Dec 7.

17. Satarkar S, Munshi M, Kotwal M, Bobhate S. Muir Torre syndrome: a case report. Indian J Pathol Microbiol. 2007 Oct;50(4):804-5.

18. Ponti G, Ponz de Leon M. Muir-Torre syndrome. Lancet Oncol. 2005 Dec;6(12):980-7.

19. Song A, Carter KD, Syed NA, Song J, Nerad JA. Sebaceous cell carcinoma of the ocular adnexa: clinical presentations, histopathology, and outcomes. Ophthal Plast Reconstr Surg. 2008 May-Jun;24(3):194-200.

20. Ho VH, Ross MI, Prieto VG, Khaleeq A, Kim S, Esmaeli B. Sentinel lymph node biopsy for sebaceous cell carcinoma and melanoma of the ocular adnexa Arch Otolaryngol Head Neck Surg. 2007 Aug;133(8):820-6.

21. Spencer JM, Nossa R, Tse DT, Sequeira M. Sebaceous carcinoma of the eyelid treated with Mohs micrographic surgery. J Am Acad Dermatol. 2001 Jun;44(6):1004-9.

22. Muqit MM, Roberts F, Lee WR, Kemp E. Improved survival rates in sebaceous carcinoma of the eyelid. Eye. 2004 Jan;18(1):49-53.

23. Chao AN, Shields CL, Krema H, Shields JA. Outcome of patients with periocular sebaceous gland carcinoma with and without conjunctival intraepithelial invasion. Ophthalmology. 2001 Oct;108(10):1877-83.

24. Shields CL, Naseripour M, Shields JA, Eagle RC Jr. Topical mitomycin-C for pagetoid invasion of the conjunctiva by eyelid sebaceous gland carcinoma. Ophthalmology. 2002 Nov;109(11):2129-33.

25. Tumuluri K, Kourt G, Martin P. Mitomycin C in sebaceous gland carcinoma with pagetoid spread. Br J Ophthalmol 2004 May;88(5):718-9.

26. Murthy R, Honavar SG, Burman S, Vemuganti GK, Naik MN, Reddy VA. Neoadjuvant chemotherapy in the management of sebaceous gland carcinoma of the eyelid with regional lymph node metastasis. Ophthal Plast Reconstr Surg 2005 Jul;21(4):307-9.

27. Paschal BR, Bagley CS. Sebaceous gland carcinoma of the eyelid: complete response to sequential combination chemotherapy N C Med J. 1985 Sep;46(9):473-4.

28. Stafanous SN. The switch flap in eyelid reconstruction .Orbit. 2007 Dec;26(4):255-62.

29. Henriquez A.S. Arruga A. Sebaceous Carcinoma Presenting as Dry eye Syndrome. Klinische Monatsblatter Fur Augenheilkunde 1979;175 (3):318-21.

30. Heyderman E. et al. Epithelial Markers in Primary Skin Cancer Histopathology 1984;8(3):423-34.

31. Harvey JT. Anderson RL. The Management of Meibomian Gland Carcinoma Ophthalmic surgery 1982;13(1):56-61.

32. 26. Deregibus P. Battezzati G.Su due casi di carcinoma sebaceo Minerva Medica 1982;73(5):213-7.

33. 21. Yen MT, et al. Radiation Therapy for Local Control of Eyelid Sebaceous Cell Carcinoma Ophthal Plast Reconstr Surg 2000 May, 16(3):211-5.

34. Rao NA, Hidayat AA, McLean IW, Zimmerman LE. Sebaceous Carcinoma Of Ocular Adnexa Human Pathology 1982;13(2):113-22.

Pediatric Oculoplasty—An Evidence-based Update

33

**Sunil Moreker, Milind Kirtane,
Milind Navlakhe, Mayur Moreker (India)**

INTRODUCTION

Medical science changes with time as more and more people submit their audits and personal experience to journals. These reports and studies make the understanding of diseases more clear. At times the natural history of diseases becomes clearer and at other times we realize that maybe we as humans respond differently with time. Sometimes historical mistakes are corrected but at times we might be committing newer mistakes. This chapter is an effort at looking at present updated literature on pediatric oculoplastic procedures in a critical manner with a view to applying the recent evidence to everyday clinical practice. The commonest pediatric oculolastic procedures are addressed here. Considering the unique problems presented by childhood oculoplastic conditions it seems appropriate to have pediatric oculoplasty as a separate speciality.

CONGENITAL DACRYOCYSTITIS UPDATE

The often quoted incidence of 6% was derived from a study of 200 consecutive live births in the 1940s. Actual incidences may vary from 1.2 to 30%, the disorder being commoner in children with craniofacial disorders and Down's syndrome.

Syndromes

Lacrimo-auriculo-dento-digital Syndrome (LADD)[1]

An autosomal dominant pattern of inheritance caused by FGF10 mutations with variable expressivity including cup-shaped ears, deafness, unilateral choanal atresia, bilateral nasolacrimal duct obstruction, xerostomia, alacrima due to congenital absence of lacrimal glands, agenesis of salivary glands, chronic dacryocystitis, keratoconjunctivitis sicca, ptosis, nail dysplasia of the thumb, shortness of fifth toe, temporal bone abnormality and epilepsy. Renal and urogenital anomalies may be seen variably. In the author's experience these findings do not always occur in these clusters but if one of these is seen in association with congenital dacryocystitis then the others should be looked for as they do require a multispecialty approach to management.

Microbiological Spectrum and Sensitivities

A recent study [2] conducted at Madurai, India concluded that gram-positive bacteria are the most frequent isolates with *Streptococcus pneumoniae* being the commonest. Among gram-negative bacteria the most frequent isolate was *Hemophilus influenzae*. *Candida tropicalis* has emerged as a new organism. Gram-positive bacteria are sensitive to chloramphenicol, vancomycin, and ofloxacin and gram-negative bacteria to ofloxacin and ciprofloxacin.

Treatment

Probing

Timing: In their series of 192 children with nasolacrimal duct obstruction out of 3950 children lipiec et al [3] reported that in majority of children(77%), the nasolacrimal duct obstruction did not resolve spontaneously and early probing within first few months of child's life increased the success rate of the procedure. Becker et al [4] on the basis of their 19 years experience have proposed that patients with congenital dacryocystocele should have probing on an urgent basis and as early in life as possible, unless the lacrimal sac decompresses into the nose at the time of the initial examination. According to them this approach reduces the incidence of dacryocystitis and cellulitis, and improves the success rate of surgery as they noticed that the initial probing was successful in 100% of lacrimal systems that did not have infection, but was successful in only 53% that had dacryocystitis with or without cellulitis. The mean age of probing in the surgical patients who did not develop infection in the becker et al series was 5.9 days, whereas the mean age at first probing in surgical patients who developed infection was 17.3 days. The cure rate has been reported as 89% in patients 13-24 months of age and 72% after the age of 24 months by kashkouli et al [5] in their prospective study of 169 eyes. The more important finding was a success rate of 90.2% in the membranous and 33.3% in the complex CNLDO in both late and very late probing with a high correlation between the cure rate at 1 week and final follow up suggesting that the outcome of the nasolacrimal duct probing at 1 week follow up is highly indicative of the final outcome.

Endonasal Probing and Retrograde Irrigation of Lacrimal Ducts

When endonasal probing and retrograde irrigation of lacrimal ducts is performed taking into consideration the individual peculiarities of the obstruction and the anatomical accessibility of the opening of ductus nasolacrimalis in the inferior nasal passageway, it has been reported that persistent membranes in the inferior lacrimal punctum necessitates repetition of the initial dilatation. Endonasal probing and irrigation of lacrimal ducts used in the treatment of congenital stenoses has been reported to have a high effectivity (99%) by some authors.[6] In children in whom this procedure fails endonasal dacryocysto-rhinostomy with balloon intubations may be tried

Balloon Dilatation of Nasolacrimal Duct

Balloon nasolacrimal ductoplasty is performed using the LacriCATH system (Quest Medical, Inc. An Atrion Company, Allen, TX). Becker et al[7] in their prospective series of 61 lacrimal systems reported a 95% success rate with this procedure as early as 1996. More recently Tao et al[8] reported that as a secondary procedure it was successful in 94% of those older than 24 months whereas the success rate was as low as 59.1% in those younger than 24 months. Results range from 82% (Tien at al[9]) to 95%. Yuksel et al[10] proposed on the basis of their experience with endoscopic guided balloon dacryocystoplasty in children over 36 months of age that it can be an alternative treatment in older children and can be preferred to silicone intubation and dacryocystorhinostomy performed after unsuccessful probing.

Monocanalicular Stenting

Goldstein et al[11] compared monocanalicular stenting and balloon dacryoplasty in secondary treatment of congenital nasolacrimal duct obstruction after failed primary and reported that (91%) nasolacrimal ducts responded to monocanalicular stenting, whereas 86% responded to balloon treatment. When the patient group was further stratified by age, the monocanalicular stenting was 94% successful in children younger than age 2 years and 89% successful for children older than 2 years. The balloon treatment had a success rate of 91% in the younger group and 79% in the older group.

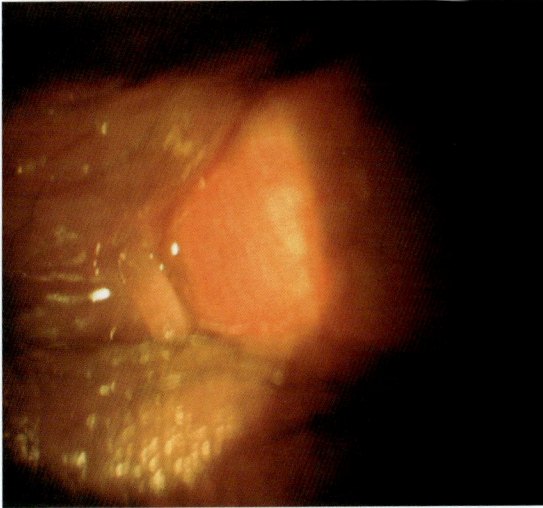

Figure 1: Stent in place

Stepwise Approach

Cassady et al[12] have proposed a treatment paradigm prescribing probing as an initial procedure regardless of age. Those who fail probing should receive balloon catheter dilation. Those who fail probing and balloon catheterization should receive silicone intubation. Dacryocystorhinostomy is reserved for patients failing the above treatments.

CONGENITAL PTOSIS

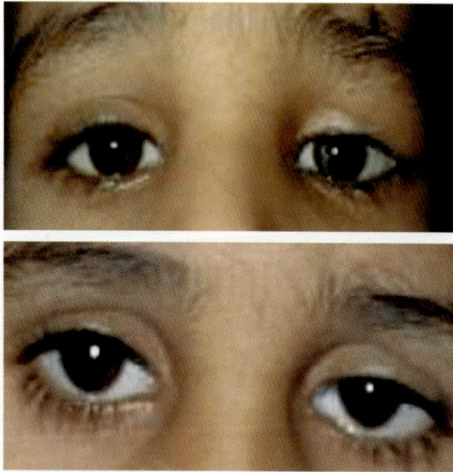

Figure 2: Pre- and post-sling

Blepharoptosis indicates the abnormal drooping of the upper lid, caused by partial or total reduction in levator muscle function. It may be caused by various pathologies, both congenital and acquired .Childhood Ptosis may be congenital or acquired. An insult, acting during the second month of gestation, may affect the development of the eye, heart, and abdomen and may lead to congenital malformations. Although congenital ptosis presenting with ocular and systemic congenital malformations is a rare condition, ophthalmologists should consider the possibility of coexisting structural defects. Congenital ptosis is more challenging than adult ptosis due to these and other co-morbidities like amblyopia and the difficulty of examination as well as the age at which surgery should be performed. Unilateral severe congenital ptosis and jaw-winking ptosis pose a challenge in the decision of the surgical procedure and whether surgery should be performed unilaterally or bilaterally. In congenital forms, these techniques were often associated with techniques to correct oculomuscular imbalance (i.e. strabismus). Surgical treatment of palpebral ptosis is complex and requires precise diagnosis and indications for surgery related to clinical examination and pathogenesis. Even if these indications are strictly followed, in some cases, the outcomes are unpredictable. In view of various newer reports the author suggests the following classifacation **(Table 1)**.

Table 1: Moreker's classification of childhood ptosis

A. Congenital
1. Simple dysmyogenic ptosis
2. Dysmyogenic ptosis with vertical strabismus
   a. Isolated superior rectus involvement
   b. Double elevator palsy (see **Figure 3**)
3. Dysmyogenic ptosis with epiblepharon
4. Childhood myasthenia
   a. Transient neonatal
   b. Congenital
   c. Juvenile
5. Syndromic ptosis
   a. WARG
   b. Partial trisomy
   c. Congenital fibrosis syndromes with ptosis
   d. With ocular and systemic congenital malformations including mild microphthalmia, microcornea, cataract, iris and chorioretinal coloboma, ectopic kidney, and ventricular septal defect
6. Ptosis with synkinesis
   a. Oculomotor abducens synkinesis—requires overcorrection
   b. Marcus Gunn jaw winking phenomenon
7. Ptosis with muscular dystrophies

B. Acquired
1. Muscle infections, e.g. Myocysticercosis
2. Traumatic—aponeurotic disinsertion or dehiscence
3. Mechanical—neurofibromatosis, lid infections

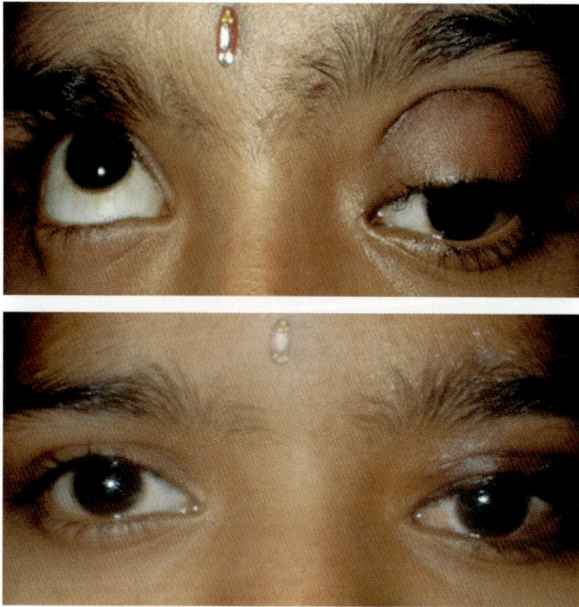

Figure 3: Ptosis with double elevator palsy—pre- and postoperatively

Diagnosis Differentiating Congenital from Aponeurotic Ptosis

Upgaze Eyelid Position[13]

Upgaze eyelid position allows differentiation between congenital and aponeurotic blepharoptosis according to the neurophysiology of eyelid retraction.Upgaze with stretching of the mechanoreceptor of Mueller muscle increases involuntary reflex contraction of the levator slow-twitch muscle fibers. Worsening of ptosis on upgaze is common in congenital ptosis and is an abnormal differentiating sign, lacking the involuntary reflex contraction. Improvement of ptosis on upgaze is common in aponeurotic blepharoptosis and likely represents a normal physiological process, restoring the involuntary reflex contraction

Ultrasound Biomicroscopy

The thickness of the levator aponeurosis can be measured with ultrasound biomicroscopy. The most common pathology in aponeurotic blepharoptosis is thinned-out aponeurosis. The levator aponeurosis of the ptotic eyelid is thinner than the normal eyelid in congenital ptosis. The thickness of the levator aponeurosis correlates with the levator function in congenital dysmyogenic blepharoptosis.[14]

Unconventional Ptosis

Childhood Myasthenia

Serum acetylcholine receptor antibody may be negative frequently, girls with onset after 11 years being more likely to be antibody positive.

Types: Three distinct groups of patients are generally reported:[15]
a. **Transient neonatal myasthenia gravis**: 6.8% of childhood myasthenia. Usually do not have ocular involvement.
b. **Congenital myasthenia** 17.2% of cases. These patients have an onset of symptoms from 1 to 12 months of age. The most frequent symptom in this group is bilateral blepharoptosis. Myasthenic crisis do not occur. Spontaneous remissions are rare
c. **Juvenile myasthenia** 76% of the patients. The onset of symptoms in this group ranges from 13 months to 14 years presenting purely with ocular symptoms. Myasthenic crisis may occur and spontaneous remissions are observed. Good

response to anticholinesterase drugs is slightly more frequent in juvenile myasthenia.

Since patients with autoimmune myasthenia and a young age of onset are often seronegative, clinical features such as changing distribution of weakness, fluctuating severity, or response to treatment might be considered as supportive criteria for differentiating Juvenile from congenital forms.

Mutations:[16] Mutations of the acetylcholine receptor (AChR) delta subunit gene (CHRND) may lead to sporadic congenital myasthenic syndrome (CMS). Mutations in various genes encoding proteins expressed at the neuromuscular junction may cause CMS. Mutations of AChR subunit genes lead to end-plate AChR deficiency or to altered kinetic properties of the receptor. Mutations in the alpha, beta and delta subunits of the AChR are less frequent than mutations of the epsilon subunit; mutations in these subunits leading to AChR deficiency are often associated with a severe phenotype. The cytoplasmic loop of the AChR subunits is known to be essential for AChR-rapsyn co-clustering. Impairment of AChR-rapsyn co-clustering—a well-known molecular mechanism for rapsyn mutations—could also result from mutations in the delta subunit. Introduction of the same mutation in the epsilon subunit has no effect on AChR clustering indicating a special role of the delta subunit in AChR-rapsyn interactions.

Treatment: Prednisone dose is slowly increased to 50-60 mg (0.4 to 1mg/kg) and then gradually reduced to 10 mg, followed by further reduction as tolerated.

The pyridostigmine dose is begun at 180 mg daily and increased as tolerated.

WARG Syndrome and Ptosis

Lennon et al [17] recently reiterated that ptosis may be associated with WARG syndrome which consists of Wilms' tumor, aniridia, genitourinary abnormalities, and mental retardation. The aniridia and predisposition for Wilms' tumor seen in WAGR are caused by haploinsufficiency for PAX 6 and WT1, respectively.

Partial Trisomy and Ptosis

Doco-Fenzy et al[18] reported a pure de novo direct duplication dup(12)(q24.1 → q24.2). She had developmental and growth retardation, facial dysmorphism with upslanting palpebral fissures, wide downturned mouth, short neck, and Marcus Gunn phenomenon, single transverse creases, hypoplasia of the corpus callosum, and cardiac malformations consisting of a bicuspid aortic valve, multiple ventricular septal defects, and kinking of the aorta.

Management

In a recent literature review clauser et al [19] concluded that the most widely used surgical techniques were levator muscle recession and frontalis suspension. It is used in the repair of ptosis with poor levator function. The materials used include tissue such as autologous or banked fascia lata or permanent suture material. The procedure involves connecting the frontalis muscle and the upper eyelid. Some authors [20] have recently reintroduced the technique of a dynamic frontalis muscle flap tunneled into the eyelid that directly attaches to the tarsal plate but its role in clinical practice remains to be defined. Some authors[21] have reported that habituation of the pterygoid-levator synkinesis and control of the ptosis with jaw positioning can occur as early as two and a half months and that surgery can be delayed until a safer time in Marcus Gunn jaw winking syndrome with severe ptosis if there are no objective signs of amblyopia but the author has in his experience seen several cases with refractive changes (reduction of astigmatism) occurring with correction of ptosis which are highlighted further in the chapter.

Recent Concepts from Evidences in Terms of Management

Refractive changes: Kumar et al [22] studied twenty-three patients between 4 and 12 years old with severe congenital blepharoptosis and poor levator function who underwent frontalis brow suspension surgery and compared them with the non-ptotic eyes and observed changes in the postoperative best corrected visual acuity, binocularity, relevant refractive parameters, lid position, lagophthalmos, lid lag, and tear break-up time for 12 weeks and found significant differences in the baseline characteristics and the postoperative changes in the eyes with and without ptosis and concluded that retinoscopy, manual keratometry, and corneal videokerato-scopy are simple and effective methods to evaluate the sequential refractive changes occurring in these eyes.

Kao SC et al published (Zhonghua Yi Xue Za Zhi 1998 Dec;61(12):689-93) their findings of astigmatic change following congenital ptosis surgery. Their incidence of high astigmatism (> 2.5 diopters, D) in congenital ptosis was 25.3% and following surgery 27.5% showed a decrease of more than 0.5 D. An average decrease of 0.18 D in astigmatism was observed.

Synkinetic ptosis-oculomotor abducens: These are extremely rare and usually require and overcorrection—a fact that has been recently highlighted by burroughs et al.[23] One usually needs to do excess levator correction or a two staged procedure for this extremely rare condition.

Role of steroids in childhood myasthenia: Kupersmith et al [24] studied recently the effect of treatment of myasthenia and found that children receiving prednisone showed resolution in primary gaze diplopia, downgaze diplopia, unilateral ptosis, and bilateral ptosis in 73.5%, 75.5%, 85.7%, and 98%, respectively at 1 month. The benefit persists at 3-6, 12, and 24 months except for the bilateral ptosis. The pyridostigmine group shows resolution in primary gaze diplopia, downgaze diplopia, unilateral ptosis, and bilateral ptosis in 6.9%, 17.2%, 50%, and 76.7% of patients after 1 month of treatment. Among the prednisone responsive patients, there are recurrences suggesting that 50-60 mg daily prednisone followed by lower doses (10 mg or less) has the benefit of resolving ptosis and diplopia that lasts for at least 2 years in approximately 70% of patients.

Comparison of silastic and banked fascia lata in pediatric frontalis suspension: Hersh et al [25] studied 131 frontalis suspension operations using either Silastic or banked fascia lata during the past 12 years at Children's Hospital at Westmead, Sydney, Australia and found that functional success rates for primary frontalis suspension procedures were not significantly different for banked fascia lata and silastic (60% versus 67.2%, respectively). Infection and granuloma rates also were not significantly different (7.1% for banked fascia lata versus 15.2% for silastic). They however found a statistically significant difference between the two materials in ptosis recurrence (35.3% for banked fascia lata versus 13% for silastic) and concluded that silastic was significantly better than banked fascia lata in terms of ptosis recurrence. But more prospective data would be required as this study was a retrospective analysis.

Frontalis lobe suspension: A Croatian group [26] recently reported in a retrospective study their long-term results in 146 patients operated by frontal muscle lobe shaping with or without shaping of corrugator muscle lobe attached to the tarsal plate in children with congenital dystrophic ptosis.

Their criteria of postoperative success (defined as a situation with eyes open in which upper eyelid covers the cornea at 12 o'clock position by 1-2 mm; there is a good contour of the eyelid margin; there is no lagophthalmos; and there is symmetry with the other eye) was met by 91% patients at 6 months, 85% at one year, and 83% at 5 years after resurgery for undercorrection being done in 18% of patients.

Advancement of Whitnall's ligament –conjunctival approach: Bajaj et al [27] recently did a prospective study of ptosis correction by advancement of Whitnall's ligament by plication of the levator aponeurosis via the conjunctival route and found that good correction, i.e. within 1 mm of the normal fellow eye in primary gaze, can be obtained in 80% of patients and that patients with more than or equal to 8 mm levator function give better results. It has the advantages of shorter surgical time, minimal dissection of tissue planes and reversibility, with the conjunctival approach being cosmetically more acceptable as there is no visible scar on the lid.

Autogenous palmaris longus frontalis sling in children with congenital ptosis: Wong et al [28] investigated the long-term outcome of using autogenous palmaris longus tendon sling for correcting congenital ptosis in children with age ranging from 2 to 7 years with a mean follow-up of 92 months (range,

80-104 months), and noted found that all eyelids were successfully corrected with good lid height. No recurrence or other postoperative complications were encountered except one patient who developed a small skin fold over the harvest site. It could be a good alternative to autogenous fascia lata, and further studies, to compare these two sling materials seem warranted.

Complication of surgery—inverse Bell's phenomenon: Betharia et al [29] reported three patients who underwent levator resection and showed an inversion of the Bell's phenomenon in the postoperative period, with the eye going down instead of up, during eyelid closure. This highlights the need for evaluating the bells phenomenon not only preoperatively but also postoperatively.

ORBITAL IMPLANTATION IN CHILDREN

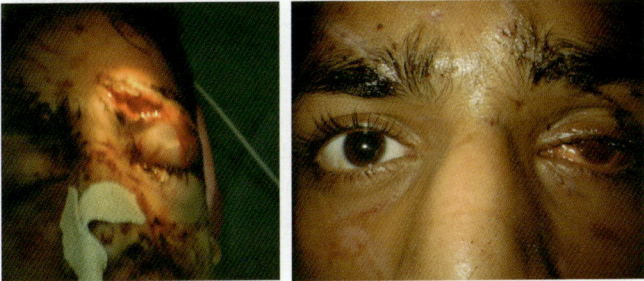

Figure 4: Traumatic globe rupture and orbital implant with cornea preserving evisceration

Orbital implants are used regularly in pediatric patients at the time of enucleation. The commonest indications for enucleation are retinoblastoma, blind eye following trauma and end stage retinopathy of prematurity. Controversy regarding the rate of complications with newer implants in the pediatric population continues to confuse clinicians.

Size of Implant[30]

The average percent volume replaced by the implants in adult patients is 68%. The average percent volume replaced by the implants in pediatric patients is 21%. Up to seventy-one percent of pediatric patients undergo secondary implant surgery to augment volume and eliminate superior sulcus deformity and enophthalmos. The placement of an adequately sized implant in pediatric patients may obviate the need for secondary augmentation of socket volume in adulthood. Some authors suggest an implant 2 mm less in diameter than the axial length of the eye in pediatric patients.

Primary Orbital Implants in Children–Hydroxyapatite

Christmas et al[31] studied 120 child eyes implanted and found that implant exposure rate was 0.8%, implant extrusion was not seen and implant migration rate was 2.4%. Of all patients 96% had good cosmesis and 98% had good motility and concluded that orbital implantation after enucleation is successful in the pediatric population and complications are minimal. Hydroxyapatite implants are not associated with unacceptable complications in the pediatric population.

Porous Polyethylene Implant in a Child

Iordanidou et al[32] studied prospectively the incidence of complications of primary insertion of porous polyethylene orbital implant in the pediatric population who underwent primary placement of an anteriorly wrapped spherical porous polyethylene orbital implant with at least 17 months of follow-up weeks and found that there were no cases of implant extrusion, superior sulcus syndrome, orbital cellulitis, or significant inflammatory response.

The spherical implant size used may be 16 mm, 18 mm or 20 mm. The prosthesis is generally fitted after an interval of 5 weeks and usually the porous polyethylene orbital implant is now not drilled for peg placement. Anteriorly wrapped primary porous polyethylene orbital implant in the pediatric population appears to be well tolerated with few complications even in the author's experience. Kim et al[33] have noted a 33% exposure rate in eyes that had conventional enucleation and porous poly ethylene implantation, and none if a free orbital fat graft in addition suggesting that a free orbital fat graft is a simple, effective way to prevent orbital implant exposure in patients requiring enucleation and implantation.

Autogenous Dermis-fat Graft Orbital Implant

Mitchell et al[34] studied autogenous dermis-fat graft orbital implants and found that all implants maintained appropriate volume allowing proper prosthetic fit and facial symmetry. Soome children experience excessive growth of their implants but that can be managed by surgical debulking. Some children develop a central graft ulcer, which can be managed by superficial revision and reclosure. It is indeed a promising implant for the pediatric anophthalmic socket.

Moreker's Expandable Balloon Implants

These can be used in severe anophthalmic sockets which are contracted, so as to expand them.

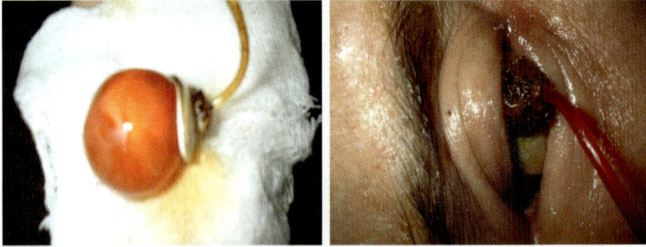

Figure 5: Moreker's expandable balloon implants

ORBITAL FRACTURES IN CHILDREN

Inferior wall involvement is the most commonly seen, and the trapdoor type fracture is the most common with soft tissue entrapment associated with nausea/vomiting. The trapdoor fracture is described as a pure orbital-floor fracture, linear in form and hinged medially, which allows herniation of orbital contents through the fracture and then entraps these herniated contents. Management of blowout fractures involving the orbital floor has been controversial over the past several decades. One school of thought recommends conservative treatment for 4 to 6 months while another recommends a 'wait and watch' period of 2 weeks before intervention.

Baek et al[35] suggested that early diagnosis, and prompt surgical intervention are required for patients with oculocardiac reflex. Grant et al [36] too in their series reported that in the cases with trapdoor fracture and restricted ocular movement, early intervention was associated with better postoperative function and thus recommended that the symptomatic trapdoor orbit fracture be considered an urgent indication for surgical intervention. Cohen et al [37] reported in their series that the positive predictive value of nausea/vomiting with a trapdoor fracture for entrapment was 83.3%.

and that patients with trapdoor fractures who present with nausea/vomiting are at a high risk of inferior rectus entrapment and poor outcome. Egbert et al [38] reported that preoperative nausea and vomiting are immediately relieved after surgery. The median time for improvement of preoperative duction deficits and diplopia is 4 days for patients receiving surgery within 7 days and 10 days for those undergoing surgery after 14 days. Resolution of duction deficits or diplopia is not dependent on time of surgery if performed within 1 month of injury. For patients with severe limitation of ductions, early surgical repair within 7 days of injury results in more rapid improvement of ductions and diplopia than surgery performed later. Jordan et al [39] called it the "white eyed fracture" and reported that a 2-week waiting period has been found to be of little benefit in these persons and possibly harmful to their motility. They advocated surgery within the first few days after injury as it may help to avoid permanent motility restriction.

We (authors) perform orbital wall reconstruction with Prolene/Medpor barrier sheet implantation (thickness 1mm) through transconjunctival approach under endoscopic guidance and at times whenever possible we do a **complete endoscopic correction**

Endoscopic Fracture Reduction and Mesh Implantation with Tissue Glue

A completely endoscopic approach transnasally with reduction of the trapdoor fracture fragments with endoscopically guided mesh kept in place by fironectin glue is done by the authors (Dr Milind Kirtane and Dr Sunil Moreker) at their institute (P.D Hinduja National Hospital and MRC,Bombay) and videos of the same were presented at the Eye Advance 2006 and the Annual conference of Asia Pacific Academy of Ophthalmology at Singapore 2006.

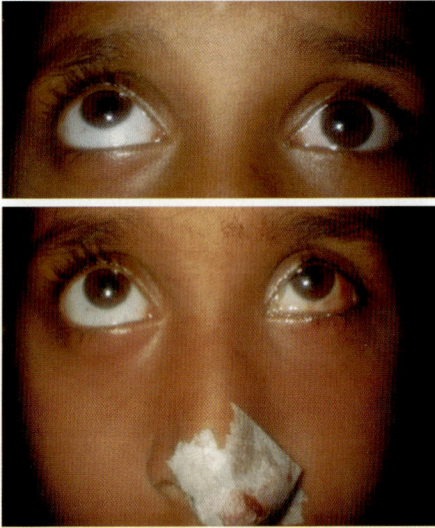

Figure 6: Pre- and post-endoscopic fracture correction

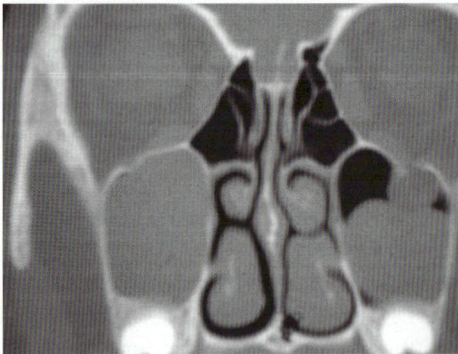

Figure 7: Trap door fracture of orbital floor (above)
(*Courtesy:* Dr Milind Kirtane)

LID AND ORBITAL TUMORS

Most pediatric orbital tumors are benign; developmental cysts comprise half of orbital cases, with capillary hemangioma being the second most common orbital tumor. The most common orbital malignancy is rhabdomyo-sarcoma. The most common intraocular malignant lesion is retinoblastoma. Choroidal melanoma, which is common in adults, is extremely rare in children. The orbit is the most common location for metastases in children, whereas the choroid is the predominant site in adults. Metastases to the orbit in childhood may be due to solid tumors such as a neuroblastoma or Ewing's tumor. Orbital cysts are quite common and varied.

Shields Classification of Orbital Cysts[40]

The major categories in the classification include

a. Cysts of surface epithelium,
   i. Simple epithelial cyst (epidermal, conjunctival, respiratory, and apocrine gland), and
   ii. Dermoid cyst (epidermal and conjunctival).
b. Teratomatous cysts,
c. Neural cysts—include those associated with ocular maldevelopment (congenital cystic eye and colobomatous cyst) and those associated with brain and meningeal tissue (cephalocele and optic nerve meningocele).
d. Secondary cysts—most common mucocele that can occur in children with cystic fibrosis.
e. Inflammatory cysts, generally due to parasitic infestations and are more common in tropical areas of the world.
f. Noncystic lesions with cystic component—include adenoid cystic carcinoma, rhabdomyosarcoma, lymph-angioma, and others.

Epidermal dermoid cyst (dermoid) is by far the most common orbital cystic lesion in children, accounting for over 40% of all orbital lesions of childhood and for 89% of all orbital cystic lesions of childhood that come to biopsy or surgical removal. Dermoid cysts are unusual neoplasms that often present in childhood, with the orbit being the area most commonly affected in the head and neck region. Imaging studies help rule out an intracranial or intraorbital extension. With complete excision, recurrence is unusual.[41]

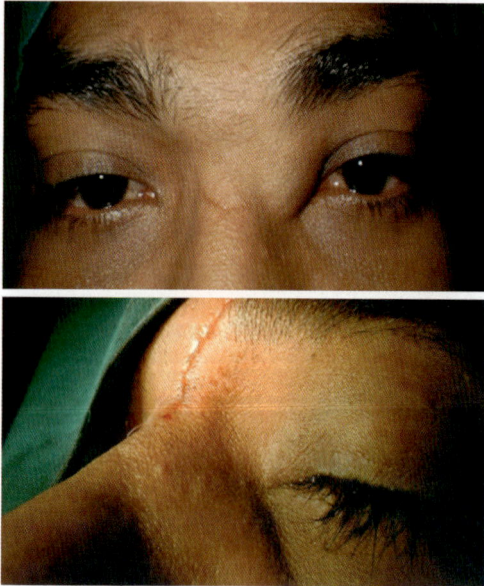

Figure 8: Dermoid—pre- and immediate postoperatively

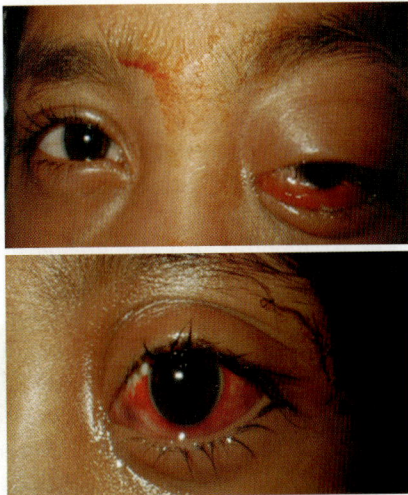

Figrue 9: Lateral orbitotomy for hemangioma (intraconal)

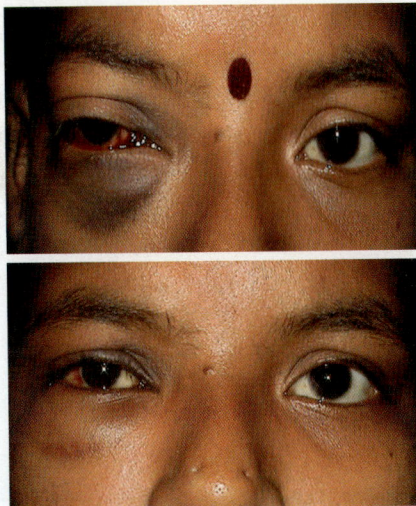

Figure 10: Complete endoscopic management of orbital tumor—hemangioma (*Courtesy:* Dr Milind Navlakhe)

Capillary hemangiomas are the most common orbital tumors of childhood and can cause amblyopia secondary to occlusion of the pupil, anisometropia, or strabismus. Hemangiomas were classified based on size. Presence of aniosometropic astigmatism, ptosis, pupillary occlusion, lid margin change, proptosis, globe displacement, and strabismus need to be recorded.

Schwartz et al[42] reported that size greater than 1 cm in largest diameter is an important predictor of amblyogenic factors and approximately half of these patients require treatment. Diffuse hemangiomas and hemangiomas in patients with PHACES syndrome cause amblyopia in the majority of cases. Periorbital hemangiomas can cause amblyopia secondary to anisometropia, induced astigmatism, strabismus or occlusion of the visual axis. Oral and intralesional steroids are considered to be the most accepted form of primary treatment. Surgery is a safe, effective treatment for selected lesions, provides a definitive early treatment, and prevents astigmatism and occlusion-related amblyopia and so some authors[43] favor early surgery.

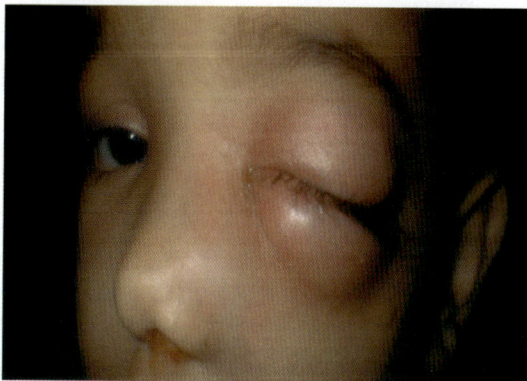

Figure 11: Orbital cellulitis (*Courtesy:* Dr Milind Kirtane)

Preseptal cellulitis is the most common orbital disease in children older than 3 years.[44] Awareness of orbital diseases in childhood, as a rare entity, is crucial for timely diagnosis and appropriate treatment, to save the vision and lives of affected children.

Endoscopic Management of Orbital Diseases

Both hemangiomas and orbital cellulites are amenable to treatment by endoscopy and have excellent results in the authors experience.

Nd: YAG Laser and Corticosteroids

Some authors[45] have tried local Neodymium: YAG-laser therapy and in patients with large subcutaneous eyelid hemangiomas and involvement of the orbita tried with interstitial Neodymium: YAG-laser therapy in combination with systemic corticosteroids with good results.

Orbital Lymphangioma and AV Malformations

Orbital lymphangioma and AV malformations are uncommon, benign cystic appearing lesions, generally manifest in childhood. They usually present with a slowly progressive proptosis, displacement of the globe, ptosis and restriction of eye movements. Occasionally, focal lesions may remain asymptomatic. Spontaneous intraorbital hemorrhage may cause acute proptosis, compressive optic neuropathy and

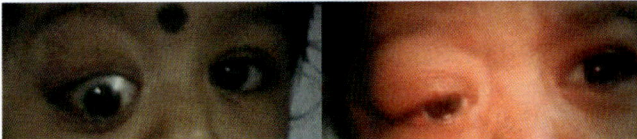

Figure 12: Pre- and post-decompression

loss of vision. Surgical decompression of the optic nerve may be performed if there is progressive decrease in visual acuity.[46]

CONGENITAL EYELID RETRACTION AND CHILDHOOD THYROID

Congenital eyelid retractions may affect either the lower or the upper eyelid. They make up a rare condition and most cases are associated with craniofacial syndromes such as Crouzon or Apert syndromes or childhood thyroid. Burroughs et al [47] have proposed that thyroid eye disease may be present in children and even neonates with both mother and child being euthyroid. Upper eyelid retractions may spontaneously improve in some cases, but lower eyelid retractions do not. Treatment requires surgery, depending on the corneal consequences.

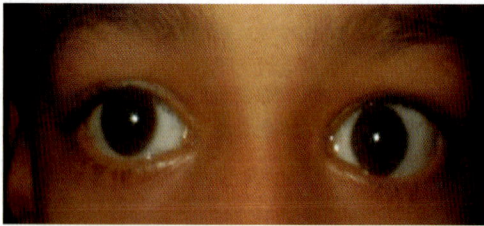

Figure 13: Congenital eyelid retraction

EYELID MALPOSITIONS

Ruban's Classification (Ruban JM, Baggio E). Surgical treatment of congenital eyelid malpositions in children .J Fr Ophtalmol. 2004 Mar;27(3):304-26.)

It is important to separate eyelid malpositions, which are topographical disorders, from eyelid malformations, which are constitutional morphological disorders.

Eyelid malpositions can be as follows:

A. **Static–including**

i. Epiblepharon—Epiblepharon is characterized by the absence of adhesion between the lower eyelid retractors and the orbicularis-skin layer, which allows the anterior lamella to roll over

ii. Congenital ectropion and entropion,

iii. Epicanthus—Epicanthus involves a semi-lunar fold of skin extending from the upper eyelid across the medial canthal area to the margin of the lower eyelid. Four types

a. Supra-ciliaris,

b. Palpebralis,

c. Tarsalis and

d. Inversus of epicanthus are described. Treatment requires surgery.

iv. Telecanthus—defined as an increased distance between canthi.

a. Primary telecanthus results from attenuation of the medial canthal tendons and is usually associated with other soft tIssue abnormalities such as epicanthus or blepharophimosis, or is seen after trauma.

b. Secondary telecanthus is caused by underlying bony malpositions with an abnormal separation between the orbits because of an increased thickness of the interorbital bones such as that seen in hypertelorism or in other complex craniofacial syndromes

v. Centurion syndrome.

B. **Dynamic disorders:** Ptosis and congenital eyelid retractions. Euryblepharon is distinguished by an enlargement of the horizontal palpebral fissure associated with enlarged eyelids.

Congenital Entropion

When the eyelid margin is rolled inward against the globe,at birth, the condition is referred to as congenital entropion. Upper eyelid involvement is commonly associated with a tarsal abnormality, while lower eyelid entropion is often associated with epiblepharon. Entropion does not resolve spontaneously, and may cause corneal pathology if untreated. Serafino et al[48] studied patients with lower bilateral congenital entropion to compare the results of incisional versus rotational surgery. The authors consider both techniques satisfactory, but the procedure of choice, considering the age of the patients and previous studies, remains rotational sutures because of its simplicity, quickness, and low risk of complication. Some authors[49] have tried the pretarsal orbicularis muscle injection with 5 units of botulinum toxin with resolution of entropion four days after treatment and no recurrence of the entropion 7 months after botulinum toxin injection suggesting that injection of botulinum toxin may effectively treat certain cases of congenital entropion.

Surgical Correction of Entropion in Congenital Cutis Laxa[50]

Congenital cutis laxa is a rare generalized inherited elastosis, characterized by the appearance of premature aging and skin laxity with mild to severe systemic anomalies. Ocular manifestations include excess skin in the eyelids, ptosis and lower lid ectropion. Of the hyperelasticity syndromes—Ehlers Danlos, pseudopxanthoma elasticum and cutis laxa—only cutis laxa has normal skin wound healing. The diagnosis must therefore be established before surgical options for treatment are considered.

Congenital Ectropion

Congenital eversion[51] of the upper eyelids is a rare condition, the exact cause of which remains unknown. It is more frequently associated with Down's syndrome and black babies. If diagnosed early and treated properly, the condition can be managed without surgery conservatively by lubricants, antibiotics and eyelid patching.

Congenital ectropion in congenital ichthyosis[52] which is a generalized hyperkeratinization of the skin at birth. Depending on clinical aspects and severity, three forms of congenital ichthyosis have been defined: mitis, tarda, and gravis. Desquamation of the parchment-like hyperkeratinized skin begins shortly after birth and may require several weeks to complete. Skin alterations in the eyelid cause shortening of the anterior lamella, subsequently resulting in ectropion. This affects the upper eyelid more often than the lower and can lead to complications such as chronic palpebral or bulbar conjunctivitis and keratinization or exposure keratopathy. In mild forms of congenital ichthyosis surgical treatment of eyelid ectropion is not required. In more severe cases a skin graft may become necessary.

CRYPTOPHTHALMOS

Cryptophthalmos, a very rare congenital anomaly of the eye, is characterised by skin passing continuously from the forehead to the cheek over a malformed eye.

It is genetic disorder with systemic involvement (sometimes life threatening) and if not leaves the family devastated and unsatisfied with treatment and fearful of one more such occurrence in the family. Thoughtful and methodical approach can alleviate some aspects.

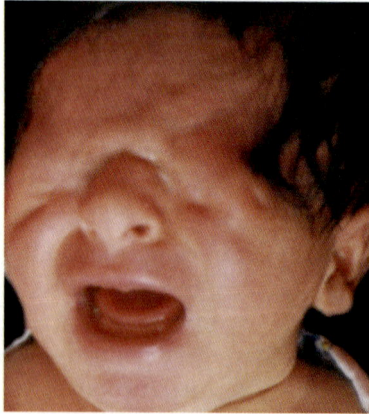

Figure 14: Cryptophthalmos

Parental Age

The average paternal age is 27 years of age and the average maternal age is 24 years of age.

Known Risk Factors

Oligohydramnios is the most frequent complication during pregnancy.

Pathogenesis

Fras,[1] that is specifically detected in a linear fashion underlying the epidermis and the basal surface of other epithelia in embryos. Loss of Fras1 function results in the formation of subepidermal hemorrhagic blisters as well as unilateral or bilateral renal agenesis. Homozygous Fras1 mutants have fusion of the eyelids and digits and unilateral renal agenesis or dysplasia. Modifier genes are important determinants of phenotypic variation. (The pathogenesis of phenotypic modules could include disruption to a morphogenetic field or a developmental field, mutation specific effects, or malfunction of temporally distinct genes).

- Triallelic inheritance
- Autosomal recessive inheritance
- Dominant mode of inheritance

The loss of a cytoplasmic multi-PDZ scaffolding protein, glutamate receptor interacting protein 1 (GRIP1), leads to the formation of subepidermal hemorrhagic blisters, renal agenesis, syndactyly or polydactyly and permanent fusion of eyelids (cryptophthalmos). GRIP1 can physically interact with Fras1 and is required for the localization of Fras1 to the basal side of cells. Grip1 is disrupted by a deletion of two coding exons .GRIP1 is required for normal cell-matrix interactions during early embryonic development and that inactivation of Grip1 causes cryptophthalmos.

Classification

A. Nouby's classification of congenital upper eyelid coloboma and cryptophthalmos.
  - Grade 1: Coloboma without cryptophthalmos.
  - Grade 2: Coloboma with abortive cryptophthalmos.
  - Grade 3: Coloboma with complete cryptophthalmos.
  - Grade 4: Classic cryptophthalmos (absence of all eyelid structures and the eye is completely covered with skin).
  - Grade 5: Severe cryptophthalmos (with severe deformity of the nose and ectropion of the upper lip).
B. Moreker-Agashe classification:
  - Grade 1-Frasers syndrome
  - Grade 2-Congenital orbito-palpebral cyst
  - Grade 3-Bilateral cryptophthalmos
  - Grade 4-Unilateral partial crytophthalmos

- Grade 5-Symmetrical partial lateral 'cryptophthalmos'
- Grade 6-Symmetrical medial cryptophthamos
- Grade 7-Asymmetrical hemi cryptophthalmos
- Grade 8-Congenital symblepharon associated with meningoencephalocele.
- Grade 9-Bilateral abortive cryptophthalmos associated with oculocutaneous albinism
- Grade 10-Congenital symblepharon (abortive cryptophthalmos)
- Grade 11-Cryptophthalmos solum corneae
- Grade 12-Ablepheron macrostomia syndrome.

Treatment

Complete Cryptophthalmos

Weng et al[53] described a three-stage reconstructive procedure in which a conchal cartilage 'sandwich' graft is first placed between the skin flap and the globe, mucous membrane subsequently grafted onto the inner surface of the cartilage graft, and lid level adjusted as the third stage. Ferri et al [54] have discussed the steps in more details.

Incomplete Cryptophthalmos

Dibben et al[55] described that incomplete cryptophthalmos can be corrected by dissection of the eyelids from the cornea, reconstruction of the conjunctival fornices with buccal mucosa, and repairing the upper lid coloboma if present in a flap reconstruction using the inferior eyelid margin is the usual procedure.

Role of Amniotic Membrane

Stewart et al[56] reported successful creation of a superior fornix in a case of partial cryptophthalmos after an amniotic membrane graft concluding that amniotic membrane is a useful resource for fornix reconstruction in cryptophthalmos.

Prenatal Diagnosis[57,58,59]

Ultrasound diagnosis in a prenatal state as well as genetic counseling seems to be the only way to control this condition.

BIBLIOGRAPHY

1. A Yuksel D, Ceylan K, Erden O, Kilic R, Duman S. Balloon dilatation for treatment of congenital nasolacrimal duct obstruction. Eur J Ophthalmol 2005 Mar-Apr;15(2):179-85.
2. Baek SH, Lee EY. Clinical analysis of internal orbital fractures in children. Korean J Ophthalmol 2003 Jun;17(1):44-9.
3. Bajaj M, Pushker N, Mahindrakar A, Balasubramanya R. Advancement of Whitnall's ligament via the conjunctival approach for correction of congenital ptosis Orbit 2004 Sep;23(3):153-9.
4. Becker BB, Berry FD, Koller H. Balloon catheter dilatation for treatment of congenital nasolacrimal duct obstruction. Am J Ophthalmol 1996 Mar;121(3):304-9.
5. Becker BB. The treatment of congenital dacryocystocele. Am J Ophthalmol. 2006 Nov;142(5):835-8.
6. Berg C, Geipel A, Germer U, Pertersen-Hansen A, Koch-Dorfler M, Gembruch U. Prenatal detection of Fraser syndrome without cryptophthalmos: case report and review of the literature. Ultrasound Obstet Gynecol 2001 Jul;18(1):76-80. Review.
7. Betharia SM, Sharma V. Inverse Bell's phenomenon observed following levator resection for blepharoptosis. Graefes Arch Clin Exp Ophthalmol 2006 Jul;244(7):868-70. Epub 2005 Sep 21.
8. Burroughs JR, Anderson RL, Elliot RL. Correction of congenital blepharoptosis in oculomotor-abducens synkinesis. Ophthal Plast Reconstr Surg 2006 Jan-Feb;22(1):64-5.
9. Burroughs JR, Bearden WH, Anderson RL, Hoffman RO, Elliot RL, McCann JD. Congenitally enlarged extraocular muscles: can congenital thyroid eye disease exist in a euthyroid infant? Ophthal Plast Reconstr Surg 2006 Jul-Aug;22(4):314-6.
10. Casady DR, Meyer DR, Simon JW, Stasior GO, Zobal-Ratner JL. Stepwise treatment paradigm for congenital nasolacrimal duct obstruction. Ophthal Plast Reconstr Surg 2006 Jul-Aug;22(4):243-7.

11. Christiansen G, Mohney BG, Baratz KH, Bradley EA. Botulinum toxin for the treatment of congenital entropion. Am J Ophthalmol 2004 Jul;138(1):153-5.

12. Christmas NJ, Van Quill K, Murray TG, Gordon CD, Garonzik S, Tse D, Johnson T, Schiffman J, O'Brien JM. Evaluation of efficacy and complications: primary pediatric orbital implants after enucleation. Arch Ophthalmol 2000 Apr;118(4):503-6.

13. Clauser L, Tieghi R, Galie M. Palpebral ptosis: clinical classification, differential diagnosis, and surgical guidelines: an overview. J Craniofac Surg 2006 Mar;17(2):246-54.

14. Cohen SM, Garrett CG. Pediatric orbital floor fractures: nausea/vomiting as signs of entrapment. Otolaryngol Head Neck Surg 2003 Jul;129(1):43-7.

15. Dibben K, Rabinowitz YS, Shorr N, Graham JM Jr. Surgical correction of incomplete cryptophthalmos in Fraser syndrome. Am J Ophthalmol 1997 Jul;124(1):107-9.

16. Doco-Fenzy M, Mauran P, Lebrun JM, Bock S, Bednarek N, Struski S, Albuisson J, Ardalan A, Collot N, Schneider A, Dastot-Le Moal F, Gaillard D, Goossens M. Pure direct duplication (12)(q24.1—>q24.2) in a child with Marcus Gunn phenomenon and multiple congenital anomalies. Am J Med Genet A 2006 Feb 1;140(3):212-21.

17. Dzhambazov KB, Gyulev IA, Traikova NI, Yovchev IP. Endonasal treatment of postsaccal stenoses of lacrimal ducts: intranasal retrograde probing in congenital stenosis Folia Med (Plovdiv). 2005;47(3-4):28-32.

18. Egbert JE, May K, Kersten RC, Kulwin DR. Pediatric orbital floor fracture direct extraocular muscle involvement. Ophthalmology 2000 Oct;107(10):1875-9.

19. Ferri M, Harvey JT. Surgical correction for complete cryptophthalmos: case report and review of the literature. Can J Ophthalmol 1999 Jun;34(4):233-6.

20. Gamio S, Garcia-Erro M, Vaccarezza MM, Minella JA. Myasthenia gravis in childhood. Binocul Vis Strabismus Q 2004;19(4):223-31.

21. Goldstein SM, Goldstein JB, Katowitz JA. Comparison of monocanalicular stenting and balloon dacryoplasty in secondary treatment of congenital nasolacrimal duct obstruction after failed primary probing Ophthal Plast Reconstr Surg 2004 Sep;20(5):352-7.

22. Grant JH 3rd, Patrinely JR, Weiss AH, Kierney PC, Gruss JS. Trapdoor fracture of the orbit in a pediatric population. Plast Reconstr Surg 2002 Feb;109(2):482-9; discussion 490-5.

23. Gurelik M, Ozum U, Erdogan H, Aslan A. Orbital lymphangioma and its association with intracranial venous angioma. Br J Neurosurg 2004 Apr;18(2):168-70.

24. Hersh D, Martin FJ, Rowe N. Comparison of silastic and banked fascia lata in pediatric frontalis suspension. J Pediatr Ophthalmol Strabismus 2006 Jul-Aug;43(4):212-8.

25. Hirasawa C, Matsuo K, Kikuchi N, Osada Y, Shinohara H, Yuzuriha S. Upgaze eyelid position allows differentiation between congenital and aponeurotic blepharoptosis according to the neurophysiology of eyelid retraction. Ann Plast Surg 2006 Nov;57(5):529-34.

26. Hosal BM, Ayer NG, Zilelioglu G, Elhan AH. Ultrasound biomicroscopy of the levator aponeurosis in congenital and aponeurotic blepharoptosis. Ophthal Plast Reconstr Surg 2004 Jul;20(4):308-11.

27. Inan UU, Yilmaz MD, Demir Y, Degirmenci B, Ermis SS, Ozturk F. Characteristics of lacrimo-auriculo-dento-digital (LADD) syndrome: case report of a family and literature review. Int J Pediatr Otorhinolaryngol 2006 Jul;70(7):1087-14.

28. Iordanidou V, De Potter P. Porous polyethylene orbital implant in the pediatric population. Am J Ophthalmol 2004 Sep;138(3):425-9.

29. Jordan DR, Allen LH, White J, Harvey J, Pashby R, Esmaeli B. Intervention within days for some orbital floor fractures: the white-eyed blowout. Ophthal Plast Reconstr Surg 1998 Nov;14(6):379-90.

30. Kaltreider SA, Peake LR, Carter BT. Pediatric enucleation: analysis of volume replacement. Arch Ophthalmol 2001 Mar;119(3):379-84.

31. Kashkouli MB, Beigi B, Parvaresh MM, Kassaee A, Tabatabaee Z. Late and very late initial probing for congenital nasolacrimal duct obstruction: what is the cause of failure?

32. Kim NJ, Choung HK, Khwarg SI, Yu YS Free orbital fat graft to prevent porous polyethylene orbital implant exposure in patients with retinoblastoma. Ophthal Plast Reconstr Surg 2005 Jul;21(4):253-8.

33. Kumar S, Chaudhuri Z, Chauhan D. Clinical evaluation of refractive changes following brow suspension surgery inpediatric patients with congenital blepharoptosis. Ophthalmic Surg Lasers Imaging 2005 May-Jun;36(3):217-27.

34. Kupersmith MJ, Ying G. Ocular motor dysfunction and ptosis in ocular myasthenia gravis: effects of treatment. Br J Ophthalmol 2005 Oct;89(10):1330-4.

35. Lelli GJ Jr, Nelson CC. Early habituation of severe blepharoptosis in Marcus Gunn jaw-winking syndrome. J Pediatr Ophthalmol Strabismus 2006 Jan-Feb;43(1):38-40.

36. Lennon PA, Scott DA, Lonsdorf D, Wargowski DS, Kirkpatrick S, Patel A, Cheung SW. WAGR(O?) syndrome and congenital ptosis caused by an unbalanced t(11;15)(p13;p11.2)dn demonstrating a 7

megabase deletion by FISH. Am J Med Genet A 2006 Jun 1;140(11):1214-8.

37. Lipiec E, Gralek M, Niwald A. Evaluation of therapy outcome in congenital nasolacrimal duct obstruction in own material. Klin Oczna 2006;108(4-6):174-7.

38. Maheshwari R, Maheshwari S. Congenital eversion of upper eyelids: case report and management. Indian J Ophthalmol 2006 Sep;54(3):203-4.

39. Menke TB, Moschner S, Joachimmeyer E, Ahrens P, Geerling G. Congenital ectropion in ichthyosis congenita mitis and gravis Ophthalmologe 2006 May;103(5):410-5.

40. Mitchell KT, Hollsten DA, White WL, O'Hara MA. The autogenous dermis-fat orbital implant in children. J AAPOS 2001 Dec;5(6):367-9.

41. Muller JS, Baumeister SK, Schara U, Cossins J, Krause S, von der Hagen M, Huebner A, Webster R, Beeson D, Lochmuller H, Abicht A. CHRND mutation causes a congenital myasthenic syndrome by impairing co-clustering of the acetylcholine receptor with rapsyn. Brain 2006 Oct;129(Pt 10):2784-93. Epub 2006 Aug 17.

42. Pryor SG, Lewis JE, Weaver AL, Orvidas LJ. Pediatric dermoid cysts of the head and neck. Otolaryngol Head Neck Surg 2005 Jun;132(6):938-42.

43. Ramirez OM, Pena G. Frontalis muscle advancement: a dynamic structure for the treatment of severe congenital eyelid ptosis. Plast Reconstr Surg 2004 May;113(6):1841-9; discussion 1850-1.

44. Rousseau T, Laurent N, Thauvin-Robinet C, Lionnais S, Durand C, Faivre L,Sagot P. Prenatal diagnosis and intrafamilial clinical heterogeneity of Fraser syndrome.Prenat Diagn 2002 Aug;22(8):692-6.

45. Schwartz SR, Blei F, Ceisler E, Steele M, Furlan L, Kodsi S. Risk factors for amblyopia in children with capillary hemangiomas of the eyelids and orbit. J AAPOS 2006 Jun;10(3):262-8.

46. Serafino M, Bottoli A, Nucci P. Correction of congenital entropion of the lower eyelid: incisional versus rotational surgery. Eur J Ophthalmol 2005 Sep-Oct;15(5):536-40.

47. Shah-Desai SD, Collins AL, Tyers AG. Surgical correction of entropion and excess upper eyelid skin in congenital cutis laxa: a case report. Orbit 1999 Mar;18(1):53-8.

48. Shields JA, Shields CL. Orbital cysts of childhood—classification, clinical features, and management. Surv Ophthalmol 2004 May-Jun;49(3):281-99.

49. Slaughter K, Sullivan T, Boulton J, O'Reagan P, Gole G. Early surgical intervention as definitive treatment for ocular adnexal capillary haemangioma. Clin Experiment Ophthalmol 2003 Oct;31(5):418-23.

50. Sterker I, Frerich B. Orbital diseases in childhood Klin Monatsbl Augenheilkd 2006 Jan;223(1):59-67.

51. Sterker I, Grafe G. Periocular hemangiomas in childhood—functional and esthetic results. Strabismus 2004 Jun;12(2):103-10.

52. Stewart JM, David S, Seiff SR. Amniotic membrane graft in the surgical management of cryptophthalmos. Ophthal Plast Reconstr Surg 2002 Sep;18(5):378-80.

53. Stiglmayer N, Tojagic M, Juri J. Long-term results of frontal lobe suspension in children with congenital dystrophic ptosis. Coll Antropol 2004 Jun;28(1):349-56.

54. Tao S, Meyer DR, Simon JW, Zobal-Ratner J. Success of balloon catheter dilatation as a primary or secondary procedure forcongenital nasolacrimal duct obstruction.Ophthalmology 2002 Nov;109(11):2108-11.

55. Tien DR, Young DJ. Balloon dilation of the nasolacrimal duct AAPOS. 2005 Oct;9(5):465-7.

56. Usha K, Smitha S, Shah N, Lalitha P, Kelkar R. Spectrum and the susceptibilities of microbial isolates in cases of congenital nasolacrimal duct obstruction. J AAPOS. 2006Oct;10(5):469-72.

57. Vijayaraghavan SB, Suma N, Lata S, Kamakshi K. Prenatal sonographic appearance of cryptophthalmos in Fraser syndrome.Ultrasound Obstet Gynecol 2005 Jun;25(6):629-30.

58. Weng CJ. Surgical reconstruction in cryptophthalmos. Br J Plast Surg 1998 Jan;51(1):17-21.

59. Wong CY, Fan DS, Ng JS, Goh TY, Lam DS.Long-term results of autogenous palmaris longus frontalis sling in children with congenital ptosis. Eye 2005 May;19(5):546-8.

Periocular Applications of Botulinum Toxin

34

Pelin Kaynak-Hekimhan (Turkey)

INTRODUCTION AND HISTORY

In this chapter, botulinum toxin's application modalities on eyelid and periocular area, treatment doses, interactions, its side effects and secondary effects are discussed. Extraocular muscle procedures, such as treatment of strabismus and nistagmus are out of the scope of this chapter.

Botulinum toxin is a powerful toxin, which prevents muscular contraction by blocking acetylcholine release in neuromuscular junction. This toxin, which is used predominantly in treatments of muscle dystonias with spasms and for cosmetic reasons, was first used by Scott et al in 1973 in strabismus patients.[1] Food and Drug Administration (FDA) approved botulinum toxin use for strabismus patients in 1979. FDA approval for the treatment of hemifacial spasm and blepharospasm was in 1989 although botulinum toxin was utilized for blepharospasm treatment since 1982. Cosmetic effects of botulinum toxin, which were discovered accidentally during treatments of facial dystonia, were first reported in 1989[2] and Carruthers and Carruthers published a number of studies including systemic effect evaluations related to cosmetic applications of botulinum toxin, proving that it decreases the depth and appearance of the kinetic facial lines.[3-5] In 2002, FDA approved the use of botulinum toxin A for the removal of glabellar lines, however botulinum toxin is used extensively for areas such as crowsfeet, perioral area, nose, chin, neck, etc. along with glabellar lines.[6]

Intramuscular botulinum toxin injections, frequently applied in treating spastic facial dystonias are still the most preferable treatment methods today due to undesired effects of alternative treatment methods.[7-14]

Botulinum toxin is successfully used in temporary treatment of idiopathic and thyroid dysfunction induced upper eyelid retraction.[15-18]

In addition to the rare applications of periocular botulinum toxin, treatments such as lacrimal gland blockage and temporary ptosis-intended chemodenervation in facial paralysis , the areas of use for this toxin is quite wide, including hyperhidrosis, migraine, tension-type headaches, and paralitic spasticity.[10]

WHAT IS BOTULINUM TOXIN?

Botulinum toxin is the poisonous exotoxin of *Clostridium* species. The bacterium *Clostridium* botulinum produces eight antigenically distinct exotoxins. Serologic types include A, B, C, D, E, F, and G. Type E is also produced by *Clostridium butyricum*. Type F is produced by *Clostridium baratii*.[19]

Type A, B and E botulinum toxins are colorless, odorless, and tasteless. Only these three types of toxins affect humans and can cause systemic botulismus. Type A is the most potent toxin, followed by types B, and F. Each botulinum toxin is synthesized as a single chain protein, which is inactive until it is cleaved by bacterial proteases into its active form. The active botulinum toxins are composed of two chains: one heavy chain joined to one light chain by a relatively weak disulfide bond, which is shown to be highly responsible for the unstability of the molecule. The toxin is inactivated by heat, 85°C (185°F) or greater in 5 minutes. [19-23]

MECHANISM OF ACTION

Botulinum toxin prevents muscular contraction by inhibiting the release of acetylcholine from vesicles at the presynaptic nerve terminal at the neuromuscular junction. It also inhibits release of acetylcholine at the autonomic gangliae, postganglionic parasympathetic and sympathetic nerve endings. The different serotypes bind to different sites on the motor neuron terminal and within the motor neuron. The heavy chain functions both as a channel and a companion to bring the light chain across the endosomal membrane and then into the cytosol in the presynaptic region. The light chain acts inside the cell on synaptosomal associated protein receptor proteins (SNARE) to block the release of the vesicle-bound neurotransmitter acetylcholine from nicotinic and muscarinic nerve endings. Muscle weakness becomes evident in 2 to 4 days due to the continued release of acetylcholine from vesicles that have not been blocked by the toxin. Recovery of muscle activity typically begins 3 to 4 months after injection and is thought to occur due to the regeneration of new end plate units.[23]

Doses of all commercially available forms of botulinum toxins are expressed in terms of units(=mouse units). The standard measurement of the potency of the toxin is one international unit (IU), which is the amount of toxin that kills 50% of a group of 18–20 female Swiss-Webster mice (LD50) when injected intraperitonally. The LD50 in humans is estimated to be approximately 2,730 IU.[19-21]

COMMERCIAL PREPARATIONS

BOTOX® (Allergan Corporation, Irvine, CA, USA) is a dry, protein crystalline complex of botulinum toxin A and it contains 100 units (MU = U) per bottle. One unit of BOTOX®

COSMETIC equals to the calculated median intraperitoneal lethal dose (LD50) in mice.[19] The product is unstable so it must be kept frozen before constitution. The recommended doses are usually prepared by diluting the contents of bottle with 2 ml of sterile saline without preservative, leaving 25U for each 0.5 ml of solution . One nanogram contains 2.5 IU.[21]

The onset of paralysis takes 24-48 h and reaches maximum at 7-10 days .The effect usually lasts 4-6 months. Repeated injections may delay the onset of paralysis but sometimes a more protracted paralysis will occur.[20]

Dysport (Ipsen, Slough, UK) which is another trademark of botulinum toxin type A. Four units of Dysport is approximately equivalent to one unit of BOTOX®.[22]

Myobloc® (Neurobloc) (Elan Pharmaceuticals, San Diegoo, CA, USA) contains a liquid formulation of purified botulinum toxin type B. When reconstituted, Myobloc® has a shelf life of more than 12 months which is longer than BOTOX®. It has a faster onset of action and better diffusion to tissues however the injections are more painful due to the acidity of the product.

Botulinum toxin A is 50-100 times more potent than botulinum toxin B.[24]

Table 1 lists the most commonly used preparations and the storage conditions.

RECONSTITUTION AND STORAGE

Botulinum toxin A is recommended to be reconstituted with sterile nonpreserved 0.9% NaCl solution before injection and must be kept at 4°C until injection. It has to be injected in 4 hours after reconstitution for maximum activity. The weak disulfide bonds between the two chains of the toxin renders it fragile under mechanical stress such as frothing when diluting and agitating the liquid inside the vial.

Table 1: Botulinum toxin: storage and preparation conditions

| | Storage temperatures | | Duration of activity |
	Before reconstitution	After reconstitution	
Botulinum Toxin A			
Botox®	–5 °C	2-8 °C	4 hours
Botox Cosmetic®	–5 °C	2-8 °C	4 hours
Dysport®	2-8 °C	2-8 °C	1 hour
Botulinum Toxin B			
Neuroblock®	2-8 °C	Room temperature	8 hours
Myoblock®	Room temperature	Room temperature	Up to 30 months

The concentration of the botulinum toxin depends on the amount of diluent in the vial determined by the physician. In our clinical application, preferred dilution is generally 50 U/ ml when used for the management of blepharospasm and hemifacial spasm and 100U/1ml for cosmetic applications around the eye 0.5 or 1U/ml. Table 2 shows the toxin concentration in 0.1 ml of two common used commercial forms of botulinum toxin A with various volumes of diluent. Tuberculin syringes with 30 gauge needle are preferred which allow more painless and accurate injections at intended sites, and less bleeding.

When botulinum toxin is injected in the periocular area both icepacks and EMLA® cream can be applied for topical anesthesia .

Elibol et al reports that EMLA® cream for periocular anesthesia works slightly better than icepack skin cooling when botulinum toxin A is injected.[25]

Table 2: Botulinum toxin a concentration with various volumes of diluent used

0.9% NaCl added (ml)	Botox® dose (U/0.1 ml)	Dysport® dose (U/0.1 ml)
1	10	50
2	5	25
4	2.5	12.5
8	1.25	6.25
10	1	5

Table 3: Essential equipment for botulinum toxin applications (Fig. 1)

Alcohol and betadine swaps

Gause swabs and dry paper tissue

2 cc syringes with 25 gauge needles for reconstitution of botulinum toxin

Sterile, preservative free(?)* 0.9% saline for dilution

0.5-1ml tuberculin syringes

Frozen gel or icepacks or,

EMLA® cream for anesthesia

*Some collegues use normal saline with preservatives for less painful injections without increasing the dose.

In Table 3 the equipment needed for practical preparation, dilution and injection for botulinum toxin is listed.

THERAPEUTIC USES OF BOTULINUM TOXIN

Facial muscle dyskinesias such as benign essential blepharospasms, hemifacial spasms, Meige syndrome, apraxia of eyelid opening and orbicularis myokimia, synkinetic eyelid movements are manageable with botulinum toxin injections.

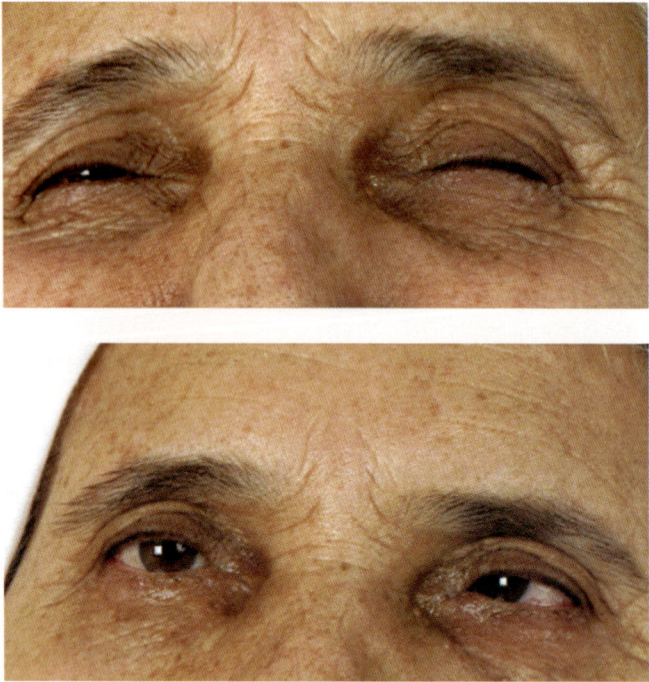

Figure 1: Photographs of a patient with blepharospasm before
(upper) and after (bottom) botulinum toxin A injection

CNS depressants,[26] orbicularis myectomy and selective
facial nerve neurectomy are alternative treatments. Botulinum
toxin injections in orbicularis oculi, corrugator superciliaris
and occasionally into frontalis muscles are effective for
treatment of blepharospasm.[6-13]

Muscles involved in facial dyskinesias must be correctly
evaluated in physical examination. Accompanying pathologies have to be consulted with neurologist. Electromyographic examination may be a helpful tool in localizing the

Table 4: Periocular therapeutic and cosmetic applications of botulinum toxin

Therapeutic applications of botulinum toxin in eyelids and periocular area:
- Essential blepharospasm
- Hemifacial spasm
- Meige syndrome
- Treatment of apraxia of eyelid opening
- Orbicularis myokimia
- Aberrant regeneration of 7th nerve
- Control of synkinetic eyelid movements
- Eyelid retraction
- Lower eyelid entropion
- Lacrimal gland blockage
- Pharmacologic tarsorrhaphy for corneal protection
- Treatment of dry eye
- Adjunct to facial wound healing

Cosmetic applications of botulinum toxin on eyelids and periocular area:
- Glabellar lines
- Lateral orbital lines (crawsfeet)
- Hypertrophic orbicularis oculi
- Narrow palpebral vertical aperture
- Dermatochalasis
- Browlift
- Asymmetric features of the face
- Adjunctive procedures for other antiaging methods

involuntarily contracting muscles occasionally, when the muscle to be injected is not localized accurately.

Video documentation before and after treatment is more useful than documentary photographs.

Periocular therapeutic and cosmetic applications of botulinum toxin are summarized in Table 4.

Botulinum Toxin Use in Blepharospasm and Hemifacial Spasm

Benign essential blepharospasm is the involuntary, repetitive contractions of orbicularis oculi muscle. Depressor muscles of eyebrows as corrugator superciliaris, procerus are also involved. Reflex blepharospasm due to dry eye must not be mistakenly diagnosed as benign essential blepharospasm. Meige syndrome is a cranial dystonia with bilateral blepharospasm accompanied by dystonia in the lower face. Involountary contractions of orbicularis oris, buccinator and masseter muscles are prominant. Hemifacial spasm is characterized by unilateral repetitive contractions of facial muscles. It may result from compression of fibers of 7th nerve root. Posterior fossa tumors may be underlying this condition. Orbicularis myokimia denotes a condition in young individuals with involuntary twitches of some orbicularis oculi muscle fiber bundles. Stress and fatigue and caffeine and alcohol intake may exacerbate the frequency and severity of spasms.

The usual dose and muscles injected for blepharospasm treatment in our practice is about 5U in each of the 3 points laterally in orbicularis oculi muscle 1 cm lateral to the lateral orbital rim. Subcutaneous injections of 2U botulinum toxin A into medial to upper and lower eyelids in the orbicularis oculi preseptal fibers, especially not into the pretearsal fibers in this area, are given. The injection sites must be at least 5 mm far from lacrimal punctae to avoid lacrimal pump failure. Botulinum toxin A injections of 1-3 units into frontalis muscles centrally and 5-10 U in the corrugator supercilii muscles and 1-2U procerus muscles administered in these group of patients generally stop contractions for 4-6 months (see Fig. 1). Patients are seen in the second week post injection, for evaluation of the efficacy, side effects and secondary effects of the treatment. Reinjections may be done at this visit. Doses and modifications for the future injections are noted.

Patients with hemifacial spasms need botulinum toxin injections in mid face muscles, and occasionally in the lower facial muscles. Dose vary individually , being lower than those for blepharospasm. Meige syndrome is treated with higher doses where orbicularis myokimia treatment requires lower dose injections of the toxin.

Response to the treatments with botulinum toxin continues after repeated injections in majority of the cases followed up for more than 10 years.[8] For patients who are not responding to botulinum toxin A botulinum toxin B may be effective in treating the spasms.[9] Injecting higher doses of toxin may also stop unvoluntary contractions, that do not respond to lower doses.[27]

Temporary eyelid and facial ptosis, lagophthalmus and epiphora are the undesired effects of the treatment. Diplopi a may occur as a result of diffusion of toxin into extraocular muscles.

Botulinum Toxin Use in Apraxia of Eyelid Opening

Apraxia of eyelid opening is the inability to initiate to open the eyelids. It may be noted in patients with blepharospasm due to pretarsal fibers of orbicularis oculi muscle activity.

We inject 0.5-2U of toxin A at 2 sides medially and laterally 5 mm. away from the lid margin aiming the pretarsal orbicular oculi muscle.

Botulinum Toxin Use for Dysthroid and Upper Eyelid Retraction Management

In 1996 Özkan et al investigated effect of botulinum toxin in cases with dysthyroid upper eyelid retraction, which was one of the first studies conducted for this subject.[15] Botulinum toxin administered for temporary correction, particularly in ascending stage of Randal's curve and during the period when stabilization is expected, and radical surgical management is delayed for more accurate outcome.

We inject 1-10 U of botulinum toxin A subconjunctivally at the upper border of tarsus divided into two, medially and laterally to minimize eyelid ptosis complication due to levator muscle paralysis. Despite multiple administrations of botulinum toxin A the effect is temporary and whenever the upper eyelid retraction persists, although the patient becomes euthyroid for more than a year, levator recession surgery with or without spacer materials is performed.[28-29]

In Figure 2 photographs of two patients with upper eyelid retraction before (left) and after (right) botulinum toxin A injection are seen.

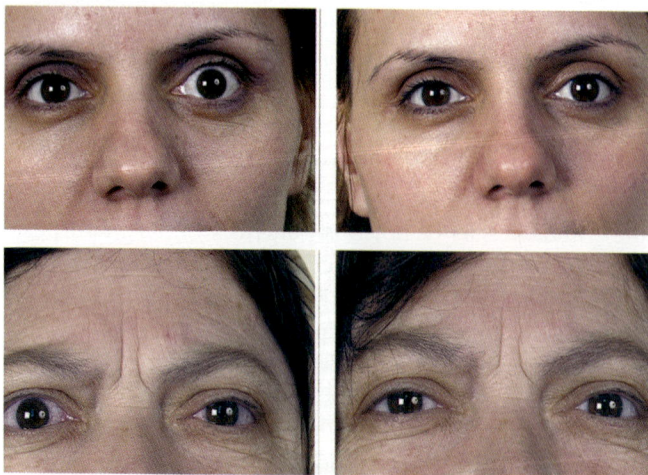

Figure 2: Photographs of two patients with upper eyelid retraction before (left) and after (right) botulinum toxin A injection

Morgensten et al have achieved decrease in eyelid aperture in 94% of the cases by administering 2,5-10 U botulinum toxin A injections transconjunctivally in 1 or 2 points of levator-Müller's muscle complex from the upper side of the tarsus.[18] Shih, Liao and Lu have also achieved similar results by injecting botulinum toxin A through skin into levator muscle.[30] Upper eyelid ptosis is the most frequently seen undesired effect of such injections, and it is temporary. Olver has also reported successful results in decreasing the activity of corrugator supercilii muscles in cases with dysthyroid ophtalmopathy by injecting botulinum toxin in these muscles.[16]

Botulinum Toxin Use for Entropion Treatment

Botulinum toxin injection decreases the tonus of lower pretarsal and preseptal fibers of orbicularis oculi overriding , therefore correcting entropion temporarily. 1-5 U injections to the central portion of the subciliary orbicularis muscle 3-5 mm inferior to the eyelid margin in lower eyelid trets the spastic component of entropion for 4-5 months.

Christiansen et al injected botulinum toxin A on sub-eyelid of a 3-week old congenital entropion patient, and treated corneal ulcers of the infant without any undesired effects.[31]

We do not prefer to inject botulinum toxin in infants in our practice.

Botulinum Toxin Use for Lacrimal Gland Blockage

Gustatory lacrimal gland function (crocodile tear syndrome) can be controlled by 2,5-20 U botulinum toxin A injection administered in lacrimal gland, however side effects such as eyelid ptosis and dry eye symptoms might be experienced.[31-34]

Botulinum Toxin Use for Cornea Protection in Facial Paralysis

For cases with facial paralysis, particularly for patients for whom a surgical procedure seems to be difficult, lagophthalmus can be decreased by achieving eyelid ptosis with 2-10 U botulinum toxin A injection in levator palpebrae superioris muscle instead of tarsorrhaphy and/or gold weight implantation, so that corneal ulcers can be prevented.[35]

The patients who receive radiation therapy near the face are also good candidates for this application of botulinum toxin because the atrophied eyelid skin would not tolerate an eyelid implant for a long time.

We inject 5-15 U of botulinum toxin A in the levator muscle subconjunctivally 5-6 mm above the tarsus to prevent diffusion into orbicularis oculi muscle fibers and worsen the lagophthalmus in these patients.

Control of Synkinetic Eyelid Movements

Synchronic movements of eyelid retractor and protractors as well as extraocular muscles can be seen after aberrant regeneration of especially 3rd or 7th cranial nerve palsies. The muscle contraction can be seized by customized doses of botulinum toxin injections and in these muscles.

Chua et al administrated 40-120U botulinum toxin A (Dysport) injections on orbicularis oculi muscle of 5 cases in order to limit the synkinetic eyelid movements occurring after aberrant 7th nerve paralysis, and observed that synkinetic movements descreased for 3 months both objectively and subjectively in all cases. Ptosis was observed in 2 patients, but this side effect was not seen in patients treated with lower doses such as 40 U.[36]

COSMETIC ADMINISTRATION OF BOTULINUM TOXIN ON EYELIDS AND PERIOCULAR AREA

Glabellar Area

Corrugator superciliaris muscle originates at the junction of the nasal and frontal bones close to the supramedial orbital rim. A transverse line drawn coronally through the middle of the eyebrow identifies the horizontal position of the bulk of the muscle. Injections between 4 and 20 U of botulinum toxin A in the belly of the muscle at one or two points decrease or erase the glabellar frown lines. Area lateral to the midpupillary line is avoided to prevent botulinum toxin induced blepharoptosis.

The procerus muscle is located vertically in the midline of the nose. The optimal injection site is the midline just caudal to the nasal root. 1-3 U is injected at one or two points to treat the horizontal lines located at the superior part of the dorsum nasi.

In Figure 3 photographs of a patient with glabellar furrows before (left) and after (right) botulinum toxin A injection. Upper and lower row photographs demonstrate the static and dynamic wrinkles before and after treatments,respectively.

Based on the multi-centered, double-blinded, randomized, placebo-controlled study conducted by Carruthers et al, 20 U botulinum toxin A injected into corrugator and procerus muscles of glabella caused the lines to disappear, and this effect achieved its peak within 30 to 60 days, and was permanent for 90 days in 50% of the patients, and for 120 days in 25% of the patients. These effects are statistically significant when compared to placebo group (p< 0.003). The most frequently seen complication was mild eyelid ptosis observed in 1-5.4% of the patients.[37,38] In another study, 30 cases were administered 10 U botulinum toxin A at the

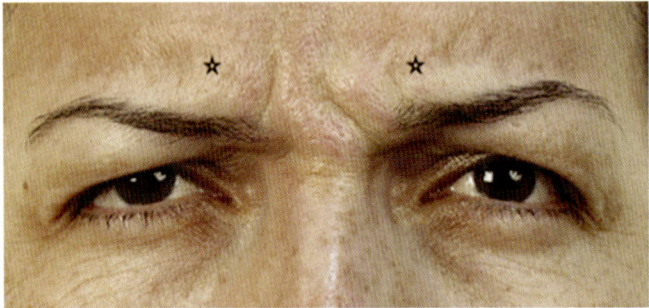

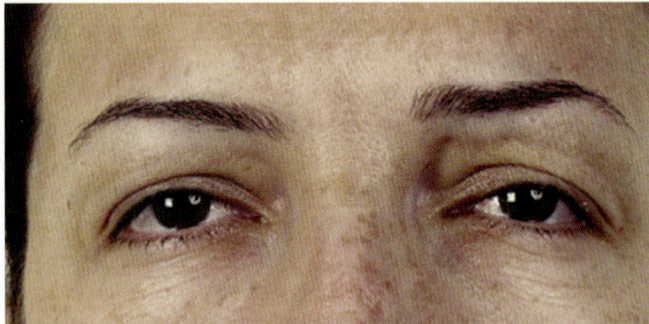

Figure 3: Photographs of a patient with glabellar furrows before (upper) and after (lower) botulinum toxin A injection. Upper and lower row photographs demonstrate the static and dynamic wrinkles before and after treatments, respectively. "Star"s in the upper photograph, indicate the preferred injection sites for treating glabellar furrows in most of the cases (doses and sites are customized for each patient)

glabella, a significant decrease in lines was recorded in 2 to 12th weeks, and the effect continued for 17.8 weeks.[39] Better improvement is reported in patients receiving the injections accompanied by EMG,[40] however we find EMG not easily applicable and practical in cosmetic use. Cosmetic cases prefer less complicated, fast applications of botulinum toxin.

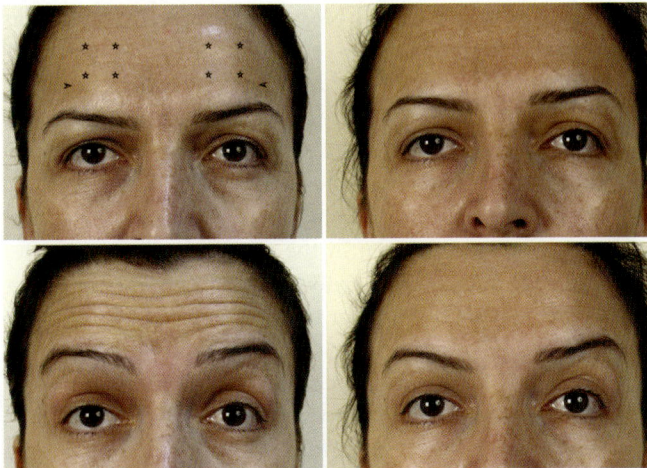

Figure 4: Photographs of a patient with horizontal forehead lines before (left) and after (right) botulinum toxin A injection. Upper and lower row photographs demonstrate the static and dynamic wrinkles before and after treatments,respectively. "Star"s in the upper-left photograph, indicate the preferred injection sites for treating forehead lines in most of the cases (doses and sites are customized for each patient). "Arrows" shows the points wher we occasionally prefer to inject to prevent the angry "V" look of the eyebrows

The effect of injections of botulinum toxin in corrugator muscles not only diminish the appearance of glabellar furrows but also broadens the distance between the eyebrows and the eyebrow upper eyelid margin (Figs 3 and 4). By administering 60 U botulinum toxin A injections on glabella and forehead lines, it was observed that frontal muscle activity decreased by 35% in the 2nd week, and aperture between eyebrows increased by 12% when digital photographs were examined.[41]

In Carruthers, Carruthers and Cohen's study, a total of 16, 32 and 48 U botulinum toxin A were injected in 8 points of glabella, frontal and orbicularis oculi muscles, the maximum eyebrow elevation was observed in 53% of the patients in high dose group. No eyebrow or eyelid ptosis was developed in the study. Positive cosmetic effects on such cases have continued even after return of muscle contractions.[42]

We observe a direct correlation between the dose and treatment of glabellar lines generally, in our practice, but there are studies that show no dose-response relations as well.[43]

Younger appearance is obtained by increasing vertical aperture of eyelid as seen in the patient in Figure 4, after injections administered in crowsfeet and pretarsal orbicular muscle; however botulinum toxin A injected too close to medial canthus, might induce functional epiphora.[44]

Eyebrow ptosis and dermatochalasis are frequently seen complications of botulinum toxin. A careful patient selection, low volume/high concentration applications and adding adrenaline in injector in order to decrease complications are recommended.[45] Cohen and Dayan also reported that a significant correction was obtained in dermatochalasis in 47% of the patients by means of infiltrating botulinum toxin into orbicularis and corrugator muscles in order to decrease dermatochalasis.[46]

Forehead

Frontalis muscles lies vertically between the orbicularis oculi muscle and inserts widely into the galea on each side of the forehead and causes the horizontal forehead rhytides when contracted.[47-48] To decrease the contraction effect, we inject the thickest portions of the muscle at 4-8 points on each side, points 1-1.5 cm apart. Doses between 0.5 and 4 U botulinum toxin A at each point is, generally injected in accordance with the severity of the wrinkles. It is recommended to laterally raise the line of the injections away from the brow to prevent lateral brow droop, however we prefer to inject that area not infrequently to prevent the "joker" look (Fig. 4).

Crowsfeet and Palpebrae

Orbicularis oculi muscle lies subdermally in a circular fashion surrounding the palpebral aperture and its main function is closing the eye. This muscle also contributes highly to the lacrimal pump mechanism in drainage of the tears down the nasolacrimal duct to the nasal cavity. Temporal injections subcutaneously target the orbicularis oculi fibers, especially causing the crawsfeet rhytides which are one of the first signs of aging.

In Figures 5 and 6 photographs of patients treated for crawsfeet wrinkles before and after botulinum toxin A injection are seen.

Injections in the upper temporal part of the orbital fibers of orbicularis oculi muscle lift the lateral end of the eyebrow and decrease the dermatochalasis at this area.[45-46,48]

Injecting 1-3 U of botulinum toxin A in the subciliary pretarsal fibers of orbicularis oculi muscles we can flatten the hypertropied orbicularis muscle which is not so infrequently confused with lower eyelid bagginess. This application must be done cautiously may lead to lower skleral show and occasional epiphora when the doses are exceeded.

Figure 6 also shows the patient flattened hypertrophic pretarsal orbicularis before and after botulinum toxin A injection.

Injections of 1-5 U botulinum toxin A at each point, at least 1 cm lateral to the orbital rim avoid the diffusion of the toxin to the extraocular muscles, thus complications like diplopia. Injecting too close to the lid margins may lead to insufficent eyelid closure, reflex tearing and sometimes corneal erosions. It was reported that botulinum toxin leaking into extraocular muscles might induce dyplopia,[49] and it might also cause decrease of lacrimal excretion, corneal ulcers and decrease in visual accuity due to high doses of botulinum

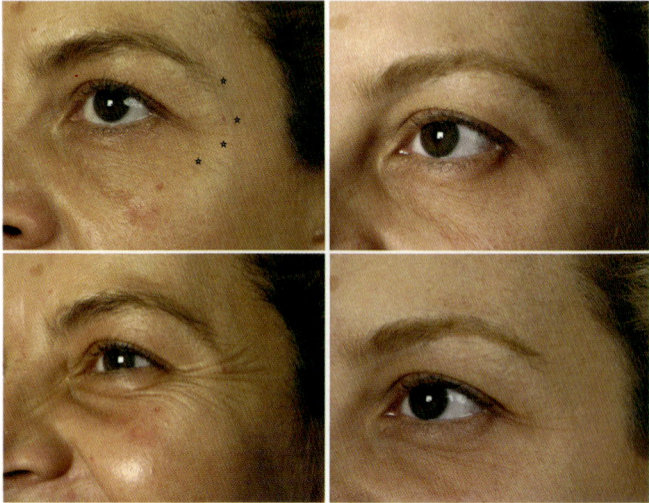

Figure 5: Photographs of a patient with crawsfeet before (left) and after (right) botulinum toxin A injection. Upper and lower row photographs demonstrate the static and dynamic wrinkles before and after treatments, respectively. "Star"s in the upper-left photograph, indicate the preferred injection sites for treating crawsfeet in most of the cases (doses and sites are customized for each patient). Note that the lateral eyebrow is also lifted and increased the distance between the lateral canthus and the tip of the eyebrow

toxin injections diffused in posterior septum, and infiltrating in lacrimal gland.[50] Another paradoxical recommendation for botulinum toxin procedures is inducing pretarsal orbicular muscle weakness to decrease lacrimal drainage effect, which is considered as a complication of botulinum toxin , therefore can be used for recovery of dry eye.[51]

These points must be kept in mind when injecting the orbicularis oculi muscles.

General and ocular complications are shown in Table 5.

In addition to the complications given in Table 5, perilabial ptosis when botulinum toxin is injected for crowsfeet

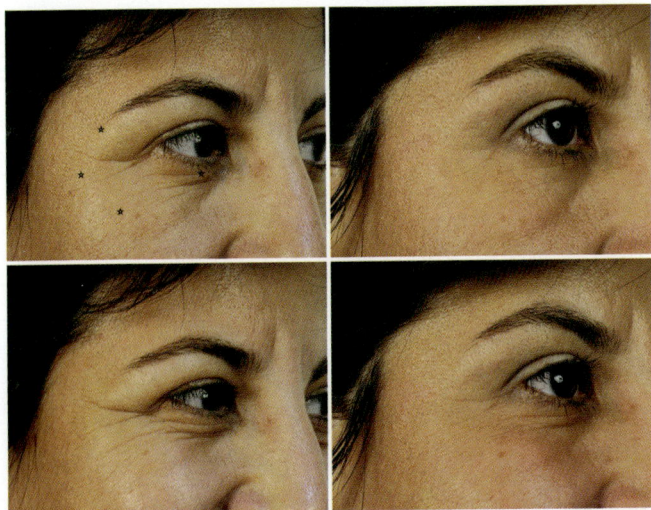

Figure 6: Photographs of a patient with crawsfeet and lower hypertrophic orbicularis muscle before (left) and after (right) botulinum toxin A injection. Upper and lower row photographs demonstrate the static and dynamic wrinkles before and after treatments,respectively. "Star"s in the upper-left photograph, indicate the preferred injection sites for treating crawsfeet and lower hypertrophic orbicularis muscle in most of the cases (doses and sites are customized for each patient). Note that the lateral eyebrow is also lifted and increased the distance between the lateral canthus and the tip of the eyebrow. Lower pretarsal fibers of orbicularis oculi muscle is flattened (upper and lower right)

treatment occurring due to zigomaticus major muscle being affected is a rarely observed complication, which requires special care.[52] Festoon formation developing in recovered cases with blepharoplasty is another reported botulinum toxin complication. The reason is decreased lymphatic drainage due to hypotony of orbicular muscles of the patients involved, and fluid accumulation in loose soft tissue on zigoma.[53]

Another complication that could be caused by anticholi-nergic effects of botulinum toxin is high intraocular pressure

Table 5: Complications of botulinum toxin in periocular procedures

General complications
- Pain,
- Ecchymosis, rash, hematoma
- Headache
- Flu-like symptoms,
- Nausea, dizziness

Ocular complications
- Undercorrection
- Asymmetrical features
- Change in and/or loss of facial expression (overcorrection)
- Lower eyelid laxity
- Dermatochalasis
- Ectropion
- Epiphora
- Eyebrow and eyelid ptosis
- Lagophthalmus in closing due orbicularis muscle weakness
- Keratitis sicca
- Dyplopia
- Photophobia
- Decrease in visual accuity
- High intraocular pressure?[54]

due to possible angle closure occurring as a result of anticholinergic effects when reaced to ciliary ganglion.[54]

Other applications of botulinum toxin that can be adjuncts to the periocular applications in this chapter are listed in Table 6.

Extensive use of botulinum toxin for as an adjunct to CO_2 laser cosmetic surgery and non-surgical procedures are reported.[55] Dehiscence and scar formation was observed less in patients who were injected with botulinum toxin in order to limit the movement of the surgically interfered area when compared to patients not treated with injection.[56]

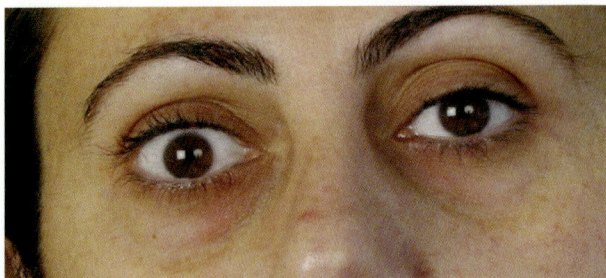

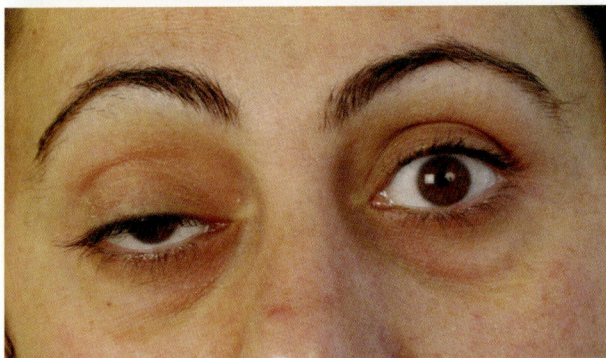

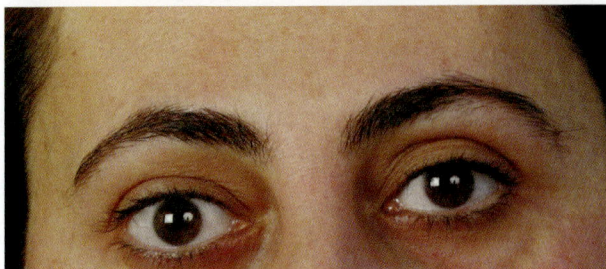

Figure 7: Patient with lagophthalmus (upper) had ptosis complication (middle) after botulinum toxin injections and returned to normal after 4 weeks with the correction of lagophtalmos (lower)

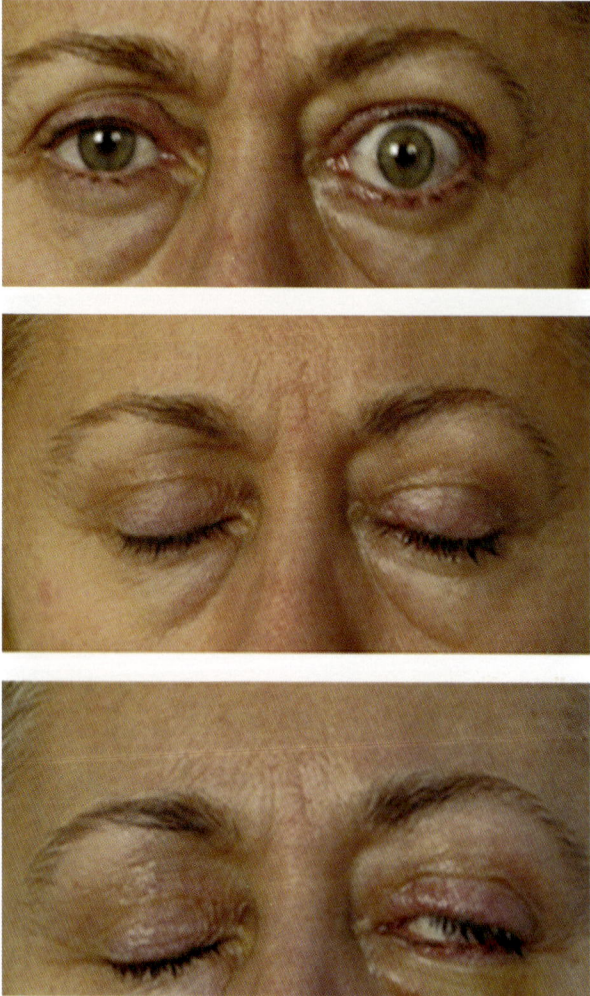

Figure 8: Patient with lagophthalmus (upper) who had good closure of upper eyelid (middle) had insufficient eyelid closure complication (lower) after botulinum toxin injections, due to diffusion of the toxin into orbicularis oculi muscle

Table 6: Other therapeutic and cosmetic applications of botulinum toxin

- Nose wrinkles (bunny lines)
- Perilabial wrinkles
- Low lip corners
- Orange peel look on the chin
- Platismal bands
- Horizontal neck wrinkles
- Décolletage wrinkles
- Rhinoplasty
- Scar revision
- Adjunct procedures for other anti-aging methods and surgery

Table 7: Contraindications of botulinum toxin injections

- Pregnantcy and lactation
- Neuromuscular junction disorders (Myasthenia gravis)
- Peripheral motor neuropathies
- Active infection
- Hypersensitivity to any of the contents

Botulinum Toxin, Botulismus and Antibody Development, and Non-responder Cases

As the doses are low and intervals are relatively long in cosmetic procedures, there is only one reported case in the literature who was reported for botulismus development after injection, and this 47-year old female patient was completely cured, despite a long-term healing period.[57]

One of the most important issues to be faced in relation with increasing number of cosmetic procedures in the future is antibody development against botulinum toxin, and the concern for not receiving proper response after the treatment.[58] For cases refractory to botulinum toxin A injections, other botulinum toxin subtypes might receive responses.[59-61] However, pharmacological effects and duration of activity of such various subtypes are different from botulinum toxin A, and Botox and Dysport are still considered as the most effective and reliable preparations.[62]

Cross tolerance may occur between various subtypes of the toxin. In a study published by Berwick et al, it was reported an 8-year old child who did not respond to the treatment after receiving botulinum toxin B injections three times in salivary glands. He also became refractory against botulinum toxin A preparations. His botulinum toxin A antibody titration was 0; this situation induced an idea that botulinum toxin B antibodies engaged in a cross-reaction with botulinum toxin A molecules, and a clinical response was prevented as these complexes were destroyed by phagocytes.[63]

Dutton found in his meta-analysis study in 1996 that 6% of the cases did not respond although this was the first injection of botulinum toxin A.[64] Unlike these cases, patients who responded when the dose was increased or who did not respond though they did to former treatments develop secondary antibodies and neutralized botulinum toxin molecules. This phenomenon should not be confused with non-responder cases, and such patients can be treated with different botulinum toxin subtypes.[65]

QUESTIONABLE ISSUES ABOUT DILUTION AND STORAGE?

According to recommendations of producer companies, one of the paradoxical issues about botulinum toxin is, the toxin's activity decreases significantly within a certain period after reconstitution, and breaks into pieces due to fracture of protein chains, whose molecular structure is connected with weak disulphide bonds, as a result of heat and agitation. Therefore, the toxin should be transported in a cold chain and without vibration. However, Trinidade et al reported in their controlled and double blinded studies that molecular structure of botulinum toxin A was resistant to foaming and cosmetic effect lasted for the same period.[66]

Studies by various authors showed that reconstitution of botulinum toxin 1 week[67] 2 weeks[68-69] prior to injection did not decrease the efficacy of botulinum toxin.

Similarly Hexel et al reported that botulinum toxin molecule reserved its effectiveness after 6 weeks post-constitution.[70]

The botulinum toxin producer companies recommend, injection of botulinum toxin type A with the nonpreserved preparation. However, less painful injections were noted with the use of the preserved saline compared the nonpreserved preparation (P<0.0001). The preserved reconstitution appeared to have no effect on clinical outcome reports Kwait and coauthors.[71] Studies by van Laborde et al[72] and Alam, Dover and Arndt[73] also proves that use of preservative-containing saline to further dilute botulinum toxin type B and A, respectively can significantly decrease patient discomfort on injection. The effect does not change with the preservative content of the diluent.

Vadoud-Seyedi and Simonart reported that short- and long-term results show the equal effectiveness of botulinum toxin A, whether reconstituted in saline or in lidocaine. Injections of botulinum toxin A reconstituted in lidocaine are associated with significantly reduced pain, lidocaine-reconstituted botulinum toxin A may be preferable for treating axillary hyperhidrosis.[74]

CONCLUSION AND FUTURE RESEARCH

The therapeutic and cosmetic use of botulinum toxin for periocular area pathologies are repeatable, safe and temporarily effective. Potential complications should be discussed with the patient before cosmetic procedure, patient should be selected carefully.

Determining optimum doses for certain anatomic areas, ideal concentrations, dose responses between different botulinum toxin serotypes, prevention of antigen formation , possible efficacy changes in long-term treatments, and long-term reliability are the areas that require more research.

REFERENCES

1. Scott AB, Rosenbaum A, Collins CC. Pharmacologic weakening of extraocular muscles. Invest Ophthalmol 1973;12:924-7.
2. Clark RP, Berris CE. Botulinum toxin (a treatment for facial asymmetry caused by facial nerve paralysis). Plast Reconstr Surg 1989;84:353-5.
3. Carruthers J, Carruthers A. Botulinum toxin (botox) chemodenervation for facial rejuvenation. Facial Plast Surg Clin North Am 2001;9:197-204vii.
4. Carruthers J, Carruthers A. BOTOX use in the mid and lower face and neck. Semin Cutan Med Surg 2001;20:85-92.
5. Carruthers A, Carruthers J. Botulinum toxin type A (history and current cosmetic use in the upper face). Semin Cutan Med Surg 2001;20:71-84.
6. Harrison AR. Chemodenervation for facial dystonias and wrinkles. Curr Opin Ophthalmol 2003;14:241-5.
7. Silveira-Moriyama L, Goncalves LR, Chien HF, Barbosa ER. Botulinum toxin a in the treatment of blepharospasm: a 10-year experience. Arq Neuropsiquiatr 2005;63(2A):221-4.
8. Mauriello JA Jr, Dhillon S, Leona T, Pakeman B, Mostafavi R, Yepez MC. Treatment selections of 239 patients with blepharospasm and Meige syndrome over 11 years. Br J Ophthalmol 1996;80:1073-6.
9. Colosimo C, Chianese M, Giovannelli M, Contarino MF, Bentivoglio AR. Botulinum toxin type B in blepharospasm and hemifacial spasm. Journal of Neurology Neurosurgery and Psychiatry 2003;74:687.

10. Naik MN, Soparkar CN, Murthy R, Honavar SG. Botulinum toxin in ophthalmic plastic surgery. Indian J Ophthalmol 2005;53:279-88 .

11. Frueh BR, Felt DP,Wojno TH, Musch DC. Treatment of blepharospasm with botulinum toxin. A preliminary report.Arch Ophthalmol 1984; 102:1464.

12. Cakmur R, Ozturk V, Uzunel F. Comparison of prseptal and pretarsal injections of botulinum toxin in the treatment of patients with blepharospasm and hemifacial spasm. J Neurol 2002;49:64-8.

13. Horwath-Winter J, Bergloeff J, Floegel I, Haller-Schober E-M, Schmut. Botulinum toxin A treatment in patients suffering from blepharospasm and dry eye. British Journal of Ophthalmology 2003;87:54-6.

14. Forget R, Tozvolanu V, Iancu A, Bogden D. Botulinum toxin improves lid opening delaysin blepharospasm associated apraxia of eyelid opening. Neurology 2002;58:1843-6.

15. Ozkan SB, Can D, Soylev MF, Arsan AK, Duman S. Chemo-denervation in treatment of upper eyelid retraction. Ophthal-mologica 1997;211:387-90.

16. Olver JM. Botulinum toxin A treatment of overactive corrugator supercilii in thyroid eye disease. Br J Ophthalmol 1998;82:528-33.

17. Uddin JM, Davies PD. Treatment of upper eyelid retraction associated with thyroid eye disease with subconjunctival botulinum toxin injection. Ophthalmology 2002;109:1183-7.

18. Morgenstern KE, Evanchan J, Foster JA, Cahill KV, Burns JA, Holck DE, et al. Botulinum toxin type a for dysthyroid upper eyelid retraction. Ophthal Plast Reconstr Surg 2004;20:181-5.

19. Allergan (2005) BOTOX® COSMETIC (botulinum toxin type A) purified neurotoxin complex. http://www.botoxcosmetic.com/resources/pi.aspx. Cited 11 April 2007.

20. Dysort Slough, Berkshire, England Ipsen Ltd. 2000.

21. Quinn N, Hallett M. Dose standardization of botulinum toxin. Lancet 1989;1:964.

22. Odergren T, Hjaltason H, Kaakkola S, Solder S, Hanko J, Fehling C, et al. A double blind, randomized, parallel group study to investigate the dose equivalence of Dysport and Botox in the treatment of cervical dystonia. J Neurol Neurosurg Psychiatry 1998;64:6-12.

23. Lipham WJ. What is botulinum toxin and how does it work? In Lipham WJ (Ed): Cosmetic and Clinical Applications of Botox and Dermal Fillers. Slack incorporated, Thorofare NJ 2004;6-9.

24. Lipham WJ. Getting started, commercially available products, basic equipment and supplies, reconstitution and dilution recommen-dations and clinical implementations. In Lipham WJ (Ed): Cosmetic

and Clinical Applications of Botox and Dermal Fillers. Slack incorporated, Thorofare NJ 2004;23-37.

25. Elibol O, Ozkan B, Hekimhan PK, Caðlar Y. Efficacy of skin cooling and EMLA cream application for pain relief of periocular botulinum toxin injection. Ophthal Plast Reconstr Surg 2007;23:130-3.

26. Wirtschsfter JD. Clinical doxorubicin chemomyectomy. An experimental treatment for benign essecial blepharospasm, hemifacial spasm, and eyelid fasciculations. Ophthalmology 1991;98;357-60.

27. Levy RL, Berman D, Parikh M, Miller NR. Supramaximal doses of botulinum toxin for refractory blepharospasm. Ophthalmology 2006;113:1665-8.

28. Yýldýrým Y, Kaynak-Hekimhan P, Demirel B, Kaya V. Treatement of upper eyelid retraction with botulinum toxin A. presented at TOD 42. National Ophthalmology Congress 19-23 nov 2007 Belek, Antalya.

29. Kaynak-Hekimhan P. Botulinum toxin applications in periocular pathologies (review). Turkiye Klinikleri Cerrahi Týp Bilimleri Oftalmoloji (J Surg Med Sci) 2007, 3:56-61(article in turkish).

30. Shih MJ, Liao SL, Lu HY. A single transcutaneous injection with Botox for dysthyroid lid retraction. Eye 2004;18:466-9.

31. Christiansen G, Mohney BG, Baratz KH, Bradley EA. Botulinum toxin for the treatment of congenital entropion. Am J Ophthalmol 2004 ;138:153-5.

32. Nava-Castaneda A, Tovilla-Canales JL, Boullosa V, Tovilla-y-Pomar JL, Monroy-Serrano MH, Tapia-Guerra V, et al. Duration of botulinum toxin effect in the treatment of crocodile tears. Ophthal Plast Reconstr Surg 2006;22:453-6.

33. Montoya FJ, Riddell CE, Caesar R, Hague S. Treatment of gustatory hyperlacrimation (crocodile tears) with injection of botulinum toxin into the lacrimal gland. Eye 2002;16:705-9.

34. Keegan DJ, Geerling G, Lee JP, Blake G, Collin JR, Plant GT. Botulinum toxin treatment for hyperlacrimation secondary to aberrant regenerated seventh nerve palsy or salivary gland transplantation. Br J Ophthalmol 2002;86:43-6.

35. Ellis MF, Daniell M. An evaluation of the safety and efficacy of botulinum toxin type A (BOTOX) when used to produce a protective ptosis. Clin Experiment Ophthalmol 2001;29:394-9.

36. Chua CN, Quhill F, Jones E, Voon LW, Ahad M, Rowson N. Treatment of aberrant facial nerve regeneration with botulinum toxin A.Orbit 2004;23:213-8.

37. Carruthers JA, Lowe NJ, Menter MA, et al. BOTOX Glabellar Lines I Study Group. A multicenter, double-blind, randomized, placebo-

controlled study of the efficacy and safety of botulinum toxin type A in the treatment of glabellar lines. J Am Acad Dermatol. 2002;46:840-9.

38. Carruthers JD, Lowe NJ, Menter MA, et al. Botox Glabellar Lines II Study Group. Double-blind, placebo-controlled study of the safety and efficacy of botulinum toxin type A for patients with glabellar lines. Plast Reconstr Surg 2003;112:1089-98.

39. Lowe NJ, Maxwell A, Harper H. Botulinum A exotoxin for glabellar folds (a double-blind, placebo-controlled study with an electromyographic injection technique). J Am Acad Dermatol 1996;35:569-72.

40. Pribitkin EA, Greco TM, Goode RL, Keane WM. Patient selection in the treatment of glabellar wrinkles with botulinum toxin type A injection. Arch Otolaryngol Head Neck Surg 1997;123:321-6.

41. Heckmann M, Schon-Hupka G. Quantification of the efficacy of botulinum toxin type A by digital image analysis. J Am Acad Dermatol 2001;45:508-14.

42. Carruthers A, Carruthers J, Cohen J. A prospective, double-blind, randomized, parallel-group, dose-ranging study of botulinum toxin type A in female subjects with horizontal forehead rhytides. Dermatol Surg 2003;29:461-7.

43. Lowe NJ, Lask G, Yamauchi P, Moore D. Bilateral, double-blind, randomized comparison of 3 doses of botulinum toxin type A and placebo in patients with crow's feet. J Am Acad Dermatol. 2002; 47:834-40.

44. Flynn TC, Carruthers JA, Carruthers JA. Botulinum-A toxin treatment of the lower eyelid improves infraorbital rhytides and widens the eye. Dermatol Surg 2001;27:703-8.

45. Kaltreider SA, Keneddy RH, Woog JJ, Bradley EA, Custer PL, Meyer DR. Cosmetic Oculofacial Applications of Botulinum Toxin: a report by the American Academy of Ophthalmology. Ophthalmol 2005;112:1159-67.

46. Cohen JL, Dayan SH. Botulinum toxin type a in the treatment of dermatochalasis: an open-label, randomized, dose-comparison study. J Drugs Dermatol 2006;5:596-601.

47. Redaelli A, Forte R. How to avoid brow ptosis after forehead treatment with botulinum toxin. J Cosmet Laser Ther 2003;5:220-2.

48. Huang W, Rogachefsky AS, Foster JA. Browlift with botulinum toxin. Dermatol Surg 2000;26:55-60.

49. Aristodemou P, Watt L, Baldwin C, Hugkulstone C. Diplopia associated with the cosmetic use of botulinum toxin a for facial rejuvenation. Ophthal Plast Reconstr Surg 2006;22:134-6.

50. Northington ME, Huang CC. Dry eyes and superficial punctate keratitis: a complication of treatment of glabellar dynamic rhytides with botulinum exotoxin A. Dermatol Surg 2004;30(12Pt 2):1515-7.
51. Sahlin S, Chen E, Kaugesaar T, Almqvist H, Kjellberg K, Lennerstrand G. Effect of eyelid botulinum toxin injection on lacrimal drainage. Am J Ophthalmol 2000;129:481-6.
52. Matarasso SL, Matarasso A. Treatment guidelines for botulinum toxin type A for the periocular region and a report on partial upper lip ptosis following injections to the lateral canthal rhytids. Plast Reconstr Surg 2001;108:208-14.
53. Goldman MP. Festoon formation after infraorbital botulinum A toxin: a case report. Dermatol Surg 2003;29:560-1.
54. Lachkar Y, Bouassida W. Drug-induced acute angle closure glaucoma. Curr Opin Ophthalmol 2007;18(2):129-33.
55. West TB, Alster TS. Effect of botulinum toxin type A on movement-associated rhytides following CO_2 laser resurfacing. Dermatol Surg 1999;25:259-61.
56. Choi JC, Lucarelli MJ, Shore JW. Use of botulinum A toxin in patients at risk of wound complications following eyelid reconstruction. Ophthal Plast Reconstr Surg 1997;13:259-64.
57. Souayah N, Karim H, Kamin SS, McArdle J, Marcus S. Severe botulism after focal injection of botulinum toxin. Neurology 2006: 28;67:1855-6.
58. Borodic G. Botulinum toxin, immunologic considerations with long-term repeated use, with emphasis on cosmetic applications. Facial Plast Surg Clin North Am 2007;15:11-6, v.
59. Greene P, Fahn S, Diamond B. Developement of resistance to botulinum toxin typeA in patients with torticollis. Mov Disord 1994;9:213-7.
60. Greene P, Fahn S. Response to botulinum toxin type F in sreo-negative botulinum toxin type A patients. Mov Disord 1996;11:181-4.
61. Barnes MP, Best D, Kidd L, Roberts B, Stark S, Weeks P, et al. The use of botulinum toxin type-B in the treatment of patients who have become unresponsive to botulinum toxin type-A initial experiences. Eur J Neurol 2005;12:947-55 .
62. Dressler D. Pharmacological aspects of herapeutic botulinum toxin preparations. Nervenarzt 2002;77:912-21.
63. Berweck S, Schroeder AS, Lee SH, Bigalke H, Heinen F. Secondary non-response due to antibody formation in a child after three injections of botulinum toxin B into the salivary glands. Dev Med Child Neurol 2007;49:62-4.

64. Dutton JJ.Botulinum-A toxin in the treatment of craniocervical muscle spazms: short- and longterm local and systemic effects. Surv Ophthalmol 1996;41:51-65.

65. Dressler D, Lange M, Bigalke H. Mouse diaphragm assay for detection of antibodies against botulinum toxin type B. Mov Disord 2005;20:1617-9.

66. Trindade De Almeida AR, Kadunc BV, Di Chiacchio N, Neto DR. Foam during reconstitution does not affect the potency of botulinum toxin type Dermatol Surg 2003;29:530-1.

67. Lizarralde M, Gutiérrez SH, Venegas A. Clinical efficacy of botulinum toxin type A reconstituted and refrigerated 1 week before its application in external canthus dynamic lines. Dermatol Surg. 2007 ;33:1328-33; discussion 1333.

68. Yang GC, Chiu RJ, Gillman GS. Questioning the need to use Botox within 4 hours of reconstitution: a study of fresh vs 2-week-old Botox. Arch Facial Plast Surg 2008;10:273-9.

69. Hui JI, Lee WW. Efficacy of fresh versus refrigerated botulinum toxin in the treatment of lateralperiorbital rhytids. Ophthal Plast Reconstr Surg 2007;23:433-8.

70. Hexsel DM, De Almeida AT, Rutowitsch M, et al. Multicenter, double-blind study of the efficacy of injections with botulinum toxin type A reconstituted up to six consecutive weeks before application. Dermatol Surg 2003;29:523-9. Dermatol Surg 2007;33:1328-33; discussion 1333.

71. Anderson ER Jr. Proper dose, preparation, and storage of botulinum neurotoxin serotype A. Am J Health Syst Pharm 2004 15;61(22 Suppl 6):S24-9. Review.

72. Kwiat DM, Bersani TA, Bersani A. Increased patient comfort utilizing botulinum toxin type a reconstituted with preserved versus nonpreserved saline. Ophthal Plast Reconstr Surg 2004;20:186-9.

73. van Laborde S, Dover JS, Moore M, Stewart B, Arndt KA, Alam M. Reduction in injection pain with botulinum toxin type B further diluted using saline with preservative: a double-blind, randomized controlled trial. J Am Acad Dermatol 2003;48:875-7.

74. Alam M, Dover JS, Arndt KA. Pain associated with injection of botulinum A exotoxin reconstituted using isotonic sodium chloride with and without preservative: a double-blind, randomized controlled trial. Arch Dermatol 2002;13:510-4.

75. Vadoud-Seyedi J, Simonart T.Treatment of axillary hyperhidrosis with botulinum toxin type A reconstituted in lidocaine or in normal saline: a randomized, side-by-side, double-blind study. Br J Dermatol 2007;156:986-9.

Index